LIVING WELL WITH

Endometriosis

LIVING WELL WITH

Endometriosis

What Your Doctor

Doesn't Tell You . . .

That You Need to Know

KERRY-ANN MORRIS

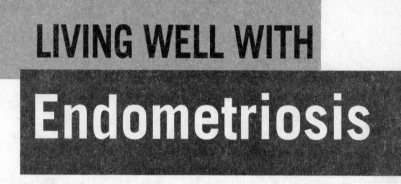

WILLIAM MORROW

An Imprint of HarperCollins*Publishers*

HarperCollins books may be purchased for educational, business, or sales promotional use. For information please write: Special Markets Department, HarperCollins Publishers, 10 East 53rd Street, New York, NY 10022.

FIRST EDITION

Designed by Joy O'Meara

Library of Congress Cataloging-in-Publication Data

Morris, Kerry-Ann.
    Living well with endometriosis : what your doctor doesn't tell you...
that you need to know / by Kerry-Ann Morris.
        p. cm.
    ISBN-10: 0-06-084426-4 (pb.)
    ISBN-13: 978-0-06-084426-4
    1. Endometriosis—Popular works. 2. Endometriosis—Alternative treatment—Popular works. I. Title.

    RG483.E53M67 2006
    618.1'42—dc22

                                                                    2005058167

        12 13 14 WBC/RRD 10 9 8 7 6 5 4

MEDICAL DISCLAIMER

*This book is dedicated to my mother,
a woman whose belief in the proverbial silver lining
fueled my passionate belief in this book's mission.
She is my tower of strength, without whom I would certainly be lost.*

CONTENTS

ACKNOWLEDGMENTS

The concept for this book really began in September 2002 in the form of the Unveiling Endometriosis Project, http://www.unveilingendometriosis.com. While learning as much as I could about this disease's intrusion in my life, I discovered a never-quenched thirst for information among the women of the international endometriosis community. A thirst for a book like the one you hold in your hands—one that teaches, empowers, and puts a face to the disease. They cried for *Living Well with Endometriosis*.

This book would not have been possible without the tireless belief of the participants of the Unveiling Endometriosis Project, participants from all across the world who contributed their stories and suggestions to the book. The wheels began turning once I found my agent, Robert G. Diforio, who took my idea and me and, within days (literally!), found us a home. Thank you so much for your tireless efforts and support, although we are hundreds of miles apart and have never met!

Our new guardian, my editor, Sarah Durand, took us under her wings and nurtured us to what we are today. Words cannot describe how much I appreciate her belief in this book and tireless efforts to make it possible.

To my family I have to say, if I could move the world just to say thanks, I would. My mother, Claudette; younger sister/typist, Kimberley; and youngest sister/occasional adviser, Kristina, gave up much of their time to work on this book with me. My mother spent many late nights and countless hours helping me reorganize the manuscript. Kimberley, statistics major/typist, never faltered in her task, typing page after page of text, complaining every now and then about my bad handwriting. Kristina, the bossy twelve-year-old, gave her well-appreciated words of wisdom to guide the writing process. By the way Kim, if you do indeed have carpal tunnel syndrome, bill me!

Spiritual encouragement was bestowed upon me by my loving grand-aunt, Ina Moore, who, like on many other occasions, prayed for the Lord's guidance on my journey. Thank you so much for your prayers, Auntie Sissy. Thanks also to my cousins, Lola (who also has endometriosis), Christine, and Allison, who encouraged me with this book project.

Many thanks to the Endometriosis Research Center (ERC) and especially Heather C. Guidone, who instantly saw the book's potential and the importance of its message to all endometriosis sufferers. They have been there with me from the very beginning, their own work in the endometriosis community inspiring me to continue with this book to help others like myself. Thanks for your support.

Special thanks to my dearest and closest friends, Nicole Patrick and Melissa Johnson, who have been there with me for over a decade, through thick and thin, high school and university, heartbreak and endometriosis, and who never faltered in their support of my decision to write this book.

Many thanks to the doctors and other professionals in the medical community who took the time out of their busy schedules to answer my queries and to contribute to the book, including: Mark Perloe, MD; Thomas L. Lyons, MD; Deborah Metzger, MD; David Redwine, MD, and the staff of the St. Charles Endometriosis Treatment Program; Robert B. Albee, MD; Donna Laux of Northside Hospital in Atlanta, Georgia, former program director of the Center for Endometriosis Care (CEC); Barbara Nesbitt, Editor in Chief of MediSpecialty.com; Dian Shepperson-Mills, clinical nutritionist, director of the Endometriosis and Fertility Clinic in the United Kingdom and author of *Endometriosis: A Key to Healing Through Nutrition* (2002); Ellen T. Johnson; Belle Browne, RN, coproducer of the best-selling documentary *Endometriosis: The Inside Story*; Diane Carlton, chair of the SHE Trust; Glenda Motta, RN; Nancy Petersen, RN; Ros Wood, chair of the Australian Endometriosis Association; Lone Hummelshøj, editor in chief of http://www .endometriosis.org/; Rollin M. Gallagher, MD, MPH, editor in chief of the National Pain Foundation (NPF); Jennifer Lobb, managing editor of the National Pain Foundation (NPF); and John Blondin, creator of MENDO, a Web site dedicated to men who love women with endometriosis.

I need to say a special thank you to the following who gave of their time, effort, advice, and stories to the Unveiling Endometriosis Project:

Errikka Aguirre, Lindsey S. Aliff, Moira Allen, Maria Bachicha, Kourtney Benoit, Patricia Bergström, Judy Birch, Antonia Boyton, Danielle Brown, Belle Browne, Keara Conness, Kimberly Crausaz, Andy Dann, Lisa-Marie Ehlert, Elisabet Eriksson, Melissa Essex, Amanda Fergusaon, Treva Frasure, Candida Greeley, Maria Gregoric, Robyn Grubbe, Heather C. Guidone, Sandy Harrison, Jimmy Hobbs, Lorie Hobbs, Johnna Howell, Julie Huffaker, Michelle Lee Impens, Yolanda Jeffries, Deborah Ann Klenzman, Melissa Kovach, Marina Kubacki, Tiffiny Lewin, Sybille Lichtenstein, Dawn Louise Sa, Seph Mackinnon, Julie McGhee, Amy Meyer, Gen Osson, Christel Palmberg, Edward Rendini, Amira St. James, Athina Marie Sanchez, Jill Anne Smeallie, Andrea Smethurst, Elizabeth Stutzman, Celina Symmonds, Jennifer Thornton, Linda Tyo, Brandilyn Vaidya, Jude West, Paivi Williams, Lynn Willers and Lori Phillips (the "Pneumothorax Twins"), Cassandra Worbanski, and Bente Zimling. While not everyone's story could be used in the book, they inspired me to continue with this project.

*   *   *

Finally, but not least, thanks to the millions of women, like myself, who suffer from this disease on a daily basis but who survive because of the strength they have to overcome. It is your strength that inspires me; it is your ability to persevere in the face of seemingly insurmountable odds that encourages me to continue with this work. I hope that *Living Well with Endometriosis* will help you and many other generations of women like us.

Thank you!

FOREWORD

Many books and publications addressing the clinical aspects of this enigmatic illness are widely available. However, *Living Well with Endometriosis* is the first of its kind, where women and their personal stories are at the core. The compilation of this book afforded those with the disease an interactive, creative outlet in which to share their own narratives, experiences, and coping strategies. As a result, an anecdotal guide for living well with—and often in spite of—endometriosis was born.

Endometriosis affects over 70 million women and adolescents worldwide. Such prevalence notwithstanding, the disease continues to be underdiagnosed and highly misunderstood. Even with today's medical advances, researchers remain unsure as to the definitive causes, and an absolute cure continues to escape us. Much of society has failed the endometriosis patient, lacking a comprehensive understanding of the potentially devastating toll this disease can exact from those living with it. As a result, many patients find themselves deficient in accurate information and support, fighting the disease alone and in silence. Through Kerry-Ann Morris's Unveiling Endometriosis Project, they have found their voices. Silent no more, contributors have shared their private perspectives on living with this enigmatic disorder.

Readers from every part of the world and all walks of life can gain immeasurable validation, encouragement, and advice through these stories of hope, courage, and inspiration, all contributed by those who know the disease best: the women and girls who battle it every day. Their poignant stories and sound suggestions for coping effectively with this puzzling illness are further complemented by the current research and educational data offered within, effectively creating a veritable manual from which everyone can ascertain crucial information to be adapted to their own lives. The edification and support found in these pages will assist readers in becoming informed, empowered patients in charge of their own health care. *Living Well with Endometriosis* is an invaluable asset to the global endometriosis community, benefiting everyone affected by the illness, from patients to loved ones to health professionals alike.

Over the course of my tenure with the Endometriosis Research Center and throughout my own personal quarter-century struggle with the disease, I have had the honor and privilege of becoming acquainted with many remarkable and resilient women from every corner of the world, several of whom are featured in these pages. These women have taught themselves—and others—how to deal effectively with the adversity of chronic illness. They are the real heroes in the fight against endometriosis, successfully overcoming the challenges they face every day. These are their stories, in their own words. May you learn from them as I have.

—Heather C. Guidone

Heather C. Guidone is the Program Director of the Center for Endometriosis Care (CEC) and Director of Operations of the Endometriosis Research Center (ERC). She struggled for years with the disease, undergoing more than twenty surgical procedures and many medical treatments. Fortunately, she was able to have a child—the child no one thought she could have—before undergoing a hysterectomy. Her own words of experience and advice are featured throughout the book.

To make aware the plight of those living with
this most puzzling disease; to educate;
to support the increasing number of diagnosed women
and teenage girls with endometriosis; and to empower
women with this disease worldwide.
We aim at bringing hope to millions worldwide.

—MISSION STATEMENT OF THE
UNVEILING ENDOMETRIOSIS PROJECT,
http://www.unveilingendometriosis.com

PART ONE

Understanding Endometriosis

1

Introduction

Picture this—you are twenty years old and lying on a gurney, trying to brace yourself for the surgery that lies ahead. You hear the dull thuds of doctors' feet rushing back and forth as they answer calls, rush to surgery rooms, and discuss cases among themselves. Suddenly, a door opens and another doctor joins the entourage at your side—an anesthesiologist (who is also your godmother), your urologist, and a fretting mother. The doctor is your gynecologist, and she has good news and bad news. The good news is the cyst they found is benign. Thank God! Unfortunately, the bad news is you have endometriosis. Huh?

I was dumbfounded and at a loss for words. The words eventually soaked in—"You have endometriosis"—surrounding me in a constricting sense of overwhelming distress. I knew nothing about the disease, although my cousin had been diagnosed with it a couple of years earlier, but the word sounded disarming, conjuring images of distressing illness, more surgeries, and even more hospital stays—a state of affairs that my already had-it-to-about-here-with-hospitals state could not endure. (I previously had major surgery to correct kidney problems.)

Since the age of twelve, my menses lasted for eight days out of each month without a hitch. Out of those eight days I spent the first three in absolute agony. For relief I took painkillers every four hours and spent numerous hours scrunched between the bathroom wall and the toilet. It was coldest there, and my logic was that the cold of the floor and the wall would freeze the pain in place and stop it from traveling from my pelvic area to the nether regions of my body. The bathroom was also a handy spot for the fits of vomiting that also accompanied the pain.

At school, when the pain became unbearable, I lived in the nurses' quarters and received Nurse Campbell's favorite remedy for pain—two cetamols, a hot-water bottle, and a bed for a couple hours of rest. Although the pills hardly worked I took to the hot-water bottle completely and held on to its comforting warmth while I struggled for sleep during these painful moments. Sometimes, I had to stay home on account of the pain.

I never considered those eight days out of each month abnormal in any way. As far as I was concerned, confirmed by the experiences of other girls I knew, those days were just another form of normal in any woman's life. The women in my family all had terrible menstrual cycles, my fellow schoolmates also experienced pain during their menses—I went to an all-girl high school—and the general female population in Jamaica suffered from pain during their menses. Did this seem abnormal in any way? No.

Pain during my menses worsened during my first year at college. In fact, the pain became worse after a humiliating defeat at a karate tournament in October 1998. Although it was mostly my pride that was injured by that fall, I started to experience burning and stabbing pains along the left side of my lower back. The pain worsened during my menses. Coupled with the pain of my menses, it felt as if bombs were exploding in every crevice of my body. Walking became an almost impossible task, and I was nauseous all the time. The pain became so bad that I was eventually rushed to the hospital.

To find out what was causing all of this pain I was sent from clinic to clinic at the university hospital, with various doctors diagnosing me with several problems that were never found to be the case. At the orthopedic clinic, doctors diagnosed me with arthritis, but at my age? I was only twenty years old! Then, almost by accident, after a routine X-ray of my left thigh and leg (as they thought the pain may be associated with the leg because it seemed to emanate from there) five objects were captured in an X-ray of my left lower back. Immediately, I was referred to the general urology (GU) clinic, with possible kidney obstruction.

At the GU clinic I was referred to one of the best urologists in the country. He examined the X-rays and explained that they were possibly kidney stones; however, to be absolutely sure, I had to have tests done on the kidney. A renal ultrasound was done, which verified the appearance of five kidney stones. Further tests revealed that the left kidney was not removing all the fluids, and thus there were also problems with the ureter. I had a blocked kidney due to the five kidney stones and a congenital disorder that had to be corrected via surgery.

During all of this time my menses were still giving me major problems and even more so with the pain from my blocked kidney. Surgery had to be done in April 1999, a few days from my end of semester exams, so I had to take a leave of absence from exams and from the first semester of the next academic year. I would return to school in January 2000. Surgery was done and a stent was left in to aid in reshaping the ureter. This was to be left in for a few weeks and then taken out.

Surgery was a success. I recovered quite well at home, and post-op visits to the GU clinic proved this. Then, during a routine renal ultrasound, the radiologist asked me: "Have you ever suffered from cysts?" What? She saw a mass in my pelvic area of such a size that it created concern. Her advice: See a gynecologist.

A follow-up visit with my urologist proved that there was indeed a mass in my pelvic area, which he felt during a pelvic and renal exam. His advice as well was to get in touch with a good gynecologist. With the help of my godmother, an anesthesiologist at the university hospital, I was able to make an appointment with one of the best female gynecologists in the country. The visit was quite comfortable; she asked me questions about my monthly cycle, and I gave her as much detail as possible. She also confirmed the presence of a mass in my pelvic area but could not determine exactly what it was just from the pelvic exam alone. She therefore recommended doing a laparoscopy to find out what this cyst was. An appointment was set for a laparoscopy at the Family Planning Clinic in July 1999.

On the day of the laparoscopy I was very nervous. I was eager to know what was going on, but at the same time I was apprehensive at the thought that there was something else wrong with me. I was given a general anesthetic and wheeled in for the operation. Afterward, my gynecologist explained that she was not able to do anything due to the size of the cyst but that she would have a more conclusive report for me at our next meeting, once she received results from the lab tests. However, she did emphasize that the cyst was chocolate brown and, although she suspected endometriosis, she would have a more definitive answer for me the following week.

The following week, while I lay on a gurney waiting for the operating theater and my surgery to remove the stent from my left ureter, I received the news that I had endometriosis.

My monthly excruciating pains were not *normal* after all.

Normal. The word constantly appears in any story you hear about endometriosis. The belief in the normalcy of excruciating pain plagues the lives of women. Maria, for instance, lived with the excruciating pain for years because of the belief, taught to her by her parents, that the pain was normal:

> *They grew up with the myth that it is normal for a woman to suffer during her period, so that became my belief, too. There*

was no need to see a doctor or a gynecologist for this. After all, what I was going through was normal. This was not something we even discussed among friends in great detail. Yeah, I got bad periods, blah, blah, blah . . . but we never said more than that. My mom had no idea what I was going through. She had never suffered from pain, even though she had migraines. Even with all my pain, it never crossed her mind, or mine, that there could be a problem.

We are taught from early on that the pain that accompanies menstruation is as normal as the sun rising. We actually prepare for the pain, just as one prepares for the inevitable hurricane season every June to November in the Caribbean. We stock up on painkillers and get the hot-water bottle ready for the days of pain ahead; we purchase wholesale supplies of sanitary napkins and tampons for the inevitable days of heavy menstrual flow; we even change the way we dress. Now does this sound normal to you?

Take Moira, for instance. For years she suffered from pelvic pain that became increasingly debilitating. While she had always had painful periods, it was not until the pain began interfering with the prospects of holding a full-time job that she revised her definition of "normal":

Let me share what "normal" meant for me. I'd always had hard periods, with lots of cramps; over the years, I switched from one pain reliever to another as each lost effectiveness. (For the record, the pain reliever that finally worked consistently was ibuprofen—and oh, my joy when it became an over-the-counter drug!) Off and on, however, I had begun to notice pain after the period—a dull ache in the abdomen, and, often, several days during which urination would be excruciatingly painful. However, no one could uncover any kidney, bladder, or other urinary problems, and since the pain didn't persist beyond those few days each month, no doctor ever seemed to consider it worth pursuing. (And yes, I did get the impression that some doctors really did think it was "all in my head," though none actually said so.) As for the "dull ache," that was attributed to ovulation, and since ibuprofen usually knocked it back, I paid it little attention.

By 1995–1996, however, that "dull ache" was becoming more pronounced. I was noticing that once my period stopped, I generally had some sort of pain for another full week—usually until, so far as I could determine, I ovulated. At that point, I would be pain-free for about a week—the "normal" week of the month! But pain would set in again about a week before the start of my next period—followed, of course, by the usual pain and debilitation of the period itself. Though ibuprofen continued to "manage" the pain, my system was always at a "low" during those three weeks, and if I wasn't cautious, I would easily get sick. My husband had noticed that if I overexerted during those weeks, I was very likely to come down with a cold, as if my immune system was just too stressed to handle "normal" life.

I also noticed how little energy I had during the "bad" weeks. Sometimes I'd just sit on the sofa for an hour or more, rubbing the ache in my abdomen. I had stopped working outside the home several years earlier and had begun freelancing—and I realized that I would quite probably not have the "energy" to hold down a full-time job anymore. Or, I'd end up being "sick" one week out of every month, which would hardly be conducive to staying employed! But since I didn't have any illness that I knew of, I often felt that my lack of stamina was simply laziness.

In 1997, "normal" suddenly became "abnormal." In addition to my usual repertoire of aches and cramps, a new pain reared a very ugly head. Within a few days of the end of my period, I would get a stabbing, absolutely intolerable pain in the right side of the abdomen. Usually, this would follow defecation—so I assumed it was something intestinal. This wasn't the sort of pain that you could grit your teeth and bear—it was a "grovel on the bed moaning until it goes away" pain. It came in spasms or waves, and no pain reliever would touch it. It usually happened only once per month. And since I couldn't control WHEN it would happen—on one occasion it occurred while I was interviewing for a part-time teaching job—I realized that my life was now out of control. It was time to get serious about seeing a doctor.

Sound familiar? Her story mirrors those of millions of women. Acceptance of debilitating pain, thinking that menstrual pain is quite the normal routine of any woman's life, is characteristic of being a woman. What makes it even worse is the fact that others believe in the normalcy of pain during menses, and hence do not believe the extent to which the pain can go from mere cramps to chronic and debilitating. The unbelievers extend from the family members and friends we turn to for support to the doctors we go to for solutions. Take Dawn, for instance. She struggled for years with the pain of her menses but lived with it because her doctors told her it was normal:

My gynecologists, whom I had been seeing since the age of thirteen, never questioned my pain; every one of them told me that ALL women have cramps with their periods. They prescribed Anaprox and birth control pills and sent me on my way. . . . When I told one of my doctors that I was in excruciating pain after I had sex, she told me that I should wait until I was married before I had "relations."

As Heather noted in her own story: *In hindsight, I know now that the real problem was not so much the pain and symptoms themselves, but that I thought they were normal. No one ever told me differently. No one ever said, "This is wrong."*

This belief in the normalcy of painful menstruation leads to delays in getting a proper diagnosis. According to a survey conducted by the Endometriosis Association (EA) in 1998, the average delay in getting a diagnosis is 9.28 years, although many experienced painful menstruation (dysmenorrhea) and their first pelvic pain at age 15 or younger. Why this reluctance to accept that painful menstruation is not normal and that endometriosis may be the reason? Dr. David Redwine, endometriosis specialist and medical director of the St. Charles Endometriosis Treatment Program in Bend, Oregon, has this to say about the state of affairs surrounding women and endometriosis in America in his article, "Endometriosis: Ignorance, Politics and 'Sophie's Choice'":

In America, it is estimated that at any one time there are up to 10 million women who are symptomatic with endometriosis. This number remains fairly constant year after year, with younger patients being added and older patients resolving their pain in some way and dropping out of the symptomatic group. In contrast, there are only about 3–4 million babies delivered each year. Thus, endometriosis outnumbers pregnancy by about 3 to 1, so perhaps in America the profession should be called Gynecology and Obstetrics instead of the reverse nomination. Endometriosis is to gynecology what delivering babies is to obstetrics. Despite the numerical burden of endometriosis and the tremendous negative impact it can have on patients, their families and friends, the disease gets no respect because sufferers are not identified as part of a recognized media victim group. Think about all the diseases or human states which have their own telethons, races, billboards and spokespersons testifying before government bod-

ies: *breast cancer, diabetes, AIDS, the elderly, gays, and so on. Endometriosis is more common than most of these, yet it is off the radar screen and many people have never heard of it. So one of the simplest things that will help is for gynecologists to recognize how common it is and make endometriosis the first diagnosis in women with pelvic pain, not the last.*

"Make endometriosis the first diagnosis in women with pelvic pain, not the last." Very fitting words, but the reality for many women is quite the opposite. Take Celina's struggle to find a doctor to diagnose her condition:

Finding a suitable doctor has been my biggest and most frustrating challenge. My family doctor when I was twelve basically ignored me, told me it was in my head and that I had a low tolerance for pain. He convinced me that I was crazy; he also convinced me that I was not strong. . . . I believe in my heart of hearts that if he had believed me and I had been diagnosed earlier, today I would be able to have children.

How do we change this attitude? Elisabet has a suggestion:

I think we need to start with a change in attitudes toward women altogether. We need to stop seeing women as more closely connected to nature and the body than men. It's not equal and leads to unfair treatment in health care. A patient needs to be taken seriously when she goes to the doctor with a complaint. Not only are women not taken seriously, within the medical establishment women are often seen as weak and they are seen as nagging for no reason. They are also seen as mentally unstable. Many women with endometriosis have been exposed to doctors who assume they are making up the pain they are feeling. This is outrageous. I think it happens

when the doctors don't know what to do. They can easily turn
it around on the patient. These doctors are using their power
position in the doctor/patient relationship to their own advan-
tage. But it often leaves women with endo doubting their own
sanity and in many cases even drives women into mental ill-
ness and depression.

Not only is endometriosis one of the leading causes of chronic
pelvic pain, it is also the second leading reason for more than
650,000 hysterectomies performed annually in the United States.
The disease is prevalent among 5 to 10 percent of women of reproductive age and is the leading cause of female infertility—as much
as 30 to 50 percent of women with endometriosis suffer from infertility. These are staggering figures, but the disease remains deep in
mystery, resulting in delays in diagnosis and a growing sense of despair among the affected. Additionally, considering how prevalent
the disease is in the general female population, it remains a significantly undertreated condition and underfunded disease in the medical research community. Only $2.7 million was earmarked for
endometriosis research by the National Institutes of Health (NIH)
in the fiscal year 2000, from an overall budget of $16.5 billion. This
approximates to only $0.40 per endometriosis patient, in sharp con-
trast to the planned allotment of $105 per patient for Alzheimer's
research and $30 per patient for lupus research.

But there is hope. The medical community recognizes the serious
nature of this disease and has invested the time and energy to find
new and better medical therapies with fewer negative side effects
and less-invasive methods of diagnosis. Currently, endometriosis
can be definitively diagnosed only via a laparoscopy, a minimally
invasive outpatient surgical procedure. Additionally, endometriosis
has gained recognition at the policy level, resulting in the passage of
the National Endometriosis Resolution Bill (H. Con. Res. 291) on
October 1, 2002, in the U.S. Congress. H. Con. Res. 291 officially

recognizes the need for endometriosis awareness and education and expresses the sense of Congress that it "strongly supports efforts to raise public awareness of Endometriosis throughout the medical and lay communities and recognizes the need for better support of patients with Endometriosis, the need for physicians to better understand the disease, the need for more effective treatments and, ultimately, the need for a cure." Several resolutions at the state level have also been passed, namely in California, Florida, Michigan, New York, and Pennsylvania.

Women are now becoming more educated about their bodies and hence more empowered about making decisions about their medical care. No longer will we accept as an explanation for debilitating monthly pain "it's all in your head" or "you just have a low threshold for pain." We can be our own enemies or our own healers, and many have decided that they are their best advocates for living well with endometriosis.

That is why I wrote this book—to engage women like Moira, Seph, Heather, Celina, you, and myself in an educational process about endometriosis; to teach you to believe your gut instincts about what is normal and, in the process, become your own best health advocate. If *Living Well with Endometriosis* had been available years ago, I am sure that thousands of women worldwide, including myself, would have been more prepared for life with this disease.

But it's never too late. As I write this, thousands of women and teenage girls are still unknowingly suffering from the symptoms of endometriosis. Of those who have been diagnosed and are living daily with this disease, many are still very ignorant of the extent to which endometriosis can affect their lives. Diagnosis is just the beginning, and it is very important that in times of confusion, unhappiness, and uncertainty with this disease, women can easily find the answers and support they need. *Living Well with Endometriosis* will do just that.

You have questions, and *Living Well with Endometriosis* has the answers.

▮ You will learn about your reproductive/endocrine and immune systems and their association with endometriosis.

▮ You will understand the various explanations about what causes endometriosis, the risk factors of developing the disease, and how to recognize if you may be at risk.

▮ You will become familiar with the disease's myriad symptoms and be able to utilize the book's Symptoms Evaluation Toolkit in chapter 11 to assess your own symptoms and evaluate any new developments for better treatment.

▮ You will gain greater knowledge and understanding of the options available to you in treating the disease—medicines, surgeries, and alternative and complementary treatments, their effectiveness and side effects—to become an empowered patient and consumer. With this knowledge you will make better-informed decisions and work closely with your doctor to create the most effective treatment strategy that is right for *you*.

▮ You will learn about the newest developments in endometriosis treatment therapies and the innovative approaches medical scientists are taking to develop effective treatments for the disease. You will also learn from endometriosis patient advocates and medical practitioners as they give advice, share information, and provide insight into the most effective measures for living well with endometriosis.

▮ You will meet the various "faces" of the disease, as well as those who live with and are indirectly affected by the disease. *Living Well with Endometriosis* recognizes that there is more to endometriosis than a disease. It is about the people who are actually affected—those women whose lives are forever altered because of endometriosis. You will learn from these women, in their own words, right throughout the book, as they give you the personal insight and advice about life with endometriosis that no medical text or doctor can provide. Most important, this book will make you aware, educate you, and support you, thus empowering you to play a more active role in your health.

In addition to all of the above, the book provides a comprehensive resources section, with a glossary of all the key words used throughout the book; information on endometriosis organizations in the United States and the rest of the world; online support groups; and books and informational Web sites about endometriosis and related topics.

Preparation. That is the key to living well with this disease, a key I give to you with *Living Well with Endometriosis*. Like preparing for the inevitable hurricane season, we have to put plans in place for the inevitable nature of endometriosis. Let each chapter serve as a jumping-off point for your personal growth and preparation for life with endometriosis. But, most especially, let this book teach you about how to live well with your condition.

2

The Female Reproductive System and Endometriosis

L et's start at the beginning. In order to better understand living with endometriosis, you need to educate yourself about the disease. In this chapter you will learn about endometriosis's association with your reproductive system, how it looks, and where in your body the disease often manifests itself. Additionally, the chapter will review the prevalence of the disease and the costs of treatment, and will present an overview on how endometriosis is diagnosed and treated.

▌ The Female Reproductive System

The primary structures in the female reproductive system are the following:

- ▌ *Uterus:* A pear-shaped organ settled between the lower intestine and the bladder. The uterus has two parts: the body and the cervix.
- ▌ *Body:* This section of the uterus is about the size of a fist when a woman is not pregnant. In this state the uterine walls are flattened against each other. The walls push apart during pregnancy as the fetus grows.

- *Cervix:* This is the base of the uterus that opens into the vagina. This opening, called the os, allows menstrual blood to flow out of the uterus and into the vagina.
- *Fallopian tubes:* These two tubes lead off each side of the body of the uterus. Each tube is about 4 inches (10 centimeters) long. At the end of each is an ovary.
- *Ovaries:* A woman's eggs are produced in these two ovaries. Each ovary is about 1.25 inches (3 centimeters) long and 0.75 inch (2 centimeters) wide and contains between 200,000 and 400,000 follicles or sacs. These contain the materials needed to reproduce ripened eggs or ova.
- *Endometrium:* This is the inner lining of the walls of the uterus. "Endo" is Greek for inside and "metrium" is Greek for uterus. During the menstrual cycle it becomes enriched with blood vessels and thickens, preparing for a possible pregnancy. If pregnancy does not occur, it is shed and flows out of the uterus and into the vagina, along with blood and mucus from the cervix, as menstruation.

The Menstrual Cycle

The menstrual cycle varies for many women, but twenty-eight days is generally the normal cycle. During ovulation, the process of discharging a mature egg or ovum, the female body develops and releases one or more eggs. The inner lining of the uterus thickens and becomes enriched with blood vessels to prepare for the possible implantation of a fertilized egg and to support the developing fetus. If fertilization and pregnancy do not occur, the uterus sheds the endometrial lining, and a new menstrual cycle begins.

Shedding of the endometrial lining is called menstruation. This menstrual bleeding—menses or period—can last five to seven days and present symptoms such as cramping, bloating, nausea, diarrhea, constipation, breast tenderness, headaches, irritability, and other mood changes.

The Endocrine System and the Menstrual Cycle

The endocrine system is the control panel for many of the body's functions. It is made up of several glands and the hormones they release, which influence various functions such as ovulation and menstruation. The major endocrine glands are the hypothalamus, pituitary, thyroid, parathyroids, adrenals, pineal body, and the ovaries.

The menstrual cycle is closely regulated by three major glands in the endocrine system. These are the hypothalamus (a region in the brain), the pituitary gland (at the base of the brain), and the ovaries (the main female reproductive organ). The hypothalamus controls the hormonal secretions from the pituitary gland, either stimulating or suppressing hormone secretions. The pituitary gland is considered the most important part of the endocrine system. Often referred to as the "master gland," it produces and secretes into the bloodstream hormones that control several other endocrine glands such as the ovaries. The ovaries also produce their own hormones in response to hormonal stimulation from the pituitary gland, which are involved in the menstrual cycle.

Hormones of the Menstrual Cycle

There are six key hormones in the menstrual cycle.

Gonadotrophin Releasing Hormone (GnRH)

This hormone is released by the hypothalamus to stimulate the pituitary gland in a series of pulses or positive and negative feedback loops to release the follicle-stimulating hormone (FSH) and luteinizing hormone (LH) into the bloodstream.

Follicle-Stimulating Hormone (FSH)

FSH and a little LH are secreted by the pituitary gland into the bloodstream to trigger the onset of ovulation. Under the influence of FSH, a number of immature follicles grow to maturity. The maturing follicles in turn produce estradiol, a powerful form of estrogen that prepares the endometrial lining for a possible pregnancy. This is called the follicular phase of the menstrual cycle.

Estrogen

The estrogen produced by the maturing follicles, estradiol, initiates the development of a new layer of endometrium (the inner lining of the uterus) to accommodate the possible implantation of a fertilized egg. As the follicles continue to ripen, they secrete more and more estradiol into the bloodstream until it reaches a certain point. At this point the estrogen sends a negative feedback loop to the pituitary gland to reduce secretion of FSH. The largest follicle secretes inhibin, which also reduces the secretion of FSH to the follicles. Testosterone is also released by the ovaries in small amounts.

Luteinizing Hormone (LH)

When the follicle has fully matured, it secretes enough estradiol into the bloodstream to cause the hypothalamus to release luteinizing hormone releasing factor (LHRF). This stimulates the pituitary gland to release a large amount of LH to begin the luteal phase of the menstrual cycle. This LH surge weakens the follicular wall and releases the now mature egg.

Progesterone

After ovulation the burst follicle remains in the ovary to form the corpus luteum (Latin for "yellow body"), which secretes estradiol and, in larger amounts, progesterone. This hormone prepares the inner lining (endometrium) of the uterus for pregnancy. If fertilization and implantation do not occur, progesterone levels fall, leading to the breakdown of the endometrial lining and shedding (menses or period).

A Word About Estrogen and Progesterone

The two major hormones in females are estrogen and progesterone. Estrogen is the umbrella name for a group of hormones that control female sex organs and secondary sexual characteristics. The three major human estrogens are estradiol, estrone, and estriol. One of the primary functions of estrogen is to control the development of the uterus. And, as we learned above, estrogen specifically initiates the development of the endometrium for possible pregnancy. Estrogen, therefore, stimulates cell growth.

The other hormone of importance to us is progesterone. This hormone is secreted by the corpus luteum after the egg is released, and it's responsible for preparing the endometrium for pregnancy. It also affects other tissues such as the cervix and vagina and functions of the body such as fat metabolism and energy production, as well as the endocrine and immune systems. Most important for women, however, is progesterone's ability to balance or oppose estrogen. Progesterone is needed in women to counter the effects of too much estrogen in our bodies. The effects of estrogen excess, or what Dr. John Lee (1929–2003)—pioneer and expert in the use of natural progesterone cream and natural hormone balance, and author of *What Your Doctor May Not Tell You About Premenopause*—refers to as "estrogen dominance," include:

- Acceleration of the aging process
- Allergy symptoms such as asthma rashes and sinus congestion, all common in as much as 61 percent of women with endometriosis
- Autoimmune disorders such as lupus erythematosus, Sjögren's syndrome, and thyroditis, also common among women with endometriosis

- Tenderness of the breasts
- Early onset of menstruation, a common occurrence among women with endometriosis, many experiencing menarche (first menstrual flow) at eleven years of age
- Irregular menstrual periods, also common among women with endometriosis
- Headaches
- Infertility, with as much as 30 to 50 percent of endometriosis patients experiencing infertility
- Irritability
- Mood swings
- Water retention (bloating)
- Premenstrual syndrome (PMS)

Estrogen, therefore, has both beneficial and harmful effects, which Dr. Ercole Cavalieri, head of cancer research at the Eppley Institute for Research in Cancer, University of Nebraska Medical Center, described as the "angels of life and the angels of death." Unfortunately for women with endometriosis, the disease thrives on estrogen for its development. Thus, hormonal/medical treatments aim to reduce the amount of estrogen in the body, ultimately suppressing the disease and leading to symptom relief. But this is not a cure.

What Is Endometriosis?

Endometriosis is one of the most commonly occurring gynecologic conditions today, affecting 5 to 10 percent of women of reproductive age, or up to 11 million American women. While there is no clear definition of endometriosis, the experts agree that the disease is estrogen-dependent for its survival. Aberrant production of estrogen has thus been implicated in the pathogenesis (development) of the disease, pointing toward a possible endocrine dysfunction, which would allow for this aberrant production of estrogen.

Endometriosis is described as a painful reproductive and immunological disease, characterized by the presence of pieces of the lining of the uterus (endometrium) outside the uterus, in other areas of the body. The condition is a leading cause of chronic pelvic pain, female infertility, and gynecologic surgery. Yet, despite its prevalence, endometriosis is still a very misunderstood and baffling disease. Interestingly, the disease first appeared in scientific literature in 1860 in a review by Austrian pathologist Karl Freiherr von Rokitansky, who referred to the disease in his writings as simply an adenomyoma.

The Endometriosis Disease Process

The disease is named after endometrium, the tissue that lines the inside of the uterus, which builds up and sheds each month during menstruation. In women with endometriosis, endometrial tissue with endometrial glands and stroma (supportive connective tissue of the endometrium) is found and develops outside the uterus (extrauterine) in other areas of the body. These ectopic endometrial implants behave similar to the endometrial lining of the uterus. Implants respond to estradiol in the bloodstream and grow just like the endometrium. And, similar to the endometrium, they break down and bleed at the end of the menstrual cycle.

Menstrual shedding from implants provokes an inflammatory reaction in the peritoneal surface. This in turn triggers the formation of a scar that encloses the implants and traps menstrual debris. This also deforms the surrounding peritoneum (smooth surface lining that covers the entire abdominal wall and folds over the organ in the pelvic area) and triggers the formation of adhesions (the medical term for scar tissue that unites two normally separate structures). Trapped menstrual debris in these ectopic locations develops into collections of blood referred to as growths, implants, lesions, and/or nodules. Implants can also interfere with organ functions if they are located in areas such as the bowel and bladder. The implants respond to estrogen produced by the ovaries, much like the endometrial lining does.

Most implants, however, have varying levels of hormone receptors, unlike the endometrial lining of the uterus. The level may be caused by the direct effect of the scarification process that reduces the implants' ability to receive estrogen. Additionally, implants may be deficient in estrogen receptors or may be hormonally independent of the ovaries. This means these implants may have the ability to create their own estrogen to continue growing. The disease, therefore, does not necessarily respond every month/cycle; it may bleed unpredictably and noncyclically. The frequency of bleeding will determine the appearance of the implants.

Endometrial Implants

Endometrial implants vary in size, shape, and color. Early implants are usually very small and look like clear pimples. These may decrease in size or disappear over a period of time. They may also grow to sizes from as small as a pea to larger than a grapefruit. Implants commonly appear clear, red flame–like, as powder-burn lesions, dark brown, yellow, and white. Red flame–like lesions are indicative of active disease surrounded by stroma. Powder-burn lesions or burned-out lesions are less active. Blue-black lesions get their color from trapped menstrual debris.

Dark brown lesions are found on the ovaries. These, referred to as chocolate cysts, are known as endometriomas; they are also filled with trapped menstrual debris from past menstrual sheddings.

Location of Implants

Endometrial implants are most commonly found in the pelvic cavity and the peritoneum: These include the fallopian tubes, vagina, cervix, vulva, outer surface of the uterus, cul-de-sac or pouch of Douglas (the area between the rectum and the back of the uterus) and the ligaments/connective tissue that support the uterus (the uterosacral ligaments).

Implants have also been reported in nearly all organs in the abdominal cavity as well as in the thoracic cavity, skin, muscles, peripheral nerves, spinal column, and surgical scars. In fact, endometrial implants have been found in all areas of the body except the heart and spleen. Within the abdominal cavity between 12 and 37 percent of patients have gastrointestinal tract (bowel) involvement, and about 20 percent have urinary tract disease. Thoracic and diaphragmatic endometriosis, while rare, has been seen in less than 0.5 percent of patients.

Stages of Endometriosis

The American Society for Reproductive Medicine (ASRM), formerly the American Fertility Society, defines staging as the criteria given to a disease based on its location, size, depth, and amount. These factors are classified from I through IV and are graded on a point system.

Stage I (Minimal)

At this stage of the disease, there is evidence of superficial (close to the surface) endometrial implants located in the peritoneum and on one ovary. Implants are between 1 and 3 centimeters in size with filmy adhesions, for a total of 4 points.

Stage II (Mild)

At this stage, endometrial implants in the peritoneum are above 3 centimeters deep. Filmy adhesions and superficial implants are also located on both ovaries, for a total of 9 points.

Stage III (Moderate)

At this stage, implants above 3 centimeters deep are present in the peritoneum and ovaries. Superficial implants are also present in the peritoneum with filmy and dense adhesions in the fallopian tubes. There is also partial obliteration of the cul-de-sac, for a total of 26 to 30 points.

Stage IV (severe)
Stage IV endometriosis show signs of deep implants above 3 centimeters in the ovaries and peritoneum. There is also superficial endometriosis along the peritoneum, dense adhesions along the fallopian tubes and the ovaries, and complete obliteration of the cul-de-sac, for a total of 53 to 114 points.

This is not a perfect staging of endometriosis. The stage of the disease is not indicative of the level of pain, infertility, or presence of other symptoms. Therefore, a woman with stage IV endometriosis may be asymptomatic while another, classified with stage I endometriosis, may experience debilitating pain.

Endo Incognito—The Mistress with Many Faces
It is very important to note that the symptoms of endometriosis are inconsistent and unique to each individual. The nonspecific nature of the disease allows it easily to mask itself as any of a number of other conditions, which results in late diagnosis for many women.

At the 1999 World Congress on Endometriosis, Dr. David Barlow from the University of Oxford pointed out that those patients with chronic pelvic pain *not* diagnosed with endometriosis were more likely to have multiple diagnoses. In his own studies, those diagnosed with endometriosis had previously been diagnosed with irritable bowel syndrome (20 percent), pelvic inflammatory disease (13.8 percent), interstitial cystitis (12.9 percent), and ovarian cysts (10 percent).

Chronic pelvic pain is the most common symptom associated with endometriosis. It is also a very common disorder among the general female population, with a prevalence of 15 percent in women aged eighteen to fifty years. Additionally, endometriosis is just one of many other conditions that cause chronic pelvic pain. Disorders of the reproductive tract, gastrointestinal system, urological organs, musculoskeletal system, and neurological system may also be associated with chronic pelvic pain.

The table on the following page includes other conditions in these five areas that also mimic symptoms of endometriosis, and that are also associated with chronic pelvic pain in women.

Prevalence of Endometriosis

The ERC estimates that up to 11 million women and teen girls are afflicted with endometriosis in the United States while the EA estimates as many as 87 million worldwide struggle with the disease. The disease affects an estimated 10 to 15 percent of all premenopausal women and 25 to 35 percent of infertile women. Endometriosis does not discriminate and is present in all ages and all racial and socioeconomic groups. Approximately four out of one thousand women, ages fifteen to sixty-four years, are hospitalized annually for endometriosis.

Despite these figures, the disease remains a puzzle. Little is known about the true prevalence of the disease, although it is a major public health problem, recognized as the third leading cause for gynecologic hospitalization and the second leading cause of hysterectomy.

Costs of Treatment

In 1991, the estimated total cost of inpatient treatments for women with endometriosis as the primary diagnosis in the United States was $504 million. This increased to $579 million in 1992. These figures, though dated, are expected to be far greater today. The annual direct medical cost of chronic pelvic pain is estimated at $2.8 billion, with an additional $600 million in indirect medical costs. Up to 97 percent of women with chronic pelvic pain also have endometriosis.

Gynecological

Uterine

Adenomyosis
Cervical stenosis
Cervical polyps
Chronic dysmenorrhea
Intrauterine contraceptive device (IUD)
Leiomyomata
Symptomatic pelvic relaxation (genital prolapse)
Uterine fibroids

Extrauterine

Adhesions
Adnexal cysts
Chronic ectopic pregnancy
Chronic pelvic inflammatory disease (PID)
Endosalpingiosis
Neoplasia of the genital tract
Ovarian retention syndrome (residual ovary syndrome)
Ovarian remnant syndrome
Ovarian dystrophy or ovulatory pain
Pelvic congestion syndrome
Postoperative peritoneal cysts
Residual accessory ovary
Tuberculosis salpingitis

Urological

Bladder neoplasm
Chronic urinary tract infection (UTI)
Interstitial cystitis
Radiation cystitis
Recurrent cystitis
Recurrent urethritis
Stone/urolithiasis
Uninhibited bladder contractions (detrusor dyssynergia)
Urethral diverticulitis
Urethral syndrome
Urethral caruncle

Gastrointestinal

Carcinoma of the colon
Chronic intermittent bowel obstruction
Colitis
Constipation
Diverticular disease
Hernias
Inflammatory bowel disease
Irritable bowel syndrome (IBS)

Musculoskeletal

Abdominal wall myofascial pain (trigger points)
Chronic coccygeal pain
Compression fracture of lumbar vertebrae
Degenerative joint disease
Disk herniation or rupture
Faulty or poor posture
Fibromyalgia
Fibromyositis
Hernias
Low back pain
Muscular strains and pains
Neoplasia of spinal cord or sacral nerve
Neuralgia of iliohypogastric, ilioinguinal, and/or genitofemoral nerves
Pelvic floor myalgia
Piriformis syndrome
Rectus tendon strain

Neurological

Abdominal cutaneous nerve entrapment in surgical scar
Abdominal epilepsy
Abdominal migraine
Bipolar personality disorders
Degenerative joint disease
Disk herniation
Familial Mediterranean fever
Neoplasia of spinal cord or sacral nerve
Porphyria
Shingles
Spondylosis

Getting a Diagnosis

The only definitive method for diagnosing endometriosis is through a minimally invasive outpatient surgical procedure called a laparoscopy. Diagnosis cannot be done by an evaluation of symptoms alone; some women with endometriosis are asymptomatic, while many women with pelvic pain do not have endometriosis. A laparoscopy then is the "gold standard" of diagnosis.

A 1998 survey conducted by the EA found that the average time taken for confirmed diagnosis of endometriosis was 9.28 years. This included an average of 4.67 years for the patient to first consult a doctor plus an additional 4.61 years for the doctor to confirm endometriosis. One very important factor that significantly contributes to the delay in getting a diagnosis is the woman's own opinion about her symptoms. According to the EA's survey, 58 percent of patients thought their symptoms were normal. However, the fact that surgery is necessary to make a diagnosis may also be a factor in delays. To speed up the process, scientists are investigating noninvasive diagnostic techniques—such as immunological and genetic markers—to diagnose endometriosis. These and others are discussed in chapter 12.

Treatment Options

No treatment strategy has proven to prevent recurrence of endometriosis. The traditional treatment path is first to get a diagnosis via a laparoscopic surgery, during which the surgeon can remove all visible implants. If removal cannot be done during a laparoscopy, then the next option will be a more invasive and open form of surgery called a laparotomy.

The laparoscopy and laparotomy are conservative surgical methods and the first line of treatment for women with pain symptoms who wish to preserve their fertility and get pregnant as soon as possible. The other surgical option is hysterectomy, a more radical surgical therapy that involves removal of the uterus along with all endometrial implants. This is not a cure for endometriosis. Specifics about conservative and radical surgical management of endometriosis are discussed in chapter 6.

Hormone medical therapy is also used to suppress ovulation and break the cycle of hormonal stimulation of implants. Medical treatments suppress the menstrual cycle and reduce estrogen levels in the body. The endometrial implants eventually shrink and become inactive. The endometriosis is still there and will eventually become active and recur once medical treatment stops and the normal menstrual cycle starts again.

Hormonal therapies include oral contraceptives such as Mircette and Ortho Tri-Cyclen; progestins such as Provera (the tablet form), Depo Provera (the injection) and levonorgestrel-releasing intrauterine system (LNG-IUS) or Mirena; gonadotropin-releasing hormone agonists (GnRH agonists) such as Lupron and Lupron Depot, Synarel, and Zoladex; and synthesized testosterones such as Danocrine and Dimetriose. One major downside of these therapies is the host of serious side effects. For instance, associated with the use of Danocrine is a high incidence of weight gain, facial hair growth, decrease in breast size, acne, increased oiliness of skin and hair, and deepening of the voice, to name a few.

New therapeutic methods for managing endometriosis are on the horizon. These include aromatase inhibitors, angiostatic therapy, GnRH antagonists, selective estrogen receptor modulators (SERMs), mesoprogestins, extracellular matrix modulators (EMMs), RU-486, and others. These treatments and more are discussed in chapter 7.

3

The Role of the Immune System

We learned in chapter 2 that there is a definite connection between endometriosis and our reproductive system, resulting from the aberrant production of estrogen. This fits in with the first part of the ERC's description of endometriosis as a painful reproductive disease. The second part describes endometriosis as a painful immunological disease, indicating not only an endocrine/reproductive dysfunction that allows for the development of endometriosis but also an immune system dysfunction that supports the development of the disease.

In this chapter we will delve into the connection between endometriosis and the immune system. We will learn about the role of the immune system, its various components, and what dysfunctions scientists have observed at its cellular level that contribute to some women developing endometriosis while others do not.

■ The Immune System

Your immune system is the body's first line of defense against infections and bacterial invasions. There is no one organ that is responsible for your body's overall immune response to potentially harmful invaders. Instead, your immune system is a complex interaction between lymphoid organs, tissues, and certain cells that protect the body. If the body is invaded, these lymphoid organs, tissues, and cells mount an attack against the invaders by first isolating them and then deactivating and/or destroying them to prevent their spreading to other parts of the body.

Self and Nonself

Your immune system has the unique ability to recognize potentially harmful invaders as "nonself," while recognizing the body's own organs, tissues, cells, blood, and so forth as "self." This ability is facilitated by the presence of certain markers on self and nonself cells. The body's cells carry a marker that makes them easily recognizable as a part of self. This phenomenon is called immune tolerance, the ability of the body's immune system to ignore the body's own tissues and cells.

Bacteria, viruses, and nonliving foreign matter all carry their own markers. The immune system specifically targets antigen, a potentially harmful substance produced by bacteria and foreign matter. It is this substance that carries the markers that designate the bacteria or foreign matter as nonself and target them for isolation and destruction by the immune system.

∎ The Organs of the Immune System

As mentioned above, there is no one organ in your body that makes up the immune system. Instead, the immune system is a complex interaction between certain organs and cells. Let us take a closer look at these different components.

The Organs

The various organs that make up the immune system are called lymphoid organs, and they are positioned throughout the body. They produce lymphocytes and antibodies that make up the cellular components of the immune system. These lymphoid organs include the thymus, lymph nodes, tonsils and adenoids, spleen, bone marrow, appendix, and Peyer's patches (round masses of lymphoid tissue found on the mucous membrane lining the small intestine). These organs are connected to other organs of the body by lymphatic vessels that transport lymph, a clear fluid that bathes the tissues of the body and carries the immune cells and foreign molecules into the bloodstream. Once in the bloodstream, lymphocytes are transported to the body's various tissues, where they look out for foreign matter and bacteria.

∎ The Cellular Components of the Immune System

There are quite a number of cells that work for the immune system. These include lymphocytes, natural killer (NK) cells, phagocytes, cytokines, and a complement system.

Lymphocytes

Lymphocytes are a variety of small white blood cells that move between blood and tissues and play a very important role in the immune system.

T Cell Lymphocytes

These cells are primarily responsible for the overall cell-mediated immune response to antigens. They depend on certain cell surface antigens called the major histocombatibility complex (MHC) to recognize nonself cells. T cells are produced in the thymus.

B Cell Lymphocytes

B cells secrete substances called antibodies, which surround antigens and mark them for destruction. Each antibody is specifically produced for a type of antigen. Once an antibody matches with an antigen, it interlocks with the antigen—much like a key fitting into a lock—and designates it for destruction.

Natural Killer (NK) Cells

There are at least two types lymphocytes that are NK cells. The first type of NK cells are called cytotoxic T lymphocytes or CTLs. These specifically target cells that have antigen fragments attached to self-MHC molecules. The second type of NK cell attacks cells that do not have self-MHC molecules. These, therefore, have the ability to attack various types of foreign cells. Both types of NK cells are filled with potent chemicals that kill the cells on contact.

Phagocytes

These are large white blood cells that can swallow and digest microbes and other foreign matter. There are two different types of phagocytes: monocytes, which circulate in the blood, and macrophages, which are found in tissues throughout the body. Macrophages are large white blood cells that act as scavengers to rid the body of worn-out cells, debris, bacteria, and other foreign bodies from tissues.

Cytokines

These are chemical messengers that help the components of the immune system to communicate with one another. Cytokines also help the immune cells to communicate with cells of other types of tissue. There are four classes of cytokines:

- Interleukins (IL), which are produced by white blood cells (leucocytes), regulate the interactions between lymphocytes and other leucocytes.
- Interferons are produced by cells infected with a virus, and have the ability to inhibit or interfere with the growth of the virus.
- Tumor necrosis factors alpha (TNF-α) and beta (TNF-β) are proteins involved in the destruction of tumor cells.
- Growth factors, such as vascular endothelial growth factors (VEGF), are chemicals that stimulate new cell growth and cell maintenance. VEGFs are involved in angiogenesis, the formation of new blood vessels that are also critical to the growth and maintenance of ectopic endometrial implants.

Complement System

The complement system is made up of about twenty-five proteins that work together to complement the work of antibodies in destroying bacteria and foreign matter. They also help rid the body of antibody-coated antigens, produce inflammation at the site of infection, and regulate immune reactions.

▌ Autoimmunity

All of the above components of the immune system interact in a complex web of activity to protect the body from the harmful effects of bacteria and foreign matter. Unfortunately, the immune system sometimes becomes confused, targeting both nonself and self cells. In this case, immune cells mistake the body's own cells and tissues as the invaders, and produce antibodies against these perceived invaders. These antibodies are called autoantibodies, and the process of an immune attack against self is called autoimmunity or self-immunity.

Scientists, while still not sure about the exact cause of endometriosis, have found evidence to suggest that the disease may result from an impaired immune response to ectopic endometrial cells. The result is an autoimmune reaction to stray endometrial self cells. The following are alterations at the cellular level of the immune system, observed by scientists in women with endometriosis, and how they may contribute to the development of the disease.

Increase in Macrophage Activity

Macrophage number and activity seems to increase in the peritoneal fluid of women with endometriosis. Peritoneal fluid functions as a lubricant for the abdominal and pelvic organs in the human body. Scientists have found that instead of facilitating the clearance of ectopic endometrial cells and inhibiting the development of endometriosis, the increase in macrophage number and activity in the peritoneal fluid promotes the growth of stray endometrial cells. Scientists conclude that this may be caused by an impaired scavenger function.

Increase in Cytokines and Growth Factors

Many cytokines and growth factors are elevated in the peritoneal fluid of women with endometriosis and play a significant role in the pathogenesis of the disease. These include IL-6, IL-8, VEGF, and TNF-α. Scientists have found that these cytokines are directly involved in the growth and survival of endometriotic implants in several ways:

1. They stimulate endometrial cell proliferation (growth of new cells) and angiogenesis (growth of new blood vessels). Vascu-

lar endothelial growth factor (VEGF) has been detected at high levels in the peritoneal fluid of women with endometriosis. Normally VEGF-induced angiogenesis plays a key role in the repair of the endometrium following menstruation. Within ectopic endometrial implants, VEGF promotes the development of new blood vessels in the surrounding peritoneal area, thus recruiting adequate blood supply for disease development and maintenance.

2. They stimulate adhesion of endometrial cells to the peritoneal surface. Scientists suggest that the inflammatory cytokines TNF-α, IL-8, and IL-6 may stimulate adhesion of endometrial cells to the peritoneal surface.

Reduced Natural Killer (NK) Cell Activity

A reduction in natural killer (NK) cell activity may lead to reduced clearance of ectopic endometrial cells and facilitate the development of endometriosis. Researchers suggest that peritoneal NK cells in women with endometriosis have higher killer-inhibitory receptors. When stimulated, these receptors send inhibitory signals that override the kill function in NK cells.

Impaired T Cell Lymphocyte Activity

Researchers have found increased concentrations of T cells in the peritoneal fluid of women with endometriosis as well as in the endometriotic implants themselves. T cells help to destroy infected cells and coordinate the body's overall immune response. However, there seems to be an impaired cell-mediated immune response in the presence of ectopic endometrial cells in the peritoneal cavity.

Increase in Matrix Metalloproteinase (MMP) Presence

This type of enzyme seems to play a very important role in the invasive process of endometriosis into the mesothelium (single layer of cells) that lines the peritoneum of the abdominal cavity. Matrix metalloproteinases (MMPs) are important in tissue remodeling associated with such processes as angiogenesis. Indeed MMPs are instrumental in the remodeling of the normal endometrium after menstrual bleeding. The experts suggest that remodeling of the extra-cellular matrix (a meshworklike substance that is found outside the cells of the body that promotes cellular proliferation) is an essential prerequisite for the implantation of endometrial tissue at ectopic locations. MMPs assist in this remodeling and thus play a key role in endometriotic tissue implantation and development. Scientists have found high levels of MMP activity in endometrium from women with endometriosis compared to those without.

Altered Apoptosis
Apoptosis is the natural process of removing unwanted cells—programmed cell death—as part of the normal development, main-tenance, and renewal of cells, tissues, and organs in the body. Scientists have found altered apoptosis mechanisms in endometrial cells from women with endometriosis compared to cells from women without the disease. This altered mechanism allows endome-trial tissue to escape cell death. The exact mechanism involved is not yet known.

All these findings—both reproductive and immune system–related mechanisms—points at the complex nature of endometriosis. Several mechanisms are obviously involved, and the scientific findings therefore produce several theories that try to explain just what causes endometriosis.

4

Endometriosis Causes and Risk Factors

Although the disease has been known to the worlds of medicine and science for some time, and the number of women with endometriosis increases annually worldwide, the causes of the disease are still not conclusively known. As we learned in chapters 2 and 3, endometriosis is closely connected to dysfunctions within the endocrine/reproductive system and at the immune system level. But what accounts for these dysfunctions?

Several theories have been advanced to account for the presence of the disease, but none offers an explanation for the occurrence of the disease in some women and not others. On the other hand, a variety of risk factors have been identified that appear to increase your likelihood of developing endometriosis.

This chapter discusses two sets of theories: The first set accounts for the origin and presence/distribution of the disease in the body, and the second set explains the persistence and growth of endometriosis outside of the uterus. I believe, like Dr. Robert Albee, medical director of the Center for Endometriosis Care (CEC), that several factors and not just one may contribute to the origin, distribution, and persistence of endometriosis. Ros Wood, chair of the

Australian Endometriosis Association, discusses the various myths that exist about endometriosis in her article, "Endometriosis Myths and Misconceptions," which appears later in this chapter.

▮ Causes of Origin

Retrograde Menstruation or Transplantation Theory

This is the most popular theory that tries to explain the presence of endometriosis outside the uterus. Dr. John Sampson (1873–1946), from Johns Hopkins Hospital, first promoted this theory in the 1920s. He found that menstrual blood containing endometrial tissue flows backward through the fallopian tubes instead of out through the vagina, then deposits and grows in the pelvis and abdomen. This process is called retrograde flow.

There are several shortcomings of this theory. While it explains how endometrial cells are relocated into the pelvic and abdominal cavities, it does not explain why endometriosis occurs in some women and not in others. Scientists have found that retrograde menstruation occurs in 90 percent of all women, but not all go on to develop endometriosis. Additionally, scientists have found little evidence that endometrial cells can attach to the pelvic organs and grow. Some other trigger, such as an immune or hormonal problem, may explain the survival of endometrial cells outside the uterus in those women who go on to develop endometriosis.

Retrograde menstruation also does not account for the presence of endometriosis in those women who undergo tubal ligation (tying of the fallopian tubes to prevent pregnancy) and hysterectomy, nor does it explain the rare cases of endometriosis in men who have undergone estrogen therapy after prostate surgery.

Coelomic Metaplasia

This is another popular explanation for the origin of endometriosis. According to the coelomic metaplasia theory, certain cells can transform themselves into a different kind of cell when stimulated. It is suggested that the normal lining of the pelvis and abdomen, once stimulated, can undergo change to form endometrial implants. Researchers are not quite sure what triggers this change; however, an inflammatory response may be a factor. This may explain the rare occurrence of endometriosis in men undergoing estrogen therapy, the occurrence of the disease in prepubertal girls, and in adolescent girls, and in women who never menstruated, and the presence of endometrial implants in unusual sites such as the pleural (lung) cavity.

Embryonic Rest

Also known as estrogenic stimulation of Müllerian rest cells, this theory suggests that some adult tissues may retain the ability they had in the embryonic stage to transform into endometrial tissue in the presence of a specific stimulus, i.e., estrogen. This is a plausible explanation for rare cases of endometriosis reported in men.

Lymphatic or Vascular Transplantation

Like the retrograde menstruation theory, this theory tries to explain how endometrial cells are distributed from the uterus to other parts of the body. Researchers surmise that endometrial tissue can spread from the uterus to other parts of the body through the lymphatic and circulatory systems. These systems may pick up endometrial cells from the peritoneal cavity and transport them to other areas of the body. This may explain the presence of endometriosis under the skin and in the lungs, nose, and brain, for instance.

Cell Differentiation

This theory arose from a Yale University study that found endometrial cells in biopsy samples of four women who received bone marrow transplants to treat leukemia. This is the first known report of circulating stem cells of extrauterine origin differentiating (converting) into endometrial tissue. The study's preliminary findings suggest that bone marrow–derived cells can generate endometrium.

▮ ▮ ▮ Endometriosis Myths and Misconceptions ▮ ▮ ▮

By Ros Wood, chair of the Australian Endometriosis Association

(Reprinted with permission from Ros Wood and
www.EndometriosisZONE.org)

Gender issues and the complex nature of endometriosis have led to the creation of a variety of myths and misconceptions about the condition. This article highlights a few of the more common ones and gives some insights into their origins.

Period Pain is Normal

"Women's problems" perplexed nineteenth-century doctors, who saw them as indicative of women's unstable and delicate psychological constitutions. Even though attitudes toward women improved during the twentieth century, some of the old beliefs still linger unconsciously, and affect the medical profession's attitudes toward women's complaints, including period pain.

As a result, while seeking help for their period pain, many women with endometriosis are told that their (severe) period pain is "normal," "part of being a woman," or "in their head." Others are told that they have "a low pain threshold," or are "psychologically inadequate."

Many women and girls do experience pain at the time of their period. However, severe pain that interferes with daily life is not normal, and is often due to the presence of an underlying condition, such as endometriosis. Any girl or woman with severe period pain should go to a doctor to determine the cause of her pain.

Too Young to Have Endo

Far too many doctors still believe that endometriosis is rare in teenagers and young women. Consequently, they do not consider a diagnosis of endometriosis when teenagers and young women come to them complaining of symptoms like period pain, pelvic pain, and painful intercourse.

Unfortunately, this belief is a carry-over from earlier times. Before the introduction of laparoscopy in the 1970s, endometriosis could only be diagnosed during a laparotomy, major surgery involving a 10- to 15-centimeter incision into the abdomen. The risks and costs of a laparotomy meant it was usually done only as a last resort in women with the most severe symptoms who were past childbearing age. Because only women in their thirties or forties were operated on, the disease was only found in women of that age. Nevertheless, the "fact" arose that endometriosis was a disease of women in their thirties and forties.

It was only with the introduction in the 1970s and '80s of laparoscopy to investigate women with infertility problems that gynecologists began diagnosing the disease in women in their late twenties and early thirties, the age group being investigated. So, they revised the typical age range for endometriosis down to the late twenties and early thirties. Again, they did not consider that they might be "finding" it because they were "looking" for it. The realization that endometriosis could be found in teenagers and young women came about as a result of research by the national endometriosis support groups. The United States, United Kingdom, and Australian groups all conducted surveys of their members in the mid-1980s. The surveys asked women when they had experienced their first endometriosis symptoms and when they had been diagnosed. The study conducted by our association showed that although almost 60 percent of the women had been diagnosed when aged twenty-five to thirty-five, 43 percent had experienced their first symptoms as teenagers. The results of our study were similar to those of the U.S. and U.K. groups.

Thankfully, the research results caught the attention of some eminent gynecologists in the 1990s. Dr. Marc Laufer of the Children's Hospital Boston conducted studies of teenagers with chronic pelvic pain. One of his studies showed that adolescents whose chronic pelvic pain was not alleviated by an oral contraceptive pill and a nonsteroidal anti-inflammatory drug like Ponstan had a high prevalence of endometriosis—as high as 70 percent. Similarly, a team led by Dr. David Barlow and Dr. Stephen Kennedy of Oxford University, England, conducted a study of diagnosed women in the United States and United Kingdom. They found that the average age when pain symptoms began was twenty-two, with a range of ten to forty-six years.

So, teenagers and young women in their early twenties are NOT too young to have endometriosis.

Hormonal Treatments Treat the Condition

Synthetic hormonal drugs like the pill, progestins, androgens (danazol), and GnRH-analogues have been used for many years to "treat" endometriosis. However, recently it has become increasingly apparent that these hormonal treatments do not have any long-term effect on the disease itself. They do suppress (quieten) the symptoms, but only while the drugs are being taken. Once use of the drugs ceases, symptoms return.

This means that hormonal treatments do not have a role in treating (eradicating) endometriosis. If eradication of the disease is desired, surgery performed by a gynecologist with extensive knowledge and experience of the specialized techniques used for endometriosis is the only effective medical treatment.

It also means that hormonal treatments should not be used to improve women's chances of conceiving. Not only do they have no effect on the disease itself, but they also reduce the time available to conceive, because conception is not possible while on the drugs. If treatment is needed, surgery by a specialist gynecologist is imperative.

Pregnancy Cures Endo

Fortunately, the myth that pregnancy cures endometriosis is slowly disappearing. However, it is not disappearing fast enough! The reality is that pregnancy—like hormonal drug treatments—usually suppresses the symptoms of endometriosis but does not eradicate the disease itself. Therefore, symptoms usually recur after the birth of the child. Most women can delay the return of symptoms by breastfeeding, but only while the breast-feeding is frequent enough and intense enough to suppress the menstrual cycle.

Endo Invariably Causes Infertility

Too many young women are given the impression that having endometriosis invariably means that they will become infertile. The Association periodically has to reassure young women who have been given this impression by their doctors. Teenagers as young as eighteen have been told to "go find a husband and have children as soon as possible, because if you don't, you never will."

Unfortunately, there are no reliable statistics that indicate what percentage of women with endometriosis have no problems having children, have difficulties but eventually succeed, or never succeed. Therefore, it is impossible to give women a reliable indication of their chances of having fertility problems.

However, in general, it is believed that the likelihood of fertility problems increases with the severity of the disease.

Many women with endometriosis do go on to have children. Gynecologists generally believe that 60 to 70 percent of women with endometriosis are fertile. Furthermore, they say that about half the women who have difficulties do eventually conceive with or without treatment.

Infertility Usually Caused by Endo on Tubes

The statement that scarring of the fallopian tubes due to endometriosis is a common cause of infertility is appearing more and more frequently in lay publications. The authors of such publications are usually people who have very little understanding of the condition.

I suspect they are confusing the causes of endometriosis-associated infertility with those of pelvic inflammatory disease–associated infertility. Pelvic inflammatory disease is an infection that damages or blocks the fallopian tubes. It causes infertility by preventing movement of the egg and sperm through the tube.

The reality is that endometrial implants are rarely found on the fallopian tubes. Therefore, endometriosis does not usually cause scarring of the fallopian tubes or infertility due to scarring of the tubes.

The mechanisms by which endometriosis causes infertility are still largely unknown, despite years of research. It may be years or even decades before the riddles of endometriosis infertility and subfertility are solved.

Iatrogenic Transplantation

This theory purports that endometrial tissue can be accidentally transferred from one site to another during surgery. For instance, endometriosis has been found in laparoscopy and laparotomy scars as well as in cesarean-sections. This is highly unlikely today due to advanced measures in surgical management.

▌ Causes of Persistence and Growth

Impaired Immune Response to Endometrial Cells

It has been hypothesized that the immune system may be altered in women with endometriosis. The disease may develop as a result of an impaired immune response that leads to inadequate removal of endometrial cells.

According to this theory, endometriosis develops in women who have an impaired immune response either as an antecedent or consequential event. As an antecedent event, the theory proposes that endometriosis develops because of immune system abnormalities that allow retrograde menstruation to establish lesions within the peritoneal cavity. Several studies have found decreased natural killer (NK) cell activity in women with endometriosis, as discussed in chapter 3. NK cells detect, identify, and destroy any cells or organisms that are either abnormal or wander out of their usual domains.

As a consequential event, the immune system becomes hyperstimulated in the presence of endometriosis, having not been able to clear the extrauterine cells from the pelvic cavity. In this hyperstimulated state, the immune system loses its ability to recognize what is foreign matter and what is actually a part of the body. It launches an attack on self, targeting the cells, tissues, and organs. This induces an inflammatory environment characterized by alterations in the immune system, increase in cytokine secretions (chemical messengers) and growth factors that support the development of endometrial implants. This also increases your risk of developing autoimmune disorders.

There is a relatively high incidence of inflammatory autoimmune disorders that occur in women with endometriosis such as rheumatoid arthritis, lupus, and multiple sclerosis (MS). It is still unclear, however, whether this immunologic response is the cause of endometriosis or the result of the inflammatory reaction that endometriosis induces.

Hereditary

This theory suggests that certain families may have predisposing factors that encourage the growth of endometriosis. This means that endometriosis tends to run in families. Scientists of Iceland's deCode Genetics and National University Hospital found that a woman has more than five times the normal risk of developing endometriosis if her mother or sister has the disease. Even having a cousin with endometriosis raises a woman's risk by 50 percent. The scientists also found that the genetic factors involved in endometriosis can be inherited through paternal as well as maternal lines.

While endometriosis seems to be heritable, the exact mechanism is unclear. Studies are currently under way to uncover the genes responsible for some women developing endometriosis. These include the Oxford Endometriosis Gene Study (OXYGENE), based at the University of Oxford.

One other study, led by Professor Linda Giudice from Stanford University in California, found that certain genes are expressed differently in women with endometriosis. The research team discovered that these genes contribute to endometrial cell proliferation and angiogenesis.

Angiogenesis

Angiogenesis is the natural process of the formation of new blood vessels. While retrograde menstruation is widely accepted as a method of transporting endometrial cells into the peritoneal cavity, some other factor must be at work to render certain women susceptible to the implantation and growth of ectopic endometrium.

Researchers propose that ectopic endometrium in women with endometriosis has the enhanced capacity to proliferate, implant, and grow in the peritoneal cavity. For endometrial implants to grow, they need to recruit a new blood supply. Scientists hypothesize that the implants' superficial epithelial layer is rich in angiogenic factors that, once exposed to the peritoneal cavity, can recruit new blood vessels.

Angiogenesis is likely to have a role in the development of endometriosis based on the following observations:

- Endometriotic lesions have been found surrounded by peritoneal blood vessels.
- The peritoneal fluid of women with endometriosis contains more angiogenic factors than that of women without the disease.
- Histological studies and animal experiments found that endometriotic deposits get their blood supply from the surrounding microvasculature. These studies also found that larger endometriotic implants grow in areas with a rich blood supply.

Aromatase Prevalence

Aromatase is an enzyme that promotes the conversion of testosterone to estradiol. It has been established that endometriosis is an estrogen-dependent disease. How does the disease get its supply of estrogen to grow? The traditional explanation was that circulating estradiol in the bloodstream could be delivered to implants. Recent research by Dr. Serdar E. Bulun (chief, Division of Reproductive Biology Research, Department of Obstetrics and Gynecology, Northwestern University Feinberg School of Medicine), however, definitively shows that ectopic endometrium contains extremely high levels of aromatase enzyme, which leads to local production of estrogen by the implants themselves. Additionally, prostaglandin F_2-alpha (a hormonelike chemical that can cause inflammation and induce pain—also called inflammatory prostaglandin), one of the major mediators of inflammation and pain, also induces aromatase enzyme activity and formation of estrogen in implants. Studies have found high levels of aromatase P450 (P450 arom) in women with endometriosis but in lower levels in endometrium from women without endometriosis. P450 arom is a key enzyme for the production of estrogen in ectopic endometrium.

Researchers are using these findings to develop a new type of treatment, aromatase inhibitors, in the management of endometriosis, as well as a diagnostic marker to screen for the disease.

■ Risk Factors

How do you know if you are at risk for developing endometriosis? A simple question but, unfortunately, there is no simple answer. Although endometriosis has become an extensively studied disease, few of these studies are concerned with the factors involved in developing endometriosis. While precise risk factors have not been established, scientists have come up with several risk factors that may predispose you to developing endometriosis. Research is still being conducted to evaluate the extent of risk associated with many of these factors.

Exposure to Environmental Endocrine Disruptors

An environmental endocrine disruptor is an external agent such as a chemical pollutant that, once introduced into the body, disrupts the synthesis, secretion, and action of natural hormones. In other words, it interferes with the normal functioning of the endocrine glands. For instance, research by the EA and Dr. Sherry Rier, from the Department of Medical Microbiology and Immunology and the Department of Obstetrics and Gynecology at the University of South Florida College of Medicine, discovered that endometriosis spontaneously developed in 79 percent of a rhesus monkey colony exposed to minute quantities of dioxin (TCCD—2,3,7,8-tetrachlorodibenzo-para-dioxin), an environmental pollutant associated with chlorine bleach. The study also found that the monkeys who had the most exposure to dioxin had the most extensive endometriosis.

Rodent studies were done to test the hypothesis that overexposure to dioxins can lead to the development of endometriosis. In most of the studies, TCDD enhanced the development of implants in the mice. However, one study found that endometrial implants in the mice regressed once exposed to TCDD. The experts suggest that the time of administration and dose of TCDD may have determined its effects on the implants. A follow-up study by Rier on the original rhesus monkey colony found that, seventeen years after the exposure, endometriosis developed.

How exactly does dioxin increase your risk of developing endometriosis? TCDD is a major endocrine disruptor, as defined above. The experts have found that dioxins may directly interfere with endocrine glands and the hormones they produce and with where these hormones act. Studies have shown that dioxins reduce the number of hormone receptor sites in target cells; dioxins occupy these sites just as the natural hormones would do, and they can mimic the effect of the hormone or block the hormone's action on the target cell. These can trigger actions that affect the body's natural growth and development. Dioxins, therefore, have an estrogenic effect on the body. These exogenous estrogens are referred to as xenohormones.

Dioxin is present in chlorine-bleached paper products such as sanitary napkins, facial tissues, tampons, toilet paper, disposable diapers, and coffee filters. It is also present in food and water as a result of pesticide contamination and the burning of toxic waste.

While animal studies of dioxin exposure reveal slight to moderate increase in risk of developing endometriosis, studies involving human subjects have been contradictory.

Anatomic Abnormalities

You may also be at risk for endometriosis if you were born with an abnormally developed uterus that obstructs the normal outflow of menses. Studies have also found that an abnormal cul-de-sac (pouch of Douglas) may be a possible factor in the development of endometriosis in some women and not others. Researchers reported in a 2000 study that the depth and volume of the cul-de-sac differs in patients with endometriosis, with or without deep endometrial implants, compared to women with a healthy pelvis.

"Kissing ovaries" have also been detected as a possible marker for endometriosis. In a 2005 report published in *Fertility and Sterility,* researchers found that "ultrasound detection of kissing ovaries is strongly predictive of endometriosis and, in particular, is a marker of the most severe form of the disease." Kissing ovaries occurs when the ovaries are entirely or partly joined together and stabilized behind the cul-de-sac. This commonly occurs in women with severe endometriosis. Women with kissing ovaries also have a much higher incidence of bowel and fallopian tube involvement than those without.

Liver Disorders

Liver disorders may predispose a woman to developing endometriosis. The liver regulates and removes estrogen from the body. If the liver fails to remove the estrogen, estrogen levels in the body will increase and a woman will begin to develop symptoms such as chronic fatigue and allergies. Estrogen, as you know, stimulates endometriosis growth. Additionally, the liver is especially vulnerable to dioxin. Persons exposed to dioxin have an enlarged liver and reduced liver function.

Previous IUD and OC Use

Women who used intrauterine devices (IUDs) may be at increased risk of developing endometriosis. Menorrhagia (extensive blood loss during menstruation) is associated with the use of copper IUDs.

Findings show that menstrual blood volume increases an average of 50 to 100 percent after insertion of IUDs. The experts suggest that if retrograde menstruation is the cause of endometriosis, then IUD use would be expected to increase your risk of developing endometriosis. They also suggest that the intense inflammatory reaction caused by IUDs, with the accompanying peritoneal immunological response, may increase your risk. The findings, however, are inconclusive. Several studies have reported an increase in risk associated with former IUD use, while others have suggested that IUD use does not influence the development of endometriosis.

The risk associated with oral contraceptive (OC) use is just as problematic. Some studies have found a protective benefit of current use of oral contraceptives. Researchers suggest that oral contraceptives decrease the risk by stopping ovulation and decreasing the volume of menstrual flow. However, it is impossible to determine whether endometriosis developed before oral contraceptive use or after since they are often prescribed as a first-line treatment when women present with irregular menstrual cycles, heavy menstrual flows, and pelvic pain. Some experts believe, however, that oral contraceptive use decreases symptoms in the short term but that symptoms return once use is stopped or the disease progresses in severity.

Presence of Autoimmune Disorders

Your risk of developing endometriosis may increase if you also suffer from autoimmune disorders or if your immune system is already weakened by autoimmune disorders such as fibromyalgia and chronic fatigue syndrome. A 2002 study of 3,680 women with endometriosis conducted by the EA, the U.S. National Institute of Child Health and Development (NICHD), and George Washington University found that 20 percent of these women had more than one other disease, including chronic fatigue syndrome, fibromyalgia, rheumatoid arthritis, lupus, and allergies.

The researchers conclude that the findings suggest a strong association between endometriosis and autoimmune disorders. This would support the theory that endometriosis may be caused by abnormalities in the immune system that allows for the growth of stray endometrial cells or that the presence of ectopic endometrial cells causes the immune system to become hyperstimulated, inducing an inflammatory response that leads to multisystemic immune dysfunction, development of endometriosis, and immune disorders.

Menstrual and Reproductive Factors

Studies done in 1986, 1991, 1993, 1995, and 1997 suggest that endometriosis is associated with increased exposure to menstruation. This assumption supports John Sampson's theory of retrograde menstruation. According to these studies, those at higher risk for endometriosis have a shorter-than-normal menstrual cycle, early age of menarche (first menstrual cycle), late pregnancy as well as a long time lag between menarche and first pregnancy, and heavier and longer periods. Experts assume that the more often a woman becomes pregnant, the lower her risk of developing endometriosis; each pregnancy decreases the lifetime number of months during which she is exposed to menstruation. However, other studies found no clear association between these factors and endometriosis.

Greater Weight

Some experts have found a connection between weight and your risk of developing endometriosis. A study of eighty-eight women with endometriosis compared to eighty-eight women without the disease found that the odds of developing endometriosis were inversely related to waist-to-hip ratio. A high waist-to-hip ratio indicated peripheral fat accumulation that is associated with high estrogen levels in the body, thus increasing your risk of developing endometriosis. Studies have shown that body fat does produce estrogen.

The experts also suggest that your birth weight may be a risk factor. A high birth weight suggests greater exposure to estrogen in utero as compared to infants of average and normal birth weight.

Height

You may be at an increased risk of developing endometriosis if taller than 5.45 feet (166 centimeters). Researchers propose that taller women may have higher estradiol levels during the follicular phase of their menstrual cycle.

Hair Color

In a study of 143 women, 12 of whom had red hair, published in the September 1995 issue of *Fertility and Sterility,* scientists found 10 of the 12 (83 percent) had endometriosis, compared to only 55 of 131 non-redheads (42 percent). The researchers concluded that the results suggest an association between the occurrence of natural red hair and those factors that lead to the development of endometriosis.

Researchers like Dr. Edwin B. Liem, an anesthesiologist from the University of Louisville's Outcomes Research Institute, in a 2002 study of the anesthetic need of persons with red hair, suspect that melanocyte-stimulating-hormone receptors, which are responsible for stimulating cells to produce the skin and hair color pigment melanin, may not function normally in women with red hair. As such, people with red hair sunburn easily. By extension, Dr. Liem suggests that this malfunction may also indirectly stimulate the brain's pain sensitivity receptors in redheads.

However, an informal survey conducted by the ERC in 2001 among its support group members, ages fourteen to fifty years, found that natural red hair was the least common hair color. Medium brown was the most common hair color among sixty-two respondents (30.65 percent), followed by dark brown (14.52 percent), light brown (11.29 percent), dark blonde (6.45 percent), red (9.68 percent), and blonde and black (4.84 percent).

Lack of Exercise

Physical activity may help reduce your risk of developing endometriosis. Research findings published in the *American Journal of Epidemiology* show that women who reported frequent, high-intensity activity had a 76 percent reduced endometrioma risk compared with women who engaged in no form of high-intensity activity. However, it should be noted that while physical activity may reduce risk of the disease, once symptoms begin, you may be less likely to exercise, thus reducing the full effect of physical activity.

Overconsumption of Coffee

Drinking more than two cups of coffee daily may significantly increase estrogen levels in your body and aid the development of endometriosis. Research findings published in *Fertility and Sterility* in October 2001 report higher levels of estradiol in women who drank at least 500 milligrams of coffee daily, the equivalent of four or five cups. During the early follicular phase of their menstrual cycles, these women had nearly 70 percent more estrogen than women who consumed no more than 100 milligrams, less than one cup, of coffee daily.

Overconsumption of Dairy Products

Dairy products contain saturated fat that puts stress on the liver to eliminate the fat from the body. This leads to reduced liver function and, inevitably, excess estrogen in the body. This increases your risk of developing endometriosis.

Overconsumption of Red Meat

Italian researchers have found that eating red meat and ham may increase your risk of developing endometriosis. Their findings, published in *Human Reproduction,* showed a 40 percent relative reduction in risk of endometriosis in women with higher consumption of green vegetables and fresh fruits. However, women with a higher intake of beef, other red meat, and ham increased their risk of developing endometriosis by 80 to 100 percent.

Animal protein contains saturated fat that, like dairy products, can put stress on the liver. This can lead to excess circulating estrogen and the increased risk of developing endometriosis.

5

Endometriosis Symptoms

The symptoms of endometriosis vary, strongly suggesting the presence of the disease but also suggesting the possibility of other conditions/diseases, as discussed in chapter 2. Additionally, many women are asymptomatic, making it very difficult to obtain a clear diagnosis. The symptoms of the disease also relate to the location of endometrial implants in the body. For instance, chronic pelvic pain and dysmenorrhea (extreme pain during menstruation) are classic symptoms of endometriosis involving the reproductive organs. Nausea, bloating, vomiting, and painful bowel movements are symptoms of endometriosis involving the gastrointestinal (GI) tract.

This chapter goes into detail about the various symptoms associated with the disease, accompanied by testimonies from women diagnosed with endometriosis.

▌ Pelvic Locations of Endometriosis

Endometriosis is commonly associated with the pelvic area and involves the reproductive organs, usually the ovaries. Other common sites for implants in this area are the following:

- ▌ Cervix
- ▌ Cul-de-sac or pouch of Douglas (area between the vagina and cervix)
- ▌ Fallopian tubes
- ▌ Ligaments that support the uterus (uterosacral ligaments)
- ▌ Outer surface of the uterus
- ▌ Pelvic peritoneum (lining of the pelvic cavity)
- ▌ Rectovaginal septum (dividing wall/membrane between the rectum and the vagina)
- ▌ Vagina

The symptoms of reproductive endometriosis include:

- ▌ Chronic to intermittent pelvic pain
- ▌ Ectopic (abnormal) pregnancies
- ▌ Heavy periods usually accompanied by heavy clotting
- ▌ Infertility or problems conceiving
- ▌ Irregular menstrual cycles
- ▌ Long menstrual cycles
- ▌ Pain during and after sexual intercourse (dyspareunia)
- ▌ Pain experienced during internal examination of the vagina
- ▌ Painful menstruation (dysmenorrhea)
- ▌ Pain with ovulation that worsens over time (mittelschmerz)
- ▌ Premenstrual spotting

Endometriosis involving the cul-de-sac also present gastrointestinal symptoms such as painful bowel movements, constipation, nausea, and vomiting, among others.

▋ Extrapelvic Locations of Endometriosis

Extrapelvic endometriosis represents a minority of all forms of the disease. Some sites of extrapelvic endometriosis include the gastrointestinal tract (GI), the urinary tract, the lungs, diaphragm, sciatic nerve, and the skin.

Gastrointestinal (GI) Tract

It is estimated that endometriosis involving the GI tract or bowel occurs in 12 to 37 percent of patients. The symptoms indicative of bowel involvement will depend on the severity and location of implants. For instance, implants are commonly found on the lower rectosigmoid colon (part of large intestine) and are associated with painful bowel movements, rectal pain while sitting or when passing gas, constipation, and diarrhea, the latter occurring during menses. Other areas of the GI tract affected by implants are the ileum (small intestine), the cecum (upper part of the large intestine), and the appendix, which hangs off the cecum. Endometriosis specialist Dr. David Redwine estimates that 30 percent of patients have more than one GI area involved.

Symptoms indicative of GI involvement include:

- Abdominal bloating
- Abdominal pain
- Alternating between constipation and diarrhea
- Blood in stool (hematochezia)
- Constipation
- Intestinal cramping
- Nausea
- Pain during rectal examinations
- Pain when passing gas
- Painful bowel movements (dyschezia)
- Rectal bleeding that may occur during menses

■ Rectal pain
■ Spasms
■ Tailbone pain

Urinary Tract

Urinary tract involvement of endometriosis occurs in about 20 percent of patients. The urinary tract includes the two kidneys, two ureters (one attached to each kidney), the bladder, and the urethra. The symptoms indicative of urinary tract involvement vary and may result when endometrial implants are located directly on these areas or when adhesions pull on the bladder.

Symptoms indicative of urinary tract involvement include:

■ Abdominal pain that is constant or is present during the menstrual cycle
■ Blood in urine (hematuria)
■ Difficult or painful urination (dysuria)
■ Fever
■ Flank (fleshy part of side of torso between the ribs and hips) pain radiating toward the groin
■ Frequent urination
■ High blood pressure (hypertension)
■ Incontinence
  • Stress incontinence (urine leakage brought on by a sneeze, laugh, cough, or sudden movement)
  • Urge incontinence (urine leakage that occurs when you feel the urge to urinate but may not have enough warning to get to the bathroom on time)
■ Lower back pain
■ Low blood pressure (hypotension)
■ Pain above the pelvic bone (suprapubic)
■ Painful or burning urination
■ Rectal pain and pressure

- Retention of urine
- Tenderness around the kidneys
- Urinary urgency (urgent need to empty the bladder)

Unfortunately for many women with urinary tract endometriosis, their symptoms are often mistaken for urinary tract infections (UTIs) or interstitial cystitis (IC), which delays proper diagnosis.

Thoracic (Lung)

Endometriosis involving the lung is rare, although mention of this form of the disease in the medical literature dates as far back as 1912. Endometriosis occurs either in the lining of the lung (the pleura) or in the lung itself (parenchyma). Thoracic endometriosis more commonly occurs in the pleura than in the lung.

Symptoms indicative of thoracic/pleural endometriosis include:

- Accumulation of air in the pleural cavity that can lead to lung collapse (catamenial pneumothorax)
- Accumulation of air in the chest cavity (pneumomediastinum)
- Collection of blood in the pleural cavity (hemothorax)
- Constricting chest pain
- Coughing up blood or bloody sputum, particularly during menses (catamenial hemoptysis)
- Deep chest pain
- Difficult or labored breathing (dyspnea)
- Dizziness
- Fatigue
- Pleural masses
- Presence of pulmonary nodules in pleural cavity
- Recurrent cough
- Right or left shoulder pain associated with menses
- Shortness of breath
- Water on the lung (pleural effusion)

All of the above symptoms are collectively referred to as thoracic endometriosis syndrome (TES). Symptoms occur within forty-eight hours of the onset of menstruation. Catamenial pneumothorax is the most commonly occurring symptom of this form of the disease. It is thought that circulating peritoneal fluid distributes endometriotic tissue that is then implanted on the diaphragm. The implanted tissue produces minute holes in the diaphragm, through which endometriotic tissue and air are transported to the lungs.

The true prevalence of this form of the disease is not quite known, although 110 cases were reported in the medical literature up to 1994, with a sprinkling of other case reports since then.

Diaphragm

The diaphragm is a thin, dome-shaped muscle that separates the chest cavity from the abdominal cavity. A very small number of cases have been reported of diaphragmatic endometriosis. Patients with this form of the disease also have pelvic endometriosis. Dr. David Redwine suggests that delayed diagnosis of this form of the disease may result from two factors. First, gynecologists are not trained to perform surgery in the upper abdomen, so they may not initially examine these areas for endometrial implants. Second, pelvic pain, the main symptom of pelvic endometriosis, occurs earlier in the patient than pain associated with diaphragmatic endometriosis.

The symptoms indicative of diaphragmatic endometriosis, similar to those of thoracic endometriosis, are a gradual onset of right or left shoulder pain associated with menses and chest pain. Some patients are asymptomatic.

Scientists suggest that, as in the case of thoracic endometriosis, circulating peritoneal fluid distributes endometriotic tissue that becomes implanted on the diaphragm. Coelomic metaplasia has also been used to explain the presence of endometriotic implants on the diaphragm.

Sciatic Area

Sciatic endometriosis is another uncommon form of the disease. This involves the sciatic nerve, a major nerve of the leg that runs down behind the thigh from the lower end of the spine.

Symptoms include:

- Cramping in the left leg when walking for long distances
- Left foot drop and weakness
- Lower back discomfort that radiates to the left leg
- Difficulty walking
- Pain in the hip that radiates down the leg
- Pain that begins just before menstruation and lasts several days after menses
- Tenderness of the sciatic notch

Endometriosis Symptoms

The following discussion focuses on many of the common symptoms and complaints faced by women with pelvic and extrapelvic endometriosis. While the mechanisms involved to account for many of these symptoms are inconclusive, scientists have explanations for some. The discussion is also supported by the words of real women diagnosed with endometriosis.

Pain/Chronic Pelvic Pain

The most common symptom associated with endometriosis is chronic pelvic pain (CPP). The American College of Obstetricians and Gynecologists (ACOG) defines chronic pelvic pain as noncyclical pain that lasts for at least six months. CPP usually occurs in locations such as the pelvis, anterior abdominal wall, lower back, or buttocks, and it is serious enough to cause disability or lead to medical care. Pain associated with endometriosis results from the release of inflammatory substances at implant sites such as prostaglandins, which irritate pain receptors. Endometriosis has also been found to compress or stretch pain receptors and to act on pain receptors to make them more sensitive; the condition may cause pain by invading tissues and organs.

Recent research revealed that sensory and sympathetic nerves grow into endometrial implants. These findings indicate that endometrial implants may have the ability to develop their own nerve supply, leading researchers to conclude that this contributes to transmitting pain as well as to the maintenance of implants.

Despite these assumptions, the association between pain and endometriosis is still unclear. The paucity in the medical literature does not accurately correlate pain and endometriosis. While there are many women who exhibit severe pain but are diagnosed with minimum to moderate endometriosis, there are instances of women who exhibit no pain but have the severe form of the disease. This absence of pain may be indicative of inactive endometrial implants, i.e., those that are less likely to release the inflammatory substances that trigger pain. It is assumed that red petechial endometriotic implants produce greater amounts of prostaglandins than typical powder-burn implants, and thus more pain such as dysmenorrhea.

Additionally, women with endometriosis have an increased number of peritoneal fluid inflammatory cells, especially macrophages, as discussed in chapter 3. These macrophages release the enzyme lysosomal, which induces tissue damage and pain, leading to the formation of adhesions or scar tissue that may also cause pain.

Despite the conflicting scientific findings, 70 to 75 percent of women who have endometriosis exhibit some type of chronic pelvic pain that has a life-altering impact, yet many are not taken seriously. Athina explains how all-consuming and life-altering her pain became:

Every day became a surprise . . . "Will I be able to walk five feet without crying, or will I have to spend another day trying to stay perfectly still for fear that my next movement will be the one that sends me to the hospital?" By December 1999, I was unable to walk ten feet without help. I was unable to do anything. The pain I had been experiencing usually occurred only the week of my menstrual cycle. However, as time passed it started to come earlier and last longer. There were whole months I spent in bed crying and in pain. I rarely left my apartment except for doctor appointments and occasionally to see my family. Around this time, I also started to go to a physician that my boyfriend recommended since I was too old to continue seeing a pediatrician. I was given painkillers and instructed to go for X-rays, ultrasounds, and blood tests. I was also referred to a gastroenterologist because the pain was so close to my abdomen. In addition, I went to numerous gynecologists, and they all told me endometriosis wasn't the cause of my pain. They all sent me for ultrasounds, and they were confident the pain I was feeling was caused by a cyst on my left ovary. This pattern of test after test, specialist after specialist, lasted for over a year. I would explain to these doctors that I had experienced this pain for years and it had progressively gotten worse. However, they weren't listening. They all looked at me as if I was whining about a cramp or two, when they could see I could barely walk without being in tears.

According to an EA survey of 968 women, ages fifteen to fifty-nine, to determine specific information about women's experiences with chronic pelvic pain, 40 percent of women who suffer from chronic pelvic pain due to endometriosis or postsurgical scar tissue have been told they exaggerate their pain. Lisa-Marie describes just such an experience:

At the age of seventeen, I started bleeding one day and didn't stop until a year later. I was weak and nauseated. I actually looked as bad as I felt . . . but still no doctor would take notice of me. My mother was told that my symptoms were psychosomatic and that there was nothing wrong with me.

For Julie M., the unbelievers extended to family, friends, and doctors:

I can't remember exactly when the pain started. I really don't remember ever not having it early on. But I was so ashamed that I had started my period that I didn't really talk to anyone about it at first. Eventually the pain became so intense that I did tell my family. I don't remember their initial reaction or the exact moment that I told them, but I do know that my pain was greatly misunderstood by my family and friends. It sort of became the big joke: Julie, the hypochondriac.

    In college I tried a different doctor. He said that he felt some kind of mass, so he did a vaginal sonogram, which revealed that my ovary was enlarged. He wanted to do a laparoscopy to see what was going on. My parents were not in favor of this idea, so I went for a second opinion. This new doctor examined me; when he was finished, he explained to me that there was absolutely nothing wrong with me and that I needed to "stop thinking about the pain and move on." When I started to cry in his office, he, with a condescending tone, asked me, "Why are you crying? You are healthy. Go home." He patted me on my head and left the office.

The survey also found that:

▮ Of the 40 percent told they exaggerate their pain, 52 percent were told this by their OB/GYN and 43 percent by a friend or family member.

▮ 60 percent of these women were told their pain was normal—56 percent of them by their OB/GYN and 29 percent by a friend or family member.

▮ 43 percent described their pain as constant.

▮ 26 percent described their pain as severe, 18 percent as very severe, and 9 percent as unbearable.

▮ More than 80 percent say they have been unable to work at times due to chronic pelvic pain.

▮ 45 percent have been debilitated for two to three days or longer each month.

Chronic pelvic pain can also be caused by other conditions, as discussed in chapter 2. Dr. David Redwine suggests, however, that gynecologists should have endometriosis at the top of their lists because the condition is very common.

Pain caused by endometriosis will also manifest itself according to the location of implants. For instance, endometriotic implants located in the reproductive organs are associated with chronic to intermittent pelvic pain and dysmenorrhea (painful menstruation). Pain symptoms associated with endometriosis in the GI tract include rectal pain, tailbone pain, sharp gas pains, painful bowel movements, and pain when passing gas. Endometriosis involving the urinary tract results in painful or burning urination and pain that radiates toward the groin. Pain in the leg and/or hip that radiates down the leg is a symptom of sciatic endometriosis involving the sciatic nerve.

Painful Menstruation (Dysmenorrhea)

Dysmenorrhea, extremely painful menstruation, is very common among women with endometriosis. The pain usually comes on prior to, during, and after menses. Pain during menstruation is not normal. Many women report the inability to do normal activities such as going to work, attending school, exercising, shopping, and even walking because of dysmenorrhea, which basically disables them for the length of their menses. Christel describes her monthly periods:

> *I have always had very severe abdominal and pelvic pains (mostly during my menstruation) and heavy periods, but during the autumn of 1998 the pains became worse. I also had premenstrual spotting, but the pains were so bad that almost every time I had my menstruation I was lying on the bathroom floor shaking and cold sweating.*

The EA reports that over 96 percent of the women in their Research Registry have dysmenorrhea, yet the condition is hardly studied. Additionally, women themselves have been socialized to believe that excruciating menstrual pains are normal and just our burden for being female. Jude's religious upbringing determined her acceptance of the pain:

> *I had my first period at eleven. As I got older my periods became heavier and more painful, to the point where my friends would comment that I looked pale and unwell. I never talked about my periods with anyone, not even my mother. I thought that painful periods were a part of my lot as a woman, confirmed by strict religious upbringing that periods were Eve's punishment for tempting Adam in the Garden of Eden.*

Depression/Mood Changes

Confronted with increasingly worsening pain, long and irregular menses, problems conceiving as well as other debilitating physical manifestations of endometriosis, many women experience changes in their moods, stress, anxiety, increased irritability, feeling low, especially during menstruation; or increased depression. These emotional changes also result from the inability to make others understand that their pain is real.

Athina describes the debilitating emotional aspects of her life with endometriosis:

Even though this is a physically painful disease without a cure, the hardest part to deal with is the emotional aspect. I sometimes feel helpless and a burden on those around me. In the beginning I was literally a prisoner in my apartment, and the warden was "endo." This made it very easy to fall into a depressive state, where nothing brought me joy. I would have horrific mood swings. One second I'd be crying, and the next I'd be mad. Since my life quickly went from active to sedentary, I gained weight, which just added to my self-loathing. It was such a shock to my system that I didn't know what was up and what was down. I started to isolate myself from those around me. I began to act out of character, doing things I'd never fathom just to push people away. I tried to commit suicide twice because the pain I felt was unbearable.

Errikka also felt the emotional stresses of endometriosis:

I tried really hard to deal with all aspects of the disease. I discussed it a lot with my family and boyfriend. They have all been such an amazing part of my fight with this awful disease. My whole family became very involved in learning about endo and how to help me cope. Even though my family and boyfriend were very supportive, I was still very depressed. In the time span of a year my life changed dramatically. I wasn't able to do anything anymore. All of my energy was engulfed by my daily pain. I felt useless. I had this unexplainable weight in my heart. I couldn't help but feel sorry for myself. I suddenly didn't know how to live anymore.

My relationship with my boyfriend changed from our being a couple to him being my nurse. We never got the chance for our relationship to grow because I was always sick and he was always taking care of me. We no longer had an intimate relationship, and unfortunately things never did get back to normal for us.

I worried about never having children. I worried about finding someone who would love me in spite of my having this horrible disease. I thought about how painful it was to have a physical relationship and who would understand. I just became this person who didn't feel worthy of finding love.

In a 2004 Parade/Research! America Health poll, depression was listed as the top health issue (22 percent) that has the most impact on the quality of women's lives. In an informal poll regarding quality of life conducted by the ERC of 1,016 members of its support groups, ages fourteen to fifty, 7.09 percent suffer/suffered from depression while 10.53 percent described endometriosis as "the most painful of their medical problems."

■ ■ ■ The Link Between Pain and Depression ■ ■ ■

By Jennifer Lobb, Managing Editor,
www.NationalPainFoundation.org

(Reprinted with permission from the National Pain Foundation)

Pain and depression are inexorably linked in a complex way. Pain causes depression—depression causes pain. About 30 percent of patients with persistent pain conditions suffer from clinical depression related to their pain, and almost all persons will experience some mood changes. Seventy-five percent of patients with clinical depression present to their doctors because of physical symptoms, including pain.[1] People in pain who have symptoms of depression experience more impairment associated with pain than those who do not have depressive symptoms.[2]

To successfully treat your chronic pain, you and your physician need to examine the emotional factors that may influence your pain level and physical disability. One of the first steps to treating pain is recognizing that depression often accompanies pain and that increases in pain or widespread pain (i.e., pain in many areas of your body) can be a symptom of depression. Understanding this aspect of your pain experience may help you identify your own symptoms and seek the care you need to lessen your pain.

The Pervasiveness of Pain

Chronic pain affects all aspects of life. It affects your quality of life as it limits your physical functioning, your ability to perform activities of daily living, and your ability to work. It has social consequences for your marital and family relationships, it may limit intimacy with your partner, and it may prevent interaction with friends. Chronic pain has societal consequences in terms of increased health care costs, increased disability costs, and lost productivity that is a consequence of missed workdays.

Given the pervasiveness of pain, it's no wonder that chronic pain affects your psychological well-being as well.[3] Research indicates that as the number and severity of a patient's physical symptoms increase, the number and severity of psychological complaints increase.[4] In other words, the more places you feel pain and the more severe the pain, the more likely you are to have a depression or problems such as difficulty sleeping or anxiety and the more severe these symptoms are. Some of the signs and symptoms related to depression reported by chronic pain patients treated at pain clinics include:

- physical deconditioning
- sleep disturbance
- reduced sexual activities
- family stress
- work issues
- legal issues
- financial concerns
- decreased self-esteem
- fear of injury
- altered mood, including irritability, anxiety, and depression[5]

Why do pain and depression coexist so often? Scientists have been studying this relationship through neurosciences and epidemiology and have made important discoveries. First of all, both depression and the suffering of pain are located in the same area of the brain.[6] Second, the same chemical messengers are involved in regulating pain and mood.[7] What are the mechanisms that affect these parts of the brain and these chemical systems? We find that depression runs in families, so that the stress of having pain may trigger the chemical changes in the brain leading to depression in persons who may be vulnerable because of a family tendency (genetic) to depressive illness. More commonly, however, a person has no family vulnerability to depression, but may get "worn down" by all the stress, losses, and problems encountered by having pain over many months.[8] Either way, this "wearing down" is biochemical, such that certain important chemicals (similar to vitamins) that are responsible for regulating both pain and mood appear to be functionally depleted. This is why the same medications that are helpful in depression may also effectively treat pain, because they enhance the pain and mood-regulating effects of these chemical systems in your brain.

Approximately 40 percent to 60 percent of patients being treated at pain clinics report experiencing symptoms of depression.[9] Unfortunately, people experiencing pain do not always receive the treatment they need to combat their depression and their pain, especially if they do not see physicians with the training and background to treat both together (e.g., pain medicine specialists, psychiatrists, or primary care physicians with this training). Given the nature of today's health care system, most Americans receive mental health care by visiting their primary care physician, but research studies indicate that 50 percent of patients who are clinically depressed are not diagnosed by their primary care physicians.[10] So be on the lookout for depression in yourself and loved ones and seek treatment before the negative effects occur.

Treating Depression and Pain

Seeking help and advocating for yourself are the first steps to treating your pain. Your physician's goals in treating you are to reduce your pain, improve your physical functioning, reduce your psychological distress, and improve your overall quality of life.[11] There are many different ways to treat depression and anxiety related to pain. Your physician may suggest one or more of the following therapies to reduce your psychological distress:

- medication
- cognitive-behavioral therapy
- stress management (e.g., relaxation techniques, hypnosis, biofeedback)
- supportive counseling
- family counseling[12]

It's important to remember that being depressed is not a sign of personal weakness—depression and anxiety are related to chemical imbalances in your brain.[13] Depressive and anxiety disorders are illnesses that can be treated. Taking medication and going to therapy to treat your depression is the same as taking antibiotics to treat an infection—the necessary steps you take to get better.

It's also important to keep in mind that not every medication or therapy works immediately for even depression and pain.[14] They also require your active participation in your care and recovery. Following are some suggestions for actively participating in your care and helping you and your physician work together to treat your pain and your depression:

- Keep a diary and record changes in your pain and emotions. Visit the My Pain section of http://www.pain connection.org and keep a pain journal online. You can print it out and bring it with you to your doctors' appointments to remind yourself of how you were feeling and when you were feeling better or worse.
- Identify a support network. Support persons could include family members, friends, support groups. The National Pain Foundation's My Community area is an online support group for persons in pain (http://www.painconnection.org/MyCommunity).
- Educate yourself through books, reputable Web sites, and organizations.
- Set realistic treatment goals.
- Stay active—with your doctor's advice and approval, begin an exercise program, try yoga, or do other stretching activities.
- Try the stress management techniques you learn in counseling and use them regularly. Guided imagery, hypnosis, biofeedback, and relaxation techniques really can work if you work at using them.

Depression is an illness, and ignoring it will not make it go away. Seek the treatment you need to get better and be involved in your care.

"When you do nothing, you feel overwhelmed and power-less. But when you get involved, you feel the sense of hope and accomplishment that comes from knowing you are working to make things better."

Pauline R. Kezer

References

1. R M Gallagher, S Cariati, "The pain-depression conundrum: bridging the body and mind," 2 October 2002. Available from Medscape.com.
2. J Mossey, R M Gallagher, F Tirumalasetti, "Pain and depression reduce physical functioning in elderly residents of a continuing care retirement community: implications for health management," *Pain Medicine* 1(4): 340–350, 2000.
3. D C Turk, "Beyond the symptoms: the painful manifestations of depression." Presented at Pain and Depression: Navigating the Intersection of Body and Mind Symposium, San Diego, 20 August 2002.
4. K Kroenke, J L Jackson, J Chamberlin, "Depressive and anxiety disorders in patients presenting with physical complaints: clinical predictors and outcome," *Am J Med* (103)339–347, 1997; K Kroenke, R L Spitzer, F V deGruy III, R Swindle, "A symptom checklist to screen for somatoform disorders in primary care," *Psychosomatics* 39:263–272, 1998; D Watson, J W Pennebaker, "Health complaints, stress, and distress: exploring the central role of negative affectivity," *Psychol Rev* 96:234–254, 1989.
5. D C Turk, "Beyond the symptoms."
6. H P Rome, J D Rome, "Limbically augmented pain syndrome (LAPS): kindling, corticolimbic sensitization and the convergence of affective and sensory symptoms in chronic pain disorders," *Pain Medicine* 1(1) 7–23, 2000.
7. Ibid.; R M Gallagher, S Verma, "Managing pain and co-morbid depression: a public health challenge," *Seminars in Clinical Neuropsychiatry* 4(3) 203–220, 1999.
8. B Dohrenwend, J Marbach, K Raphael, R M Gallagher, "Why is depression co-morbid with chronic facial pain? A family study test of alternative hypotheses," *Pain* 83:183–192, 1999.

9. D C Turk, "Beyond the symptoms."
10. Depression Guideline Panel. *Depression in Primary Care: Volume 1. Detection and Diagnosis. Clinical Practice Guideline,* Number 5. Rockville, MD: U.S. Department of Health and Human Services; 1993. AHCPR Publication No. 93-0550. G E Simon, M VonKorff, "Recognition, management, and outcomes of depression in primary care," *Arch Fam Med* 4:99–105, 1995. R M Gallagher, S Cariati, "The pain-depression conundrum."
11. D C Turk, "Beyond the symptoms."
12. Ibid.
13. R M Gallagher, S Cariati, "The pain-depression conundrum."
14. Ibid.

Heavy/Long Periods and Irregular Cycles

Heavy periods, accompanied by heavy clotting, are also a common symptom of endometriosis. The menstrual flow lasts longer than seven days, with some women requiring both tampons and sanitary napkins for protection. The length of the menstrual cycle is also affected in women with endometriosis. Often the cycle is shorter than the normal twenty-eight days, and/or irregular. Gen describes her menstrual cycle:

Since I began to have a menstrual cycle I was in pain. It progressed slowly at first, but by the time I turned fifteen the pain was unbearable. I would have thirty-six-day cycles, a period that lasted ten days with extremely heavy bleeding and debilitating pain.

Celina describes how she dealt with her heavy menstrual flows as a young girl:

There would be days I would be sitting in math class, scared to get out of my desk until everyone left because there was a pool of blood in my seat. I would wipe it up, go home, change my pants, and go back to school, figuring all the time that other girls were doing the same thing.

It is believed that greater/longer menstrual flows and irregular menstrual cycles may increase your risk of developing endometriosis.

Infertility/Problems Conceiving

Infertility is another common symptom of endometriosis. In fact, endometriosis-associated infertility occurs in one in three women with the disease, or between 30 to 50 percent of women diagnosed with endometriosis experience problems conceiving. It is difficult, however, to determine if endometriosis is the primary cause of infertility, especially in women with a mild form of the disease. In stages III and IV forms of the disease extensive scarrings distort the normal anatomy of the reproductive tract, easily creating an environment that promotes infertility. However, in infertile women with moderate to mild endometriosis (stages I and II), with no anatomical distortions, the association between endometriosis and infertility is very unclear.

Despite the various medical explanations about the causal relationship between endometriosis and infertility (see chapter 8), the emotional impact is very certain. The inability to conceive is emotionally and physically distressing. Linda describes her experience:

My husband and I were desperately trying to have a child. Although my husband had raised my daughter since she was two years old he still wanted nothing more than to have a child of his own. The sex was extremely painful at times but was worth every pain if I could conceive a child. There was heartbreak every month. Because my periods were not on a perfect schedule I often found myself buying home pregnancy tests. They never turned up positive. I kept a journal of my periods; we took my temperature every morning and recorded it. I began to keep a record of boys' and girls' names that I liked. We had sex every other day; my husband started taking zinc. The doctor felt my husband should be tested since I had already had a child. My husband's test came back with a low sperm count, hence the zinc. We were told to have him tested again since sometimes if you are sick the count can be low. We did this and the test came back fine the second time. Now the pressure was on from my husband. He wanted to do anything and everything to have a child. I was falling apart. The ups and downs of every month hoping you have conceived and finding out you haven't was destroying me.

Gen also feels the same:

Dealing with infertility has been quite a challenge. At first I thought it would be easy to get pregnant, but I was so wrong. At this point in my life, I have been told that I will never be able to conceive on my own, and that with in vitro fertilization I have a 25 percent chance of success. Being infertile takes a toll on you physically and mentally. I ended up breaking up with my fiancé as a result of this. He just couldn't accept the fact that I would most likely never be able to bear a child. Accepting the fact that I may never bear a child of my own has been extremely difficult. Every time my period is late I hope and pray that it is because I am pregnant. Every time a pregnancy test comes back positive, I pray that the pregnancy will keep, and without fail I miscarry every time. Sometimes I wonder how I have made it this far, since learning that I will most likely never carry.

Miscarriages

Increased levels of inflammatory prostaglandins can result in muscular contractions or spasms that may adversely affect the egg's travel through the fallopian tube and cause a miscarriage. Women with endometriosis have a higher-than-average risk for miscarriages.

Cassandra describes the fateful events that led up to her miscarriage:

After a few intense discussions with my boyfriend at the time (he later left me for another woman when it was discovered that I was infertile) and a lot of research on my part, we decided to go ahead and try despite the fact that we were both busy in college and working as well. I was still recovering from my laparoscopy, but we went ahead anyway. A few months later we were blessed, and I was the happiest I have ever been. I had charted my basal body temperatures at my doctor's recommendation because time was important so I knew exactly when I had conceived. I had to go for weekly blood tests because my doctor said there was an increased risk for miscarriage in patients with endo, but after a few weeks all looked good. I ate right, rested, and swam for exercise.

It wasn't. At nine and a half weeks I lost the baby. I had started bleeding on the weekend and, after a visit to the ER, I was told my blood work was fine, to go home and have complete bed rest for four days, then follow up with my doctor. I did and was told my results were in fact bad and I was to go for an ultrasound because I was miscarrying. I went and my heart was shredded to the core when there was no heartbeat. The baby had died.

Dawn had a similar experience:

In June of 2001, my husband and I decided to add to our family. Dorian was about to turn two, we had just bought a house, and life was going well. I was ecstatic to discover that I was pregnant with our second child on June 22. We told Dorian that there was a baby growing in Mommy's tummy and he was going to be a big brother. He was so happy! He put his hand on my tummy and said "Baby!" all the time, and we were so excited. I began to take my prenatal vitamins and plan my maternity leave. February 24 was my due date, and we were going to have beautiful Christmas pictures of Dorian holding my huge tummy.

On the 4th of July we went to a parade, and I began to feel very sick—light-headed and nauseous. It was unbelievably hot that day, and I felt better in the air-conditioning. On the 9th, we went to see a movie. I had been cramping and, when the movie was over, I went to use the restroom. I was bleeding. My baby and all of my dreams were gone in an instant.

My miscarriage has affected not only me, but also my husband and especially my little boy. We had to tell him he wasn't going to be a big brother anymore, and I can't even describe to you the hurt in his eyes. When I told him the baby had gone to heaven, he patted my tummy and said "Baby, heaven." My heart has never broken into so many pieces as it did that day.

Painful Intercourse (Dyspareunia)

Painful intercourse or dyspareunia is also another common symptom for 59 percent of women diagnosed with endometriosis. The pain often occurs during deep penetration and is associated with implants that are located on the uterosacral ligaments or on other areas that are stretched, pushed, or pulled with thrusting.

In the first study to describe the quality of sex life in women with endometriosis, Dr. Simone Ferrero and colleagues from San Martino Hospital at the University of Genoa evaluated the sexual function of 299 women undergoing surgery for infertility or pelvic pain. The findings of the study were published in the March 2005 issue of *Fertility and Sterility*. They found that of 170 women with endometriosis, 61 percent reported deep pain during sexual intercourse. More than 50 percent of women with endometriosis have had dyspareunia their entire sex lives. The study also found that women with endometriosis had sex less often, had less satisfying orgasms, had more frequent interruption of intercourse due to pain, and felt less relaxed and fulfilled after intercourse compared to women without endometriosis.

For Jude sex was unpleasant:

Some years after I got married in 1995, I began to notice that sex was becoming painful and unpleasant. I felt tight and experienced a grating sensation. Sex became something to avoid rather than to plan and enjoy.

Johnna also had a similar experience:

The pain got so bad, all I could do was curl up in a ball with heat applied to my abdomen. I could not even have sex with my husband because I would hurt so bad. And when I did I would always end up in tears.

The effect on relationships can be devastating. Julie M. describes her situation:

I started having extreme pain at such a young age that, in some ways, I am used to it. The pain is so familiar—just a part of who I am. The biggest area where endometriosis has affected my life is in regard to sex. It has been a very long and difficult challenge for my husband and me. He is very sensitive about my having endometriosis. He's read books with me, written letters about it with me, let me sleep in when I am feel-

ing too sick to get up on the weekends to care for our boys. But it is hard for him to fully understand how this has affected me sexually. Most of the time that we are together it is painful, both during and after. I usually have cramps and bleed afterward. It is hard for me to feel sexy, to want to be with him in that way. This is very difficult for him to fully understand and appreciate. We have had many fights, many harsh words, many wounds created because of this disease. I sometimes don't know how we will ever heal this area of our lives.

Constipation, Diarrhea, Painful Bowel Movements

Many endometriosis patients complain of symptoms that are associated with their gastrointestinal (GI) tract. Drs. Robert Albee and Ken Sinervo of the Center for Endometriosis Care (CEC) estimate that many as 60 percent or more of women with endometriosis may have at least one symptom associated with their bowel. These symptoms include constipation, diarrhea, painful bowel movements, intestinal cramping, nausea and/or vomiting, abdominal pain, rectal bleeding and/or rectal pain, among others.

Some patients may have all of these symptoms or just one. Based on preoperative questionnaires issued to all patients at the CEC, Dr. Sinervo found that:

- 25 percent of patients experience intestinal cramping and painful bowel movements
- 35 percent experience constipation
- 60 percent experience diarrhea

In the majority of patients with bowel symptoms, endometriosis is not located on the bowel. In fact, the experts suggest that less than 10 to 15 percent of patients actually have endometrial implants directly on their bowel. Instead, bowel symptoms are commonly induced by irritation from implants located in adjacent areas such as the cul-de-sac, uterosacral ligaments, and rectovaginal septum. Some bowel symptoms are due to adhesions that are constricting, twisting, or pulling on the bowel.

Julie M.'s bowel symptoms were very severe:

> [During] my second year in college, the pain became increasingly worse. I could barely function during the first few days of my period. I also started to have pain while having bowel movements. It was so intense that I would sometimes just cry and cry while using the restroom. I remember, later on in college, driving from my hometown to where my mother lived. Halfway there, a pain unlike any other I've felt in my life came over my abdomen. I had to pull over. I managed to get to a restroom at a fast food restaurant. I remember throwing up and having diarrhea. I also blacked out a few times. My appendix had been removed when I was thirteen because it was inflamed and had almost burst. I kept thinking, Did my appendix grow back? I couldn't imagine what was going on inside of me.
>
> I don't know for sure how long I was in the bathroom at this restaurant, but eventually I did make it to my mother's house. I was uncomfortable for a few days after that and had some bleeding. No one really took this too seriously, so I never did anything about it. After that day, though, my bowel problems intensified, my periods became worse than ever, and my midcycle pain intensified.

Migraines/Frequent Headaches

Women with endometriosis also frequently complain of migraines and headaches. A recent study by the University of Genoa of 133 women with endometriosis and 166 without found that twice the number of women with endometriosis (30 percent) had migraines compared to those without (15 percent). While a link between the two conditions is not very clear, the researchers suggest that biomedical mediators may be involved. This includes the systemic spreading of prostaglandins that are produced by endometriosis.

Sandy describes her migraine problems:

The migraines continued with several a month, and I had problems getting my insurance company to approve enough of the Imitrex to keep me functional. Sometimes the headaches would last for days, and they were very painful. It was hard to concentrate on getting anything accomplished.

Immune System–Related Dysfunction

Women with endometriosis also complain of other conditions such as allergies, asthma, chronic fatigue syndrome (CFS), and fibromyalgia. In the 2002 EA/NICHD/George Washington University study discussed in chapter 3, they found that:

- Chronic fatigue syndrome, a condition characterized by medically unexplained fatigue, was more than a hundred times more common in women with endometriosis than in the general U.S. female population.
- Hypothyroidism, characterized by an underactive thyroid gland that causes mental and physical slowing, was found to be seven times more common.
- Fibromyalgia, a condition involving widespread body pain and tiredness, was twice as common.
- Autoimmune inflammatory diseases such as systemic lupus erythematosis, Sjörgen's syndrome, rheumatoid arthritis, and multiple sclerosis occurred more frequently in women with endometriosis.

Allergies and asthma are found in very high rates among women with endometriosis. While allergies are found in 18 percent of the general female population, they occur in 61 percent of women with endometriosis. The study found that this number increased if the women had additional diseases. If there was endometriosis plus an endocrine disease, the number for allergies increased to 72 percent. Endometriosis plus fibromyalgia or CFS increases the presence of allergies to 68 percent.

Amy had this to say:

> I am also finding myself getting other ailments much more frequently. I recently read that one theory of the cause of endometriosis is an immune deficiency, and that women with endo are more prone to allergies and other sicknesses. I have allergy problems now and get a lot of sinus infections. I never had these kinds of problems until my endometriosis got out of control. I get so sick of not feeling well. It seems like my favorite phrase has become "I don't feel good."

Brandilyn's experience mirrors Amy's:

> One thing I did notice was as my pain increased, so did my allergies and fatigue. Seemed I never wanted to do anything, and I was always on allergy medications and having sinus infections. I at first never linked the two together, but now I find more and more people with fatigue and allergies who have endometriosis.

Catamenial Pneumothorax (CPT)

This is a common symptom of thoracic endometriosis that is characterized by a recurrence of air in the lungs during menstruation that causes them to collapse. This occurs in women in their thirties and forties and almost always occurs on the right side of the body. It is estimated that catamenial pneumothorax (CPT) occurs in 75 percent of patients with thoracic endometriosis. Women who experience CPT also exhibit monthly chest pains, shortness of breath, dizziness, and fatigue, which are other common symptoms of thoracic endometriosis.

Lynn and Lori Phillips, twin sisters who call themselves the "Pneumothorax Twins," describe their experiences with CPT:

We were thirty-nine years old, a few months before our fortieth birthday, nonsmokers, and in good health, when our symptoms first started. In those months we did not experience chest pain, but did have episodes of dizziness and a "crackling sound" upon inhalation. Symptoms would last a few days, resolve, and then return later. We did not correlate the symptoms to the onset of menses at that time.

Prior to this little adventure, we were both on ovulation suppression hormones, which were discontinued about one year before. Lynn experienced shortness of breath when the crackling sound returned in December 2002. Due to a throat infection one week prior, she thought she might have bronchitis and went to the doctor for an evaluation. A chest X-ray showed a 90 percent pneumothorax. The doctor called for an ambulance. She had a chest tube inserted in the ER and spent four days in the hospital.

One month later and back to work, Lynn became lightheaded and experienced yet another exciting ride in the ambulance! An X-ray showed a 20 percent recollapse. Both collapses had occurred at the start of her period. Being made aware (after the first collapse) of a type of pneumothorax associated with menses, we thought it too coincidental. Although Lynn was never diagnosed with pelvic endometriosis, twin sister Lori was and both shared all the same symptoms.

Gratefully, the surgeon was aware of the condition. He provided the name of it, and sent Lynn home with a Heimlich valve chest tube (a one-way valve that lets air out of the pleural space, but not back in).

After one week the collapse did not resolve, and the pulmonary specialist suggested chemical pleurodesis (the standard treatment for recurring spontaneous pneumothorax: SPT). After reading about CPT, we knew that pleurodesis alone in such cases showed a high rate of recurrence, because it does not address the cause of the collapses. When this was suggested to the pulmonary specialist, he flatly dismissed the possibility, because the condition was so rare.

Lynn refused the pleurodesis and spoke to her doctor about surgical options. Gratefully, he was much more open to the idea, and she was referred for surgery. During VATS, the surgeon found and sutured holes in the diaphragm. He also found scar tissue, which may have indicated past smaller collapses that had resolved themselves. He performed the pleural abrasion with talc. Lynn spent twelve days in the hospital.

During all of this, and for the few months prior, Lori had been experiencing episodes of light-headedness, off and on. She thought it was due to the massive bleeding she had been experiencing after receiving an injection of Depo Provera (about nine months prior, for endometriosis). In March of 2003, the dizziness got very bad and she went into an urgent care facility. After explaining to the doctor that she wanted an X-ray to rule out a pneumothorax, he said that she had good breath sounds and good blood oxygenation and refused to give her one. A few days later she was back and again asked for an X-ray, which showed a 60 percent collapse. She was transported to the hospital ER, declined a chest tube, and requested to speak to the thoracic surgeon. Two days later, Lori underwent VATS, and her surgeon also found holes in the diaphragm. He repaired the holes and performed pleural abrasion.

We are still in the process of recovering. Breathing is still at times a bit labored (two months after surgery), but is getting better every day. We still have some pain (from the chest tubes), mostly a sporadic stinging kind of pain under and along the inside of the right breast. There is still numbness there as well.

Overall recovery is going well, and we feel more back to normal each day. We have a new appreciation for just being able to breath without having to think about it! We have learned a lot along the way, and were blessed to be cared for by some really wonderful doctors, nurses, and hospital staff.

Urinary Problems

Urinary problems also show up in some patients. These include frequent urination, painful or burning urination, urinary urgency, and incontinence, among others. These symptoms are indicative of endometriosis of the urinary tract but also symptomatic of interstitial cystitis (IC), a chronic inflammation of the wall of the bladder in the absence of bacteria. Many patients eventually diagnosed with endometriosis have also been diagnosed with IC.

Andy describes her monthly IC "attacks," which always coincided with her menses:

November 1996 . . . I started to suffer with monthly bouts of cystitis, . . . always just before or during my period. The attacks were frightening, horribly painful, leaving me exhausted, passing blood, and not daring to move more than a room away from the bathroom. Sometimes even that was too far, and I moved into the bathroom with a hot-water bottle, a couple of liters of water, a radio, and a book for a couple of hours.

After three attacks in four weeks in August 1997, I started to get symptoms every day. They started off as a tickle almost, an irritation, but they made traveling and sitting through lectures difficult, and woke me several times a night. By October 1997, I was depressed.

March 1998, I was at the end of my tether. I had tried cranberry juice until just the smell made me want to throw up. I was drinking three liters of water a day just to stop the burning in my bladder. I was waking up on average two or three times a night, though some nights I was peeing every ten or fifteen minutes. My friendships, my relationship, my social life, my studies were all suffering because of this.

Fatigue and Insomnia

Fatigue is also a constant complaint for many endometriosis patients. This can follow after an intense physical workout, long hours at work, or may be a chronic and consistent state of exhaustion, even after more than eight hours of sleep, that affects daily activities and state of mind.

Elisabet describes the extent of her fatigue:

I always used to need about fourteen hours of sleep per night. There seemed that there was no end to my sleeping ability and need. I never became satisfied. I never woke up feeling rested, renewed, or refreshed. I would always wake up feeling like I had just run a marathon. . . . Today, I have learned from other endo sufferers that they are overly tired, too, and that there may be a connection between fatigue and endo. Knowing this makes me feel so much better. All these years I truly thought that I was just very lazy. Now, I know there may be more to it. Looking back, this actually explains quite a few situations where I always felt that I was so much more tired than others. I'd be amazed with people for having the kind of energy that they did. I could only explain it with me being unnaturally tired and stressed out, or something.

My social life often becomes the main loser due to my fatigue. Getting out of the house makes me so exhausted. I need to prioritize my health, and that seldom leaves much room to go out and hang with friends or go to clubs, cafés, or stores. I can't really eat out anymore so for me to go out requires that I make food and bring it with me. It's a hassle. I try my best to create some kind of balance, but it's not easy. My hope is that, in time, I'll get extra energy reserves. After all, I'm in the middle of healing. That takes a lot of energy in itself.

Insomnia is also a common complaint among endometriosis patients. They find it difficult to fall asleep or to remain asleep for an adequate length of time due to the constant pain and other related problems.

Anemia

Generally, many women with endometriosis suffer from the symptoms of anemia. Women with endometriosis experience longer durations of menses and greater volume of menstrual flow. This increased blood loss reduces the quantity of iron in the body necessary for the production of hemoglobin, an oxygen-carrying pigment, needed by red blood cells to transport oxygen throughout the body.

This lack of iron is called iron-deficiency anemia. Symptoms include:

▪ Brittle nails
▪ Depression
▪ Headaches
▪ Irritability
▪ Light-headedness

■ Pale skin
■ Pounding heartbeat and/or heart palpitations
■ Shortness of breath
■ Tiredness

Shortness of breath, dizziness, and fatigue are also common symptoms of thoracic endometriosis.

The endometriosis Symptoms Evaluation Toolkit in chapter 11 will help you assess your various symptoms. The tools include a monthly symptoms chart you can use to record your symptoms on a daily basis; a pain map to pinpoint the precise locations of your pain; and a risk factors and symptoms checklist that provides a complete list of all the risks touched on in chapter 3 as well as a comprehensive listing of the symptoms discussed above, and more.

These tools offer you an organized way to better communicate with your doctor and get a quick diagnosis as well as to assess the onset of new symptoms if already diagnosed, for better treatment.

PART TWO

Endometriosis Treatment Options

6

Surgical Management of Endometriosis and Pain

My first line of treatment was surgery, a laparotomy. It came like a blessing for me, one that continues to this day. The level of my pain drastically reduced in the months after my surgery, and I was able to comfortably endure my monthly cycles. But the course I was taken on to actually have the surgery was an emotional roller coaster.

Medical advice was that the surgery to remove the cyst should be done at the same time as the procedure to remove the stent. (Remember I had the stent left in from my previous kidney surgery.) I agreed, and, while they prepared the operating theater, I was wheeled into the recovery room to wait. I stayed there for about forty-five minutes; while there, the tears eventual burst through their barrier. I watched as post-op patients slept, and I felt a sense of doom and fear. Unfortunately, the surgeon did not have the right instrument to remove the stent, so that surgery had to be rescheduled. However, my gynecologist went ahead and removed the cyst. I have the scar below my navel to prove it.

Surgery has long been established as an integral tool in the management of endometrial implants and the disease's associated pain. This is especially so in the case of moderate to severe disease and when other organs of the body are involved, such as the bowel and bladder. Surgery also has more value to the patient who needs to improve her fertility and get pregnant as soon as possible. All medical treatment options, by their nature, prevent conception.

This chapter concerns itself with the various surgical treatment options available to treat your endometriosis and its associated pain. These options belong to two categories: conservative surgery and radical surgery.

▮ Conservative Surgery

The main aim of conservative surgery is to remove all implants and endometriomas (ovarian cysts filled with endometrial tissue that are very common in the endometriosis patient), and restore the reproductive organs to normalcy in order to preserve the patient's fertility. Experts like Dr. David Redwine strongly suggest that surgery should be the first line of treatment, since hormonal suppression does not eradicate endometriosis.

Two main categories of conservative surgical techniques are available to you to treat endometriosis-associated pain. The first category of surgery is directed at removing all endometriotic implants to realize optimum pain relief. The second category is directed at interrupting the transmission of pain signals from the uterus.

▮ Surgery Directed at Endometriosis

Laparoscopy

While laparoscopy is a diagnostic method (see chapter 12), it is also used as an operative procedure. During the laparoscopy, the surgeon can remove any implants found using any of five techniques:

excision, laser vaporization, ablation, eletrocoagulation, or fulguration. The method used depends on the surgeon's preference and skill level.

Excision

This is the most popular and effective method used by surgeons to remove endometrial implants. To excise means to cut out entire endometrial implants by hand, while preserving healthy portions of the affected organ(s). There are two main advantages of excision. First, it can quickly remove large amounts of endometrial implants at one time, without damaging the underlying structures. Second, excision has a high rate of effectiveness in significantly reducing pain.

One of excision's most fervent supporters is Dr. David Redwine, who argues that excision positively identifies, through biopsy, what has been removed while, in the case of vaporization and coagulation, only the surgeon's opinion is given as to what has been destroyed and how complete that destruction was.

Excision is not limited to particular areas in the pelvic/abdominal cavity. Endometrial implants can be removed from anywhere in the body using excision, such as hard-to-reach areas like the cul-de-sac as well as from the bladder and the bowel, without high risk of damage to underlying structures. Additionally, excision has been shown to be the only surgical method effective in eradicating or reducing endometriosis for the long term. For instance, in a recent five-year study of 176 women who had confirmed endometriosis following laparoscopic excision, 67 percent experienced improvement following the surgery compared to 25 percent with worsening symptoms and 8 percent whose symptoms remained unchanged. Overall, the women reported significant improvements in pain, sexual function, and quality of life.

However, despite the advantages of using excision to remove endometrial implants, some surgeons are wary of the technique.

Many doctors are not skilled in excision, a technically difficult procedure, and thus prefer to burn away the lesions using laser vaporization and electrocoagulation. These methods remove diseased tissue only from accessible areas and, hence, do not have long-term success. A 1996 comparative study of 240 women with endometriosis who had undergone excision alone, laser coagulation alone, or laser coagulation plus medical therapy found that twelve months after surgery, 96 percent of excision patients were pain-free compared to 69 percent of those who underwent coagulation. At two years, the figures were 69 percent compared to 23 percent, respectively.

Laser Vaporization

Next to excision, laser vaporization is another popular technique used by surgeons to remove endometrial implants. This process involves the destruction of implants by instantly boiling the cellular water (water found in cells) with a high-power laser or electrosurgical tool over a short time. The laser delivers a very concentrated packet of light energy that instantly boils cellular water. The water temperature rapidly increases, resulting in vaporization and tissue destruction.

The concentrated packet of light energy allows the surgeon to remove the endometriosis layer by layer. The surgeon has the advantage of seeing the appearance of the underlying tissue to make an accurate assessment as to whether endometriosis remains or normal tissue has been reached. However, this method can remove diseased tissue only from more accessible areas. The procedure is also very subjective; it's only the surgeon's opinion regarding whether the implants removed were really endometriotic.

Ablation

This involves the destruction of endometrial implants by any surgical means.

Electrocoagulation

Electrocoagulation involves the desiccation of implants (removal of most of the water from implants) by heating and drying the affected tissues. This is done by touching a metal electrode to the affected areas and destroying the implants. The tissue is heated until the cellular proteins become damaged, resulting in cellular death. However, this technique has several drawbacks. First, the surgeon has no way of knowing whether the diseased tissues are being completely destroyed and may also risk injury to underlying structures. Additionally, deep endometriosis may be left behind. The technique depends heavily on the opinion of the surgeon, hence there is no objective way of ensuring that all endometriosis has been destroyed. Additionally, eletrocoagulation causes thermal damage to the surrounding tissues.

Fulguration

This technique involves the superficial burning of implants from any electrosurgical tool. This is only a superficial treatment, which means that deeper disease is often left behind to cause more problems later.

Laparotomy

Laparotomy is a much more invasive procedure and is considered major surgery. The patient is placed under general anesthesia, and a much longer incision is made across the abdomen. A longer hospital stay is required after a laparotomy, typically one week, dependent on the extent of and your reaction to the surgery. Recovery time also takes longer than after a laparoscopy. Women have reported as little as one to two weeks needed for full recovery, while others need more. Note, however, that the time you take to recover from the surgery will also depend on the extent of and your own response to the surgery.

Laparoscopy, on the other hand, is a minimally invasive procedure, resulting in no or shorter hospital stays and quick recovery. A laparoscopy is also less expensive and, with the help of video-magnification, facilitates a more precise treatment.

My stay in the hospital this time was miserable and dark. I did not like the ward, and the women there seemed extra ill, which said a lot about my own situation. I cried for the first three days I was there, even frightening my poor urologist, who came to visit me one evening. I just couldn't stop crying. I felt better only when my family came to visit. In my determination to prove that a whole week's stay in the hospital for me was not necessary, I begged my gynecologist to release me early and did everything necessary to prove that I was recovering quickly. In fact, I was so successful with my begging that, on the fifth day, I was released from the ward and sent home, where I recovered quite well in the coming weeks. Since I was now on summer vacation from college, I basically had the whole summer to recover from surgery.

A laparotomy, though less so, is still used to treat endometriosis patients, especially in areas where the laparoscope cannot be used, such as the diaphragm. The experts suggest that, when compared to laparoscopy, laparotomy enhances palpation (the careful feeling of parts of the body with the hands and fingertips), examination of the bowel, retroperitoneal spaces (region within the body that contains the kidneys, adrenal glands, pancreas, lumbar, spinal nerve roots, etc.), and delicate handling of deep implants.

Both methods have been found equally effective in relieving pain. In one study, scientists evaluated 47 women with confirmed chronic pelvic pain and stage IV endometriosis by laparoscopy and 108 women with confirmed chronic pelvic pain and stage IV endometriosis by laparotomy. At twenty-four months, about two-thirds of all the women were pain free. The findings were as follows:

▪ *Dysmenorrhea recurrence:* 16.4 percent to 20.3 percent in those treated laparoscopically compared to 20.3 percent to 27.7 percent in those treated via laparotomy.

▪ *Dyspareunia recurrence:* 28.6 percent to 33.3 percent in laparoscopically treated patients compared to 10.4 percent to 15.4 percent in laparotomy treated patients.

▎ *Nonmenstrual chronic pelvic pain recurrence:* 17.5 percent to 25 percent in those treated laparoscopically compared to 15.9 percent to 20.1 percent in laparotomy treated patients.

Amy describes the effects of surgery on her endometriosis:

The surgery made me feel a lot better, at least for a while. I now knew that I wasn't crazy and that my problems actually had a name. While it was scary to know I had a chronic disease, it was a huge relief to be able to at least associate a "face" with my symptoms.

Of course, as all of us with endo know, it came back, this time with a vengeance! A couple years after surgery, my pain was back, the bleeding and migraines were worse, the fatigue was unbearable, and I really started to see my quality of life decline. I no longer felt like, nor had the energy, to enjoy many of my daily activities. Many days it was a huge effort even to get ready for work. My ovaries constantly hurt. Even sitting for too long would cause me to be in pain. I would often get out of the car or out of a chair, only to have my knees buckle because of the sharp, stabbing pain. Here I was at twenty-seven years old and I felt like an old woman! I would come home from work and do nothing but lie around on the couch. Advil and the heating pad became my new best friends. I was eating ibuprofen and painkillers on a daily basis just to get through the day. The depression got much worse as well. Many days I could barely muster the emotional strength to get out of bed and face the day. I just wanted to curl up in a ball and die—anything to make the pain and misery go away.

By this time, too, I was seeing yet another doctor because the one who did my first surgery retired. My new doctor was very nice but just seemed like he didn't get it. While he knew I had endometriosis and could look through my records and surgery files to confirm it, his answer was that I needed to have a baby. He said having a baby would solve all my problems and make the endo go away. Now because I had been doing my homework, I knew there was no cure for this wretched disease. While having a baby can sometimes help, it certainly wasn't going to solve all my problems. In fact, I saw it as creating a whole new set of issues and responsibilities for me. I mentioned earlier that I was pretty set on not having children, and the older I got, the stronger I felt about not having any. I could barely take care of myself, let alone take care of a baby.

I continued to complain loudly to my doctor. He had me try yet another kind of birth control and prescribed 800 milligrams ibuprofen for the pain, and I had another vaginal ultrasound that showed no cysts or serious problems.

My doctor finally suggested I try Lupron. I was very resistant to this idea. I had read many horror stories about the side effects and worried about how I would react to it. Doc tried to reassure me that every woman was different and that I should give it a try, but I still was reluctant and put my foot down. He then suggested doing another laparoscopy so he could see how bad things were. I agreed to the lap and went back in for surgery in June of 2000.

The surgery went well, but my doctor was surprised at the findings: I had very little scarring and adhesions, but was in severe pain all the time. He explained that this just seemed to be the nature of the disease. Some women can be covered in it and never have problems while others have very few implants and are in serious pain.

Three months after surgery, the pain was back again, worse than ever. I was finally at the end of my rope and seriously considering having a hysterectomy just to be able to *have somewhat of a normal life. But a hysterectomy seemed so radical, and because I was so young, my doctor really didn't want to go to that extreme. He once again suggested Lupron, and this time I gave in.*

Melissa had few hopes that surgery would relieve her pain, but she was pleasantly surprised:

Ironically, my pain recovering from surgery was much less than the deep pain of a typical period for me. It was interesting to me that my doctor automatically prescribed narcotic pain relievers postsurgery—the narcotics my doctor had (I thought, condescendingly) refused to give me for pain for so long. I saved my pills for later use, having little faith that the surgery would reduce my pain. It had been such a part of my life—how could the pain just disappear with a little laser laceration? I had read about endometriosis growing back, or it being impossible to laser it all away with only the human eye for guidance.

After my laparoscopy, with my next period approaching, I called my doctor to ask for a refill of my usual pain pill prescription. She would not refill it because she said my pain would no longer be there. She told me to call her if I felt pain, and then she would prescribe it. I sheepishly agreed, feeling like she thought I was overly pill hungry. The first pain hit when I was in another city in hundred-degree weather hoeing rows of asparagus on a friend's farm. I was extremely angry that I did not have access to my usual prescription because my doctor had assumed that her actions had eliminated my pain. My next two periods were quite painful, and instead of taking my usual nonnarcotic painkillers, I was left to take the narcotics left over from my surgery recovery until I got my old prescription back.

Then an unexpected thing happened: my pain significantly reduced. I remember thinking, Where does pain go once it leaves me? I still had a few bad days, but my lifestyle improved and my use of prescription medication decreased a lot. I used to wonder what I would be like without pain: would I become shallow? Would I stop appreciating the healthy days? Who is the real me, the me in pain or the me without pain? What I have found is that having less pain lets me be more social, more efficient at work, and much more emotionally stable.

Other Forms of Surgery

Transvaginal Laparoscopy
Minimal or superficial endometriotic implants can be treated during a transvaginal laparoscopy (laparoscopy through the vagina). However, the procedure cannot be utilized to remove more extensive disease. Transvaginal laparoscopy is more often utilized as a diagnostic tool (chapter 12).

Microlaparoscopy
As in the case of transvaginal laparoscopy, microlaparoscopy (laparoscopy using small/micro instruments) may also be used to treat minimal disease. However, if significant adhesions and implants are found, the surgeon will have to continue with standard laparoscopic procedures. As in the case of transvaginal laparoscopy, microlaparoscopy is also more extensively utilized as a diagnostic tool (chapter 12). However, with newer instruments becoming available, more uses of microlaparoscopy will be realized.

Patient-Assisted Laparoscopy (PAL) or Pain Mapping
Patient-assisted laparoscopy (PAL) or pain mapping is another useful microlaparoscopic technique for the diagnosis and treatment of pain associated with endometriosis. The patient is awake during the

procedure (hence the name patient-assisted or awake laparoscopy) so that she can help the surgeon find the cause of her pain.

In this procedure the patient is briefly put to sleep using a combination of local numbing medications and a short-acting general anesthetic. While she is under, the surgeon inserts the microlaparoscope and other necessary instruments; then the patient is awakened so she can participate in the procedure. A 2-millimeter probe is used to gently touch various structures such as the uterosacral ligaments, the ovaries, the fallopian tubes, the uterus, the bladder, and adhesions to see if these areas duplicate the patient's pain.

Once the painful areas are confirmed, the surgeon will give the patient a general anesthetic and the lesions and adhesions treated via standard operative laparoscopy. In one study, fifty women with persistent chronic pelvic pain were tested via patient assisted laparoscopy to find the cause of their pain. Endometriosis was found in 84 percent of the women. In that number, severe endometriosis and adhesions were treated in 29 percent with operative laparoscopy under general anesthesia. Patient-assisted laparoscopy, compared to standard laparoscopy, has fewer negative findings (no explanation of their pain) compared to laparoscopy—5 percent versus 35 percent.

Patient-assisted laparoscopy gives a clearer sense of the real location of a patient's pain, which is often quite different from where she has described its source. Dr. Larry Demco, associate clinical professor of Obstetrics and Gynecology at the University of Calgary, has found that up to one-third of patients have referred pain. This means that the pain may be felt on the left while the source of the pain is actually located on the right.

Patient-assisted laparoscopy also has the advantage of showing that a painful area may extend beyond the borders of a visible endometriotic lesion. If the surgeon had treated the lesion alone, the patient would still experience pain. This information would not have been available to the surgeon if the patient were asleep.

▌Surgery to Interrupt Pain Transmission

Surgeons also perform two types of nerve-blocking surgeries in women who suffer from severe dysmenorrhea and pelvic and back pain. By severing the nerves that lead from the uterus, doctors hope that their patients will eventually experience significant pain relief. Both procedures are done via a laparoscopy.

Presacral Neurectomy

This procedure involves severing the nerves in the back of the uterus. By doing so, pain transmission from the uterus will be blocked, resulting in pain relief. One study found that women who were treated by laparoscopic surgery experience better relief from severe dysmenorrhea when they also underwent presacral neurectomy. The study assigned 141 women either to laparoscopic surgery only or to laparoscopic surgery with presacral neurectomy, then followed up with the women two years after the surgeries. In the first group only 53.3 percent of the women experienced long-lasting pain relief, while 83.3 percent of the latter group experienced long-lasting pain relief.

There are those, however, who believe that presacral neurectomy does not provide any added benefit to endometriosis patients. Overall, the procedure has been found effective in treating dysmenorrhea but seems to have no effect on other types of endometriosis-associated pain.

Some potential side effects of presacral neurectomy include constipation, urinary urgency, and increased incidence of incontinence. Some women who have previously undergone the procedure reported no pain in the first stage of labor.

Laparoscopic Uterosacral Nerve Ablation (LUNA)

Similar to presacral neurectomy, LUNA involves severing a small nerve near the back of the uterus. This procedure is more common than presacral neurectomy and also has fewer associated risks. However, studies have shown that it is the less effective of the two. In one study, LUNA was found to have no additional impact on dysmenorrhea than traditional laparoscopic surgery. The researchers studied 180 women undergoing laparoscopic surgery for endometriosis. Half of the women received surgery with LUNA and the other half (the control) received laparoscopy alone. In one year after surgery, 75 percent of those who underwent laparoscopy and LUNA showed significant pain relief as well as 74 percent of those in the control. After three years, both groups of patients showed similar reductions in pain and improvements in quality of life.

▍Treating Different Forms of Endometriosis

Surgical treatment for endometriosis may also vary depending on the location of implants.

Gastrointestinal (GI) Tract

Implants found on the bowel are normally excised. Dr. David Redwine considers it unsafe to use laser vaporization or electrocoagulation to burn implants from the bowel because this may create an unseen hole, which can cause serious complications. Excision removes implants from the bowel safely and completely, once the surgeon is sufficiently skilled in this method.

Urinary Tract

Implants found on the bladder can be excised or vaporized. However, if deep implants have penetrated the bladder, the surgeon may have to perform a partial cystectomy (removal of part of the bladder).

Diaphragm

While laparoscopy is a perfect tool to diagnose endometriosis of the diaphragm, the technique has been found inadequate to treat this form of the disease. Dr. David Redwine suggests, based on his own practice, that diaphragmatic endometriosis may present itself as a "sentinel" lesion—a small lesion on the diaphragm. The rest of the disease, however, is often found behind the liver. In this case laser vaporization or electrocoagulation will not be suitable, as these methods would only treat only a fraction of the disease. Additionally, the whole diaphragm is usually involved, which would make it necessary to burn all the way through the diaphragm in order to completely treat the disease. This creates a hole in the diaphragm and risks damage to the lungs and heart. In this scenario, a laparotomy would be best to treat the disease.

Thoracic

Thoracic endometriosis is both diagnosed and treated via a thoracoscopy, a kind of laparoscopy of the pleural cavity. During the procedure, diseased portions of the lung are resected often followed by medical therapy.

Sciatic Nerve

Implants found on the sciatic nerve are excised via laparoscopy, often followed by medical therapy.

▌ Adhesions

Adhesions are scarlike tissues that form an abnormal connection between normally separate organs of the body. They often form as a result of damage to tissues during surgery or as a result of the inflammatory response caused by endometriosis. The body's attempt to heal tissue damage and to get rid of ectopic endometrial tissue may trigger the factors that lead to the formation of adhesions.

Additionally, the introduction of foreign bodies during surgery, such as talc from the surgeon's glove, will trigger the body's immune system to get rid of the foreign material. The body's inability to do so will trigger an inflammatory response, as in the case of ectopic endometrium that leads to adhesion formation.

Wherever they are found in the body, adhesions can cause significant pain as well as other symptoms similar to endometriosis. For instance, adhesions found on the reproductive organs cause debilitating pelvic pain, infertility, and dyspareunia. Adhesions found on the bowel and bladder often result in bowel obstruction and bladder problems. Adhesions may also pull on internal organs, distort normal anatomy of organs, and trigger certain problems such as infertility.

Types of Adhesions
There are three types of adhesions:

Filmy Adhesions
These are similar to spiderwebs. These contain few blood vessels and can easily give way if the surgeon uses an instrument to "sweep" through them just like sweeping cobwebs from off a wall. Filmy adhesions do not cause pain.

Vascular Adhesions
This is a thick, ropelike adhesion that causes pain. Vascular adhesions connect two normally unconnected tissues/organs. As these adhesions mature, they progressively shorten in length, drawing the organs closer together. This results in worsening pain.

Dense Cohesive Adhesions
This type of adhesions connects two organs tightly together, gluing the organs together and leaving no space between them. This is the worst type of adhesion, the most difficult to remove, and the most likely to recur after it is removed. Pain is excruciating.

Treatment of Adhesions

The aims of treating adhesions are twofold: to remove as much of the adhesions as is possible and to prevent them from recurring during the healing process. In the first instance, adhesion removal can be accomplished only via surgery. In the second instance, adhesion barriers are used. Let us look at each in turn.

Surgery

Surgery is necessary to treat adhesions. Lysis (cutting out) of adhesions may provide some relief. However, the fact that surgery itself contributes to the formation of adhesions means that more adhesions will form. There is also the increased risk of adhesions forming at the sites of old adhesions. The surgeon must take care to excise the entire adhesion to reduce the risk of leaving behind tissue that may lead to the development of more adhesions.

Fortunately for the endometriosis patient, it has been found that laparoscopic surgery causes fewer new adhesions than laparotomy. However, once excised, adhesion formation can and does occur at old adhesion sites. Many surgeons are now doing second-look laparoscopies a week or two after the first surgery. Adhesions usually form in the first three days after surgery. During the second-look laparoscopy, these early-stage adhesions are easier to excise since they have not had sufficient time to thicken. However, this is yet another surgery, which will, in turn, inevitably increase your risk of developing adhesions.

Adhesion Barriers

Products with the sole purpose of barring/preventing adhesion formation after surgery have been used with some effectiveness. Dr. Andrew Cook, medical director of the VitalCare Institute, refers to these as supportive adhesion prevention products. These barriers are placed at the site of surgery to prevent the tissue surfaces from sticking together during the healing process. Four such adhesion barriers include Interceed, Preclude, Seprafilm, and Gynecare Intergel adhesion prevention solution.

- *Interceed:* This is a white meshlike material that eventually dissolves and is eliminated from the body. Surgeons have not found this to be a very effective adhesion barrier because Interceed combined with minimal bleeding may increase adhesion formation.
- *Preclude:* This type of adhesion barrier does not dissolve in the body and must be sutured (stitched) into place. Additionally, this is a permanent foreign body in the body that can lead to infections.
- *Seprafilm:* This looks like wax paper that, when inside the body, turns into gel. It dissolves within a month and is eliminated from the body. Seprafilm has been found effective in reducing the number and extent of adhesions in patients.
- *Gynecare Intergel:* This adhesion-prevention solution was approved as an adhesion barrier for gynecologic surgery in November 2001. This solution has been found more effective in preventing the formation of adhesions than standard irrigating solution. Gynecare Intergel is a thick gel that lubricates the tissue surfaces and keeps them from adhering together during the healing process. The body absorbs the gel after about a week and eliminates it from the body.

Radical Surgery—Hysterectomy

Within the endometriosis community, radical surgery normally implies hysterectomy, surgical removal of the uterus. Hysterectomy is the second most common surgery in the United States. Of the more than 650,000 hysterectomies performed annually, endometriosis is the second leading reason for these surgeries. Women often

∎ ∎ ∎ The Challenge of Getting Out of Bed After Surgery ∎ ∎ ∎
By Ellen T. Johnson

(Reprinted with permission from Ellen T. Johnson and
http://www.endometriosis.org)

Call me a slow learner, but after five surgeries, I finally learned
how to get out of bed after surgery. In the past, I used the "roll
out and pray" technique. It wasn't elegant, easy, or painless, but
it was effective. No one ever told me there was a better or more
effective way!

Everyone who's had surgery knows the routine. When you're
discharged from the hospital, a professional health-care worker
(or at least a trained volunteer) ensures that you're safely
transferred from the wheelchair into the vehicle that will take
you home. Once you're there, a gracious family member, loved
one, or friend helps you safely into the house and into bed.
Then, hours later, you awaken to a single thought: I have to
use the toilet! You ignore the urge for a while because you
don't want to go to the bathroom. In fact, you don't want
to get up for any reason! Why? Because getting out of bed
will require the use of abdominal muscles that have recently
been severed by a surgeon's knife! You know it's going to hurt
really, really bad! Since you're already hurting from the actual
surgery (the reason they made those cuts in the first place),
more pain is the last thing on earth you want to experience
right now.

As I lay in my bed after surgery, I waited, hoping the urge
would pass. It didn't. I fantasized about that nice automatic bed
at the hospital. Why didn't I have one of those installed when I
had the chance? Too late for that now. Then I wondered why
my husband didn't hire some Herculean nurse to lift me in and
out of bed. I imagined being gently carried to the bathroom by
someone of great strength, my bum placed neatly on the toilet,

then carried back to bed again. Sigh. Clearly, that wasn't going to happen.

As real panic set in, I began to have cross notions about my family. Up until this precise moment, they had been hanging around my bed like puppies. But now, when I actually needed them, no one was in sight! I lay there, wondering how on earth I was going to move my body from its prone position to an upright one. Then I imagined myself rising up. And then I did the most incredible thing. I grabbed up a handful of my top sheet at approximately waist level, folded it several times vertically, fan-style, and gave a test tug to see if it would hold my weight. Luckily, the sheet was tucked in tightly at the bottom of the mattress and supported me easily. I used a hand-over-hand method of pulling myself up with the sheet until I was sitting upright on the bed. It was so easy! And I was so proud of my new technique, I just sat there in amazement for a full two or three seconds before quickly making my way toward the destination that inspired this act of ingenuity in the first place. Getting all the way out of bed required a simple butt-pivot and stand. The hard part was over.

A dear friend came over a little later, and I showed her how easily I could get out of bed. She was significantly impressed and immediately informed members of our endometriosis support group about my new technique. They decided I had a civic duty to tell everyone, which is the reason for this article. It's just too bad I can't enter it in a Science Fair. Or at the very least, have it published in *Discover* magazine!

Since first writing this article, I discovered a medical device that uses the same principle as my hand-over-hand sheet method, but is more secure. It's called a "bed pull-up" and is sold by medical supply companies. The bed pull up is made of durable cotton webbing, and features four rungs of a ladder to assist in

> *pulling oneself upright in bed. It's more secure than*
> *sheets because the webbing attaches to the bed legs at the*
> *foot of the bed.*
>
> *If you use my sheet method, try it first with someone*
> *there to support you. Also, make sure your sheet is*
> *firmly tucked in between the top mattress and the box*
> *springs or foundation.*

resort to this type of surgical treatment when other types of surgery and medical treatments fail to improve pain and fertility. Hysterectomy, however, is not a cure; many endometriosis patients experience endometriosis-associated symptoms after a hysterectomy. However, the procedure can significantly improve symptoms in many patients.

Making the Hysterectomy Decision

The decision to have a hysterectomy cannot be made lightly. This procedure is usually assigned when all other treatment options—conservative surgery and medical therapy—have been exhausted without effect. While for some women a hysterectomy will be the most effective form of treatment, other women may not be that lucky. For instance, Johns Hopkins conducted an eighteen-month-long study of 138 women with endometriosis who were treated with hysterectomy. The study found of those who kept their ovaries, 31 percent had recurrence of endometriosis; 10 percent of those who had their ovaries removed experienced recurrence of the disease.

Dr. David Redwine suggests that the main reason for recurrence of disease after hysterectomy has to do with the actual locations of the disease. According to Dr. Redwine, only 3.7 percent of patients have endometriosis confined to their uterus, fallopian tubes, and ovaries. The majority of the disease is found in peritoneal surfaces away from the uterus. Therefore, the removal of the uterus, tubes, and ovaries does not guarantee eradication of the disease, since the condition may remain in other locations. Additionally, scientists have found that endometriotic implants have estrogen receptors that, facilitated by high levels of aromatase enzymes, can produce their own estrogen required for disease development.

Educate yourself about this procedure and its associated complications and benefits before signing consent forms. The more you know, the more comfortable you will be about your decision to have the hysterectomy. If you feel forced into making a decision, seek a second opinion from another doctor with whom you feel comfortable.

The following are some tips to consider when thinking about a hysterectomy:

- Define your treatment goals. Are you considering pain relief only, or are you concerned about preserving your fertility? While a hysterectomy will help in most cases to relieve endometriosis-associated pain, fertility will be irreversibly affected.

- Exhaust other treatment options to relieve endometriosis-associated symptoms. Other treatment options include hormonal treatments (chapter 7), conservative surgery (this chapter), and alternative options (chapters 9 and 10). If hysterectomy is advised as a first line of treatment, it will be in your best interest to get a second opinion.

- Work with your doctor to choose the treatment that is best for *you*. What worked for another woman may not work for you. The treatment you choose must be made with *your* needs in mind.

Types of Hysterectomies

Once you have made a decision to go ahead with a hysterectomy, you need to discuss with your doctor what exactly will be removed and the type of hysterectomy that will be done.

There are four types of hysterectomies targeted at removing specific sections of the uterus.

Complete or Total Hysterectomy

In a complete hysterectomy the uterus and the cervix are removed, but the ovaries and fallopian tubes are left. Premenstrual women still experience ovulation but no menses.

Subtotal or Supracervical Hysterectomy

In this procedure the upper part of the uterus is removed, but the cervix is left in place.

Bilateral Salpingo-Oophorectomy

In this procedure the fallopian tubes and ovaries on both sides of the uterus are removed. Oftentimes the uterus and cervix are also removed as in a total hysterectomy. The removal of the ovaries carries the risk of experiencing surgical menopause induced by the severe drop in hormone levels in the body.

Radical Hysterectomy

This is an extensive procedure that involves the removal of the uterus, cervix, the fallopian tubes, the upper part of the vagina, the surrounding tissue, the ovaries, and sometimes the pelvic lymph nodes. Again, the patient will experience surgical menopause because of the drastic drop in hormone levels.

Methods of Access

These different surgical techniques can be done abdominally, called an abdominal laparoscopy, or through the vagina, a vaginal hysterectomy. Additionally, hysterectomies can also be performed laparoscopically, called a laparoscopic-assisted vaginal hysterectomy (LAVH) and laparoscopic supracervical hysterectomy (LSH).

Abdominal Hysterectomy

In this procedure an incision is made in the abdomen, about 6 to 8 inches (15 to 20 centimeters), either horizontally, across the top of the pubic hairline (called a bikini cut), or vertically, below the belly button. The bikini cut heals faster and is much less noticeable than the vertical incision, which is used in more complicated cases. An abdominal hysterectomy requires a longer hospital stay—two to four days, depending on your reaction to the surgery—than after a vaginal hysterectomy, but it is the more common of the two. Complete recovery normally takes six to eight weeks.

Vaginal Hysterectomy

A vaginal hysterectomy is performed via an incision in the vagina through which the uterus is removed. This approach is technically more difficult than an abdominal hysterectomy; the surgeon has less operating space and reduced visibility of the pelvic organs. However, this procedure leaves no external scar and often requires a shorter hospital stay. The procedure can affect your sexual function—causing pain during sexual intercourse—because the vagina may be shortened or tightened during the surgery. A typical hospital stay after a vaginal hysterectomy is one to two days and recovery time can take one to two weeks, although recovery time is dependent on your own individual response to the surgery.

Laparoscopic-Assisted Vaginal Hysterectomy (LAVH)

Laparoscopic-assisted vaginal hysterectomy (LAVH) is a variation of vaginal hysterectomy. In this procedure, a laparoscope is used, inserted through an incision made in the belly button, to perform the hysterectomy. The uterus is then cut and can be removed through the laparoscope but is most often removed through a vaginal hysterectomy. LAVH takes longer than the other two hysterectomy procedures and is more expensive, but the hospital stay and recovery time are significantly reduced.

Laparoscopic Supracervical Hysterectomy (LSH)

In the laparoscopic supracervical hysterectomy (LSH), the uterus is removed laparoscopically, with or without the ovaries, and a portion of the cervix and the ligaments that support the cervix and vagina remain intact. Why keep the cervix? Researchers have found that the cervix plays two very important roles. First, it supports the pelvic diaphragm. Second, the cervix has an abundance of nerves that transmit not only pain sensations but also pleasurable sensations. Scientists have found that women experience two types of orgasms during sexual intercourse: an external orgasm associated with the clitoris and an internal orgasm associated within the cervix, which is popularly referred to as the G-spot. This internal orgasm results from the abundant nerve supply around the cervix. By maintaining the cervix, LSH minimizes the risk of potential vaginal prolapse at a later date and sexual dysfunction post-operatively.

Those who object to this procedure argue that by maintaining the cervix, the woman is at increased risk of developing cervical cancer. However, studies have shown that this risk is approximately 0.1 percent. The experts suggest that women who undergo LSH should continue to have annual Pap smears done to catch any cancerous cells early.

Risks and Complications of Hysterectomy

As with all surgical procedures hysterectomy carries with it some risks and complications. For instance, the uterus is located between the ureters on each side, the bladder in front, and the rectum behind. These structures may be damaged during surgery, especially if the surgery is particularly difficult. Bleeding and infections may also occur, but the latter can be avoided with the use of antibiotics. Blood clots in the veins of the legs (thrombophlebitis) may also occur and are indicated by a sudden swelling or discoloration in the leg. You should seek immediate medical attention if this occurs. Some serious complications that may occur, although rare, include perforation of the bowel and pulmonary embolism (blood clots in the lungs).

Some long-term complications include:

- Bowel problems caused by extensive adhesions that obstruct the intestines. This will require additional surgery.
- Prolapse (descent) of the bladder, vagina, and rectum caused by extensive weakening of the supporting muscles. This will require additional surgery to correct.
- Muscle weakness experienced in the pelvic area.
- Surgical menopause characterized by hot flashes, night sweats, vaginal dryness, mood swings, insomnia, and weight gain. If the ovaries are left intact, these menopausal symptoms may be brought on by the temporary blocking of blood flow from the ovaries, which thus suppresses estrogen release. Loss of estrogen increases your risk of developing osteoporosis (loss of bone density) and heart disease.

While recovering from a hysterectomy, the following should be considered:

- Get plenty of rest and avoid lifting heavy objects and small children, driving, climbing stairs, or taking baths or douches for several weeks after surgery.
- Reduce the discomfort of coughing and sneezing by holding a pillow over the abdominal wound, or crossing your legs if you have a vaginal incision.
- Relieve gas pains by walking and doing slow deep-breathing exercises.
- Return to normal activities gradually to ensure a full recovery.

Apart from the physical effects, hysterectomy can also be emotionally disabling. Early onset of menopause and its related symptoms and the loss of fertility for those who wanted to have children but can't can be psychologically crippling for many women. However, this can be significantly lessened if you educate yourself about hysterectomy before having one and make the decision *yours* and not your family's or your doctor's. Additionally, get support from loved ones and friends. Humor also helps.

Women are also very concerned about hysterectomy's effect on their sexual function, and rightly so. Wait six to eight weeks after surgery before resuming sexual activity. Studies are inconclusive on the impact of hysterectomy on women's sexual function, with some studies showing increased sexual drive and others showing no impact. The reality of the situation also varies but depends on the individual. Some women report no effect; some experience increased sex drive and better orgasms; others report problems such as vaginal dryness, pain during sex, and the diminished capacity for orgasms. If you are concerned about the potential effect of hysterectomy on your sexual function, do not hesitate to speak to your doctor and/or get assistance from a licensed therapist.

Moira describes her hysterectomy experience:

In January 1999, I went into the hospital for a hysterectomy and bilateral oophorectomy, i.e., the removal of my ovaries. The surgery went without a hitch. My husband spent the first few hours of my postsurgery recovery curled up on the visitor's bed to keep me company; I was scarcely awake, but it was wonderful to know that he was there. He also kept an ear on the various beeps from the monitoring equipment; I was having difficulty keeping my blood oxygenated, and the nurse kept wanting to wake me up to make me take deep breaths; finally, my husband asked why they didn't just put me on oxygen, which they did! By evening, I was sitting up watching comedies—so hubby went home for a much-deserved meal and some rest.

By the next day I was able to creep from the bed to the bathroom, and by evening to hobble around the hall circuit. Once my tummy began to function, one of the nurses showed me where the stash of soda crackers was in the lounge (and a good thing, too, considering the hospital food—who would believe that "black coffee" is considered acceptable as a "clear beverage"?). The day after that, I was released.

Six weeks of pampering followed. I wasn't allowed to drive for several weeks, let alone lift, bend, or carry anything heavy. My husband rented videos, and turned each evening into dinner and a movie. I learned to sleep on my back, often with a bag of frozen vegetables clutched to my aching tummy.

Recovery went smoothly. The staples were removed from my incision, and I learned that the reason my stomach ached so much wasn't from the surgery itself (i.e., the cutting), but from the expanders used to spread the opening, which pressed directly on the abdominal muscles. They ached for weeks. I was also told (after the fact) that I might or might not regain full feeling in the area around the incision—and to this day, that area is slightly numb.

What I was also told, not only by my doctor but by several women who had undergone the same surgery, was that once I had recovered from the surgery, I would feel more energy than I had in years. As I learned to deal with permanent menopause, I kept waiting for this energy to kick in. For several years I took estrogen, but finally stopped, reasoning that women had managed to cope with menopause for hundreds of years without it. I quickly found that I could cope quite easily without it as well.

Menopause definitely agreed—and agrees—with me. In fact, I've often said that if I'd only known I could get rid of all that pain and fuss so easily, I'd have done it years earlier. (Probably I wouldn't have—I wouldn't have had the courage! But I would have liked to.) I've read accounts by some women *who feel that they've lost some portion of their "femininity" by losing their womb—but to me, I felt I'd gained more than I'd lost. What I lost was organs that were causing me no end of trouble and pain. What I gained was freedom from that pain—freedom from a calendar controlled by my menstrual cycle—freedom from PMS and mood swings—freedom to live, at long last, a "normal" life!*

Hason had a different hysterectomy experience:

The mental/emotional recovery from this surgery was very, very difficult, and it took a long time, as did the physical recovery. I was sure that after such a big surgery I would recover and feel fine, but the disease has its own rules. Two years after the hysterectomy I began to have terrible abdominal pains again, more invasive examinations, and of course it was found that the sigmoid colon had a cyst—so I ended up in another laparotomy. . . .

After another six months I returned for an "exploration and resection of scar" because the wound split open. Today, three years after the last surgery, I am still walking around with an open, ugly wound in my abdomen—that wound refuses to heal—it is painful and bleeds with a lot of clotted tissue. Many doctors have examined the wound and pulled from there surgical thread that did not dissolve.

My abdominal pains are still very painful, so much so that they often stop me from leading a normal daily life. My tummy has swollen very much.

I am a thirty-three-year-old woman with a body of a seventy-three-year-old woman. I have hot flashes as if I were going through menopause, and of course I take hormones, and since having the hysterectomy I have gained about fifty-five pounds.

Estrogen Replacement Therapy (ERT) and the Endometriosis Patient

To suppress menopausal symptoms associated with hysterectomy, many doctors will prescribe estrogen replacement therapy (ERT). But this is a very controversial treatment since endometriosis is an estrogen-dependent disease. Some experts believe that even small amounts of estrogen replacement may trigger recurrence of endometriosis. Others argue that estrogen is important for women who have had a hysterectomy; small enough doses can offer protective benefits to the bones and heart without stimulating residual disease. Still others, like Dr. Mark Perloe, director of Reproductive Endocrinology, Infertility and In Vitro Fertilization at the Atlanta Reproductive Health Center, suggest that using unopposed estrogen—estrogen not accompanied by progesterone—will likely stimulate any remaining endometriosis. He therefore suggests that patients who undergo hysterectomy, with removal of the fallopian tubes and ovaries, should be placed on combined estrogen and progesterone replacement therapy.

If ERT doesn't sound appealing, yet you will undergo a hysterectomy, you may want to consider alternative treatments—such as black cohosh and chasteberry—that relieve menopausal symptoms. Those and more are reviewed at length in chapter 9. Fully discuss estrogen replacement therapy with your doctor to make sure you understand exactly the options available to you. If, after educating yourself and talking with your doctor, you feel doubts about a hysterectomy, ask about the alternative treatment option discussed below.

▮ Endometrial Ablation—An Alternative to Hysterectomy

This is an outpatient procedure that involves surgical removal of the lining of the uterus (endometrium). The procedure suppresses menstrual flow or even stops it completely. About one or two months before your scheduled surgery, your doctor will prescribe medications such as gonadotropin-releasing hormone (GnRH) agonists to decrease the endometrium. By thinning the endometrium, the basal (lower) layer of endometrial cells will be exposed during the surgery, normally between fifteen to forty-five minutes. The procedure is done through a hysteroscope (a narrow viewing tube used to inspect the uterus) that is inserted through the vagina and cervix into the uterus; no incisions are made. The hysteroscope has a tiny video camera attached to it that allows for magnification and visualization of the uterine cavity on a television monitor. The uterus is then filled with liquid and the endometrium removed using any of the following techniques:

- *Electrical or electrocautery ablation:* A wire loop or roller ball applies electrical current to the endometrial cells as it is pulled across the endometrial surface. The electricity cauterizes (burns) away the endometrial tissue.
- *Hydrothermal ablation:* In this technique heated fluid is pumped into the uterus at a high temperature, which destroys the endometrial lining.
- *Balloon therapy ablation:* A balloon catheter is inserted into the uterus and filled with fluid. This fluid is then heated to high temperatures, which eventually cauterizes the endometrial lining.
- *Laser ablation:* This procedure involves a beam of light energy that penetrates the endometrium and cauterizes the blood vessels that supply blood to the uterine wall.
- *Cryoablation (freezing):* A probe is inserted into the uterus, and cold liquid nitrogen is pumped into the uterine cavity. The liquid nitrogen instantly freezes and destroys the endometrial lining.
- *Electrode ablation:* The surgeon inserts a triangular mesh electrode into the uterine cavity. This expands and fills the uterus. Suction is then used to bring the endometrial lining into contact

with the electrode, which destroys the lining with an electrical current.

Side effects of endometrial ablation include:

▮ Cramping
▮ Bloody, watery discharge for up to six weeks after surgery
▮ Frequent urination during the first twenty-four hours after surgery
▮ Some nausea and vomiting caused by the anesthesia

This procedure is not advised for women who are trying to get pregnant. While most women cannot get pregnant after an endometrial ablation, there is still a slight possibility of pregnancy occurring. However, remaining endometrial cells lining the uterus will not be adequate for implantation of a fertilized egg.

7

Medical Management of Endometriosis and Pain

Endometrial implants and pain are presently treated by an array of hormonal/medical therapies, but no one treatment prevents recurrence of the disease. Additionally, these treatment options are associated with a multitude of negative side effects.

While I was in the hospital my gynecologist started me on a course of danazol, a synthetic testosterone (this chapter). She explained exactly what the benefits of this drug would be, but the side effects I experienced in the coming weeks deterred me from its positives. For instance, I started to grow a very pronounced beard. Second, danazol is very expensive, and the effect it was having on my pockets, or more specifically my parents' pockets, was overwhelming. I asked my gynecologist for a better and less expensive alternative. I was then prescribed Depo-Provera and have been getting injections every three months since September 1999 to present day. I do experience some of the side effects of Depo-Provera such as the inevitable weight gain, spotting, facial hair growth, and periods of depression. However, I have tried to include exercise and other lifestyle changes to curb these side effects and other aspects of endometriosis (part III).

This chapter discusses the medical therapeutic approaches to treating endometriosis, with particular emphasis on disease suppression and relief of endometriosis's main debilitating symptom: pain. Note, however, that the effectiveness of these hormonal treatments in relieving pain is directly related to their ability to induce amenorrhea (absence of menses) in patients. The chapter ends with a review of new developments in medical treatment options for endometriosis.

■ Medical Management of Endometriosis-Associated Pain

Medical treatments for endometriosis were developed on the basis that the disease is estrogen-dependent. The main aim then is to deprive the disease of the estrogen it needs to continue developing. By reducing active disease symptoms, a patient's pain will lessen. However, hormonal treatments suppress ovulation. If you wish to get pregnant immediately, then you should not consider hormonal treatments.

There are two main categories of medical treatments available. The first category of treatment induces a pseudopregnant state and includes progestins and combination estrogen-progestogen contraceptives. The second category induces a pseudomenopausal state and includes synthetic testosterones and gonadotropin-releasing hormone (GnRH) agonists.

■ Induce Pseudopregnancy

Progestins
Endometriosis symptoms often regress during pregnancy. This is due to the action of progesterone, a hormone that prepares the inner lining of the uterus (endometrium) for pregnancy. If fertilization occurs, progesterone maintains the uterus throughout the pregnancy.

Chemically synthesized progesterone, called progestogen, mimics the actions of progesterone on endometrial tissue. Progestogens chemically derived from progesterone are called progestins. These chemicals block secretion of follicle-stimulating hormone (FSH) and luteinizing hormone (LH) from the pituitary gland and, in turn, prevent follicular maturation and ovulation. This also results in the thinning of the endometrial lining of the uterus.

Long-term exposure to progestins deprives endometriotic implants of estrogen and results in their eventual shrinkage. This may be due to the direct effect of progestins on estrogen receptors in implants. Most women who use progestins for long periods—six to twelve months—eventually develop amenorrhea (absence of menstrual cycles). As such, progestins in turn have a prolonged effect on fertility. Studies have found that 68 percent of women who used progestins for long periods regain their fertility within twelve months of stopping treatment, 83 percent within fifteen months of stopping treatment, and 93 percent within eighteen months of stopping treatment.

The most commonly used forms of progestins for treatment of endometriosis are oral medroxyprogesterone acetate (Provera tablet), intramuscular depot medroxyprogesterone acetate (Depo-Provera injection) and the levonorgestrel-releasing intrauterine system (LNG-IUS), an intrauterine device (IUD) that goes by the trade name Mirena.

Medroxyprogesterone Acetate

Medroxyprogesterone acetate is administered as an oral tablet (Provera) or as an intramuscular injection (Depo-Provera). The usual dose of Provera tablets is 20 to 100 milligrams per day for three to six months. Approximately 80 to 90 percent of women reported improvements in their symptoms while taking Provera. The intramuscular Depo-Provera injection is a popular alternative to Provera. The injections are administered every three months with doses starting at 150 milligrams. One disadvantage of Depo-Provera, however, is the long delay in resumption of ovulatory cycles. It may take nine to twelve months after cessation of treatment before you can conceive.

Treatments are effective only once side effects can be tolerated. In both oral and intramuscular forms of medroxyprogesterone acetate, patients report high incidence of abnormal/breakthrough bleeding (40 to 80 percent), weight gain and fluid retention (40 to 50 percent), acne (20 percent), breast tenderness (10 percent), headaches (10 percent), and mood changes (10 percent). The full list of side effects include:

- Abnormal/breakthrough bleeding
- Amenorrhea
- Weight gain and fluid retention
- Acne
- Breast tenderness
- Headaches
- Mood changes
- Nausea
- Diarrhea
- Fatigue
- Reduced sex drive
- Decreased high density lipoprotein (HDL, also referred to as good cholesterol), which increases your risk of cardiovascular disease
- Increased levels of low density lipoprotein (LDL, also referred to as bad cholesterol), which increases your risk of cardiovascular disease
- Reversible decrease in bone density
- Muscle cramps
- Loss or increase in appetite
- Yeast infection

- Stomach discomfort
- Numbness or pain in the arms or legs
- Sudden shortness of breath
- Yellowing of skin or eyes, which is indicative of liver dysfunction
- Skin rashes

Athina describes her use of Depo-Provera:

I started my Depo treatments a week after my twenty-first birthday, and it had helped a lot in the beginning. Even though it had a few side effects (consistent bleeding for about six months; significant weight gain of fifty pounds; slight loss of hair; and breakouts on my face), I was able to do more without being in pain. One week in February 2002 was the first time that I went food shopping and didn't have to stop at every aisle because it hurt too much to walk. I didn't have to lean against the shopping cart for fear I might fall. It was a very freeing moment. However, that freedom was short-lived. The pain had gotten unbearable again. It hurt to walk or sit for too long, and I could barely stand. I was consistently taking Aleve to try to relieve the pain, but it wasn't working.

Levonorgestrel-Releasing Intrauterine System (LNG-IUS)

Another type of progestin found effective in the treatment of endometriosis and associated pain is the levonorgestrel-releasing intrauterine system (LNG-IUS) or Mirena. It became available to women in the United States in 2001, although for ten years prior to its U.S. release women in Europe and Asia used the device.

The LNG-IUS is an intrauterine device (IUD) that releases approximately 20 milligrams of levonorgestrel per day and is effective for at least five years. The Mirena IUD, unlike copper IUDs that cause menorrhagia (abnormally heavy bleeding), induces amenorrhea. In fact, an 80 to 90 percent reduction in menstrual blood loss has been reported in women who use the device. Additionally, because it releases the hormones directly into the uterus, less of the drug is needed. Thus, there is reduced impact on other organs of the body, resulting in reduced risks associated with other progestin treatments. LNG-IUS works by blocking FSH and LH secretions, suppressing ovulation, and thinning the endometrial lining of the uterus. This thinning action significantly relieves menstrual pain since fewer endometrial cells mean fewer prostaglandin secretions and, hence, less pain.

Side effects include:

■ Irregular bleedings between menstrual cycles during the first six months of use
■ Lighter periods
■ Amenorrhea
■ Increased risk of ovarian cysts
■ Increased risk of pelvic inflammatory disease (PID)

Two studies found that 85 to 95 percent of patients using Mirena were very satisfied with this form of treatment. One major advantage of Mirena is that treatment is localized in the pelvis, maximizing effectiveness and minimizing the side effects. Experts suggest that Mirena is most appropriate for women with endometriosis of the rectovaginal septum.

These progestins offer significant cost savings and are equally effective in treating endometriosis compared to danazol. However, as with other types of hormonal-suppressive medical treatments, once treatment is discontinued, symptoms do return. Additionally, progestins do not have a beneficial effect on fertility. Progestins are potent contraceptives; thus, the effect on your fertility can last a long time.

Combination Estrogen-Progestogen—Oral Contraceptive Pills (OCPs)

Oral contraceptive pills (OCPs) are a combination of estrogen and progestogen and are a common part of medical management of endometriosis. OCPs, like progestins, block FSH and LH receptors in the ovaries, leading to the suppression of estrogen production. This eventually thins the endometrial lining of the uterus, resulting in lighter, more manageable, and less painful periods. A simultaneous effect on endometrial implants occurs because OCPs block implants' estrogen receptors, leading to suppression of the disease.

Experts suggest that, for women who do not want children and who do not respond to cyclic OC therapy, continuous OC use may be the best alternative. In one study, continuous OC use significantly improved dysmenorrhea in 80 percent of fifty women assigned to continuous OC use for two years. The experts recommend that OCs should be considered the first line of therapy in the medical treatment of women with endometriosis who do not wish to conceive immediately.

The side effects of continuous oral contraceptive use include those encountered with progestins, in addition to high blood pressure, blood clots, and enlargement of the uterus.

Amy describes her experience with OCPs:

The birth control pills seemed to help, at least for a while. I still experienced painful periods, but at least my flow had slowed down, and instead of bleeding hard for eight to nine days in a row, it went down to just three to four days a month.

Johnna says:

The pill did regulate my periods and lessen the heaviness, but as far as my cramps, they did get better at first, but then eventually got worse and worse.

Julie M. had a different experience with OCPs:

> *The birth control pills were awful for me. They did shorten my periods, but they made me feel crazy inside. I was very moody, bloated, and felt like my body was holding a monster prisoner inside my belly. It didn't feel natural, so I stopped taking the pills.*

OC brand names include:

- Alesse, Apri, Aviane
- Brevicon
- Cyclessa
- Demulen, Desogen
- Estrostep
- Genora
- Intercon
- Jenest
- Levlen, Levlite, Levora, Lo/Ovral, Loestrin, Low-Ogestrel
- Microgestin, Mircette, Modicon
- Necon, Nelova, Nordette, Norethin, Norinyl, Nortrel
- Ogestrel, Ortho-Cept, Ortho-Cyclen, Ortho-Novum, Ortho Tri-Cyclen, Ovcon, Ovral
- Seasonale
- Tri-Levlen, Tri-Norinyl, Triphasil, Trivora
- Yasmin
- Zovia

Induce Pseudomenopause

It has been observed that menopause, as with pregnancy, relieves women of the symptoms of the disease. This led researchers to develop medicines that mimic menopause to treat endometriosis. These treatments include synthetic testosterones danazol and gestrinone and gonadotropin-releasing hormone (GnRH) agonists leuprolide acetate, leuprolide depot, buserelin acetate, goserelin acetate, and nafarelin.

Synthetic Testosterones

Danazol

Danazol (Danocrine), a synthetic testosterone, was the first medication approved by the U.S. Food and Drug Administration (FDA) for the treatment of endometriosis. It has been in use since the early 1970s and quickly became accepted worldwide as the standard medical treatment. In the last decade, however, its popularity has waned, mainly due to its androgenic and other negative side effects and expense compared to other more tolerable and cheaper treatments.

Danocrine has several actions that make it an effective suppressive treatment. First, it inhibits the release of gonadotropin-releasing hormone (GnRH) from the hypothalamus, and follicle-stimulating hormone (FSH) and luteinizing hormone (LH) from the pituitary gland. As discussed in chapter 2, FSH and LH are needed to begin the ovulatory cycle. Inhibition of FSH and LH prevents ovulation and blocks estrogen to implants, resulting in implant shrinkage and symptom relief. Many women who take Danocrine also experience amenorrhea due to the similar action on the endometrial lining of the uterus.

Treatment is usually for six months, 400 to 800 milligrams per day, given orally. It has been shown to relieve pain with general symptom improvement in 55 to 93 percent of women. However, Danocrine has two major drawbacks. The drug is very expensive, with a monthly cost of $120, compared to Depo-Provera injections at $35 every three months. Second, associated with its use are a plethora of negative side effects, mostly androgenic, experienced by up to 80 percent of patients. A treatment that simultaneously relieves pain and causes weight gain, acne, deepening of the voice, and facial hair growth in its users may not be perceived as beneficial from a patient perspective. Side effects of Danocrine use include:

- Hot flashes (50 percent)
- Acne/oily skin (30 to 60 percent)
- Weight gain and fluid retention (30 to 50 percent)
- Muscle cramps (30 percent)
- Decreased breast size (25 percent)
- Hirsutism (hair growth on the face, chest, upper back, or abdomen) (15 percent)
- Irreversible deepening of the voice (8 percent)
- Breakthrough bleeding (40 percent)
- Mood changes (20 percent)
- Decreased high density lipoprotein (HDL, also referred to as good cholesterol), which increases your risk of cardiovascular disease
- Increased levels of low density lipoprotein (LDL, also referred to as bad cholesterol), which increases your risk of cardiovascular disease
- Nausea

Researchers have also found that women who take Danocrine are three times more likely to develop ovarian cancer. A 2002 study of 390 women treated for endometriosis (195 women with cancer and 195 without) found that women with endometriosis were one and a half times more likely than those without endometriosis to have ovarian cancer. It is also important that barrier methods of contraception are used while on Danocrine, as it can cause birth defects.

Gestrinone

Gestrinone (Dimetriose) has been around since the 1970s but is mostly used in Europe and South America for the treatment of endometriosis. It is an anti-estrogen and anti-progesterone steroid that, like danazol, leads to the shrinking of endometrial implants and/or amenorrhea. As an anti-estrogen agent, Dimetriose works by increasing male hormones (androgens) in the body. This in turn produces a hostile environment for follicular maturation and significantly reduces estrogen production, a necessary ingredient for endometrial implant growth and development. As an anti-progesterone agent, Dimetriose blocks secretions of FSH and LH that stimulate the ovaries to produce progesterone to prepare the uterus for pregnancy. Treatment is daily, twice or three times a week, taken orally at doses of 2.5 milligrams to 10 milligrams. The side effects are also similar to danazol.

Gonadotropin-Releasing Hormone (GnRH) Agonists

An agonist is a drug that acts in a similar fashion as the body's own hormone for which it is named. Gonadotropin-releasing hormone (GnRH) agonists are named after the GnRH released by the hypothalamus. GnRH stimulates the pituitary gland to secrete follicle-stimulating hormone (FSH) and luteinizing hormone (LH) into the bloodstream to kick-start ovulation. GnRH agonists overload the pituitary gland with chemical messages to release more FSH and LH into the bloodstream. This in turn leads the ovaries to produce more estradiol, creating a hypoestrogenic state. In this first phase of treatment some women report a worsening of symptoms.

After this initial flare, the second phase begins with continuous administration of GnRH agonists. The agonists induce a down regulation of hormone receptors in the pituitary gland, essentially shutting down the messenger hormones FSH and LH that control the ovaries. This in turn shuts down the ovaries, and estradiol production rapidly decreases. Within two to four weeks women will stop menstruating and enter a state similar to menopause or pseudomenopause. Ovulation and menstruation will resume once treatment is discontinued.

GnRH agonists have become a part of the standard means of medical treatments for endometriosis, with reports of 85 to 100 percent improvement in symptoms in women under this regimen. In one study, 94 percent of women who used GnRH agonists successfully completed six months of therapy, while 77 percent of women on placebo withdrew early because of worsening pain. Comparative studies have also been conducted between GnRH agonists and danazol. In every case, GnRH agonists were found to be equally effective as danazol as a treatment for endometriosis.

GnRH agonist therapy lasts for a maximum of six months. Treatment for longer periods is not advisable due to the potentially irreversible effect on bone mineral density (BMD). In the United States, GnRH agonists are available as:

- *Intramuscular (within the muscle) and subcutaneous (under the skin) injections:* 3.75 milligrams of leuprolide depot is injected into a muscle once a month for up to six months, and 1 milligram of leupolide is injected under the skin once a day. The brand names for leupolide depot and leuprolide are Lupron and Lupron Depot.
- *Nasal spray:* 200 milligrams (one spray) inhaled into one nostril in the morning and one spray inhaled into the other nostril in the evening for six months. The nasal spray for endometriosis treatment is nafarelin acetate (Synarel).
- *Implant with slow, sustained release:* 3.6 milligrams (one implant) is injected under the skin of the upper abdomen every twenty-eight days for six months. This implant is called goserelin and goes by the brand name Zoladex.

Although these treatments are effective for the relief of endometriosis-associated pain, they have not been shown to have any effect on improving endometriosis-associated infertility. As in the case of progestins, GnRH agonists delay conception for the duration of treatment.

The side effects of GnRH agonists are well documented and are mostly associated with the hypoestrogenic state in the first phase of treatment. These menopausal symptoms include:

- Hot flashes (80 to 90 percent)
- Sleep disturbances (60 to 90 percent)
- Vaginal dryness (30 percent)
- Joint pain (30 percent)
- Breakthrough bleeding (20 to 30 percent)
- Headaches (20 to 30 percent)
- Mood changes (10 percent)
- Bone loss (5 to 6 percent)
- Decreased libido
- Mild breast swelling or tenderness
- Fatigue
- Decreased high density lipoprotein (HDL, also referred to as good cholesterol), which increases your risk of cardiovascular disease
- Increased levels of low density lipoprotein (LDL, also referred to as bad cholesterol), which increases your risk of cardiovascular disease

GnRH Agonists Add-Back Therapy

The adverse side effects of gonadotropin-releasing hormone (GnRH) agonist treatments can be effectively managed with "add-back therapy." For instance, while most patients under short courses of therapy will regain lost bone mineral density, long-term use of GnRH agonists may lead to irreversible bone mineral density loss. To prevent bone loss associated with this treatment, physicians are "adding back" small amounts of estrogen, progestin, or both, along with calcium supplements, to reduce the side effects and limit the bone mineral loss without compromising the effectiveness of the GnRH agonist. Examples of add-back therapies include:

- Norethindrone acetate—5 to 10 milligrams orally per day (OCP)
- Premarin—0.625 to 1.25 milligrams plus 5 milligrams of norethindrone acetate orally per day (estrogen)
- Medroxyprogesterone acetate—20 milligrams orally per day (progestin)

The type of add-back therapy to be used will depend on the preference of the patient and physician. However, no one therapy has been shown to be better than another. The experts strongly suggest the following:

- Estrogen doses in add-back therapies must not be too high, or this will adversely affect GnRH agonist effectiveness.
- Progestin doses must not be too high or adverse lipid changes may occur: decreased high density lipoprotein (HDL) and increased low density lipoprotein (LDL).
- Calcium supplements should also be prescribed to women who receive add-back therapy to prevent GnRH agonist–induced osteoporosis.
- Periodic assessments of bone mineral density and lipid changes should be performed, especially if the patient is on long-term GnRH agonist treatment.

Jude describes the various medical treatments she tried to relieve her endometriosis symptoms:

I have tried four different hormone treatments, Provera, Dimetriose, Zoladex, and Depo-Provera. It is my experience that none of them work, and some of the side effects are worse than the endo. I can joke about them now, but at the time the experience of taking them was awful because I felt worse.

Provera
With Provera I spotted constantly and experienced bad nausea to the point where I could barely eat. I also found that my pain got considerably worse very quickly on Provera.

Dimetriose
With Dimetriose I had an allergic reaction in which my eyelids swelled, and hives came up on my arms every time I took a capsule, and I also became an unwholesome yellow color. It didn't help my mind-set any when I saw a three-pronged symbol that looked like a swastika printed on the side of the capsule. My pain got even worse to the point where I couldn't walk straight, and I found myself feeling very depressed and frightened because all of a sudden I felt my psyche changing, like I wasn't me anymore. Dimetriose is a testosterone-based drug that kind of turns you into a bloke, which I found rather alarming, especially when my voice got deeper and I started sprouting facial hair.

Zoladex
On Zoladex (which you can have in NZ only after you have tried and failed at two other treatments) I had a number of side effects and found the application of the drug a horrible experience. The first time one of the implants was injected into my abdomen, the local anesthetic was in a different spot, so I felt the whole thing. Afterward I had a seizure and passed out in the waiting room. My husband says it was horrifying to watch because I went rigid and my leg kicked up and down. When I came to I didn't know where I was. The injections left bruising, and I could feel them like a pinching feeling in my abdomen.

Unfortunately not only did I have adhesion pain, I also had to cope with severe symptoms of the menopause; these symptoms included hot flashes, memory loss, mood swings, tiredness, insomnia, headaches, skin blemishes, facial/body hair, change in voice, vaginal dryness, and loss of sex drive. Despite all these hormone treatments I still had active endo when I finally sought a second opinion and had my third laparoscopy.

Depo-Provera

Finally I tried Depo-Provera when my specialist wanted to put me on Dimetriose. I refused to take Dimetriose and went for the Depo option. I was fine for the first two months, and then I started spotting. The spotting went on and on and lasted for a month with a break of a few days before it started up again. It was tiring spotting all the time, and then my pain started back up again.

For Erikka, Lupron treatments were intolerable:

With much hesitation, I decided to try the Lupron. It was very hard for me to make this decision, but there weren't many other options. The side effects were immediate. I was nauseous all the time and felt like I had an eternal hangover. It was very difficult for me to keep food down. I lost eighteen pounds in the first month and another ten pounds by the second month. I had severe bone pain from the loss of bone density, and my muscles ached a lot. The texture of my hair changed, and my nails became very thin and fragile. All dairy foods tasted rotten to me. I began having intense hot flashes by the third month, and I was emotionally a wreck. After the fourth month I was a mess, I was really sick and unable to function, and I still had most of my endometriosis pain. After the fifth month I decided to stop the injections of Lupron. They just didn't seem to be helping me and I couldn't take the side effects anymore.

Julie H. describes her own experience with Lupron:

When I had recovered from the surgery, I started to analyze how I felt. My pain had changed. It was more in my back, although still on my right side, with less pain in my hip. Since I still had to take Vicodin to combat pain during my cycle, I decided to do a three-month Lupron shot to ease my pain. Little did I know, it would be the hardest three months of my life.

Lupron is supposed to increase a person's pain for the first one to two weeks, and then your pain should go away with the onset of menopausal symptoms. For me, the pain increased and never went away for three months. Before Lupron, I could take one Vicodin and not be in pain for a week. While on Lupron, one Vicodin didn't even ease my pain for an entire day. At first my doctor told me to wait until a month was up. She said that I had to give the drug a month to start working. When a month was up, she told me to try add-back progesterone to see if that would help. It didn't. Then she said that I should take a one-month Lupron shot on top of the one that I already had, in effect doubling the dosage. I didn't understand how that would work, but I agreed to try it. Before I did so, I had my doctor check my hormone levels. My hormones were postmenopausal, but my pain remained. The second shot did not help me. I don't think it made things any worse. I was in pain from the beginning of the first Lupron shot and remained in pain until they both wore off three months later. I took progesterone for a few weeks after the Lupron was supposed to wear off.

Gen describes her own experience with Lupron as well:

> *In December 2000 I was placed on monthly Lupron injec-*
> *tions. . . . The side effects of the Lupron were horrible. I suf-*
> *fered from severe hot flashes, mood swings, depression,*
> *weight gain, and memory loss. To this day, I still have prob-*
> *lems with my memory, and on occasions I still have some*
> *hot flashes. I have been off the medication for a year and a*
> *half.*

∎ Endometriosis Drug Treatment Chart

The chart on the following page is your quick-look guide to the common hormonal/medical treatments for endometriosis. The chart presents information on the generic and trade names of the medications, actions, side effects, and certain things to consider before deciding to undertake any particular treatment.

∎ Analgesics

Alongside the use of hormonal therapies to treat your endometriosis and pain symptoms, your doctor may also prescribe analgesics (painkillers). Analgesic is the broad term given to medications that relieve pain. These have no impact on the disease itself and can only be used to help relieve pain symptoms of endometriosis. There are many different types of analgesics available to complement your hormonal treatments for endometriosis-associated pain. These include over-the-counter (OTC) and prescription nonsteroidal anti-inflammatory drugs (NSAIDs), acetaminophen, prescription narcotic/opioid analgesics, and topical analgesics.

Progestins					
Generic Name	**Trade Name**	**Form**	**Actions**	**Side Effects**	**Considerations**
Medroxyprogesterone acetate Medroxyprogesterone acetate depot	Provera Depo-Provera	Oral tablets Intra-muscular injection	Blocks secretion of FSH and LH from the pituitary gland, preventing follicular maturation and thinning the endo-metrial lining of the uterus.	Abnormal/breakthrough bleeding; amenorrhea; weight gain and fluid retention; acne; breast tenderness; headaches; mood changes; nausea; diarrhea; fatigue; reduced sex drive; decreased high density lipoprotein (HDL); increased levels of low density lipoprotein (LDL); reversible decrease in bone density; muscle cramps; loss or increase in appetite; yeast infection; stomach discomfort; numbness or pain in the arms or legs; sudden shortness of breath; yellowing of skin or eyes; skin rashes	This is a very potent contraceptive that, with long-term use, will delay your chances of conceiving after treatment has been stopped.
Levonorgestrel-releasing intrauterine system (LNG-IUS)	Mirena	Intrauterine device (IUD)	Blocks secretion of FSH and LH from the pituitary gland, preventing follicular maturation and thinning the endo-metrial lining of the uterus.	Irregular bleedings between menstrual cycles during the first six months of use; lighter periods; amenorrhea; increased risk of ovarian cysts; increased risk of pelvic inflammatory disease (PID)	This is a very potent contraceptive that, with long-term use, will delay your chances of conceiving after treatment has been stopped.

Progestins					
Generic Name	Trade Name	Form	Actions	Side Effects	Considerations
Levonorgestrel-releasing intrauterine system (LNG-IUS) (cont.)			Treatment is localized, maximizing effectiveness and reducing side effects.		
Combined Estrogen-Progestin					
Oral contraceptive pills (OCPs)	Alesse Apri Aviane Brevicon Cyclessa Demulen Desogen Estrostep Genora Intercon Jenest Levlen Levlite Levora Lo/Ovral Loestrin Low-Ogestrel Microgestin Mircette Modicon Necon Nelova Nordette Norethin Norinyl Nortrel Ogestrel Ortho-Cept Ortho-Cyclen Ortho-Novum	Oral Tablets	Blocks secretion of FSH and LH from the pituitary gland, preventing follicular maturation and thinning the endometrial lining of the uterus.	Abnormal/breakthrough bleeding; lighter periods; weight gain and fluid retention; acne; breast tenderness; headaches; mood changes; nausea; diarrhea; fatigue; reduced sex drive; decreased high density lipoprotein (HDL); increased levels of low density lipoprotein (LDL); muscle cramps; loss or increase in appetite; yeast infection; stomach discomfort; numbness or pain in the arms or legs; sudden shortness of breath; yellowing of skin or eyes; skin rashes; high blood pressure; enlargement of the uterus; deep vein blood clots (thrombosis)	OCP use has been associated with deep vein blood clots (thrombosis) and high blood pressure, which may increase your risks of strokes and heart attacks.

Combined Estrogen-Progestins (*continued*)

Generic Name	Trade Name	Form	Actions	Side Effects	Considerations
Oral contraceptive pills (OCPs) (cont.)	Ortho Tri-Cyclen Ovcon Ovral Seasonale Tri-Levlen Tri-Norinyl Triphasil Trivora Yasmin Zovia				

Synthetic Testosterone/Androgen

Generic Name	Trade Name	Form	Actions	Side Effects	Considerations
Danazol	Danocrine	Oral tablets	Inhibits the release of gonadotropin-releasing hormone (GnRH) from the hypothalamus, and follicle-stimulating hormone (FSH) and luteinizing hormone (LH) from the pituitary gland. This prevents ovulation and blocks estrogen to implants, resulting in implant shrinkage and symptom relief.	Hot flashes; acne/oily skin; weight gain and fluid retention; muscle cramps; decreased breast size; hair growth on the face, chest, upper back, or abdomen; irreversible deepening of the voice; breakthrough bleeding; mood changes; decreased HDL; increased LDL; nausea	Danazol is much more expensive than other treatments. Use barrier contraceptive methods while taking danazol, as it can cause birth defects. There is an increased risk of developing ovarian cancer using danazol.

Synthetic Testosterone/Androgen (*continued*)					
Generic Name	**Trade Name**	**Form**	**Actions**	**Side Effects**	**Considerations**
Gestrinone	Dimetriose	Oral tablets	Gestrinone is an anti-estrogen and anti-progesterone steroid. As an anti-estrogen steroid it increases male hormones (androgens) in the body. This produces a hostile environment for follicular maturation and significantly reduces estrogen production. As an anti-progesterone agent, gestrinone blocks secretion of FSH and LH that stimulate the ovaries to produce progesterone to prepare the uterus for pregnancy.	Hot flashes; acne/oily skin; weight gain and fluid retention; muscle cramps; decreased breast size; hair growth on the face, chest, upper back, or abdomen; irreversible deepening of the voice; breakthrough bleeding; mood changes; decreased HDL; increased LDL; nausea	Gestrinone is not available in the United States. It is mostly used in Europe and South America.

Gonadotropin-Releasing Hormone Agonists (GnRH Agonists)

Generic Name	Trade Name	Form	Actions	Side Effects	Considerations
Leuprolide acetate	Lupron	Subcutaneous injection	GnRH agonists overload the pituitary gland with chemical messages to release more FSH and LH into the bloodstream. This leads the ovaries to produce more estradiol, creating a hypoestrogenic state. After this initial flare, continuous administration of GnRH agonists induces a down-regulation of hormone receptors in the pituitary gland, shutting down the messenger hormones FSH and LH that control the ovaries. This shuts down the ovaries, and estradiol production rapidly decreases.	Hot flashes; sleep disturbances; vaginal dryness; joint pain; breakthrough bleeding; headaches; mood changes; bone loss; reduced sex drive; mild breast swelling or tenderness; fatigue; decreased HDL; increased LDL.	GnRH agonists induce a hypoestrogenic state in the first phase of treatment that causes menopausal symptoms. Symptoms often worsen during this first phase:
Depot leuprolide acetate	Depot Lupron	Intramuscular injection			
Nafarelin acetate	Synarel	Nasal spray			
Goserelin acetate	Zoladex	Monthly implant			

Nonsteroidal Anti-Inflammatory Drugs (NSAIDs)

Nonsteroidal anti-inflammatory drugs (NSAIDs) are a group of painkillers that reduce inflammation and swelling and relieve pain. NSAIDs act by directly inhibiting the enzyme cyclooxygenase (COX), which is responsible for the body's production of prostaglandins, hormonelike chemicals that can cause inflammation and pain. The pain in women with endometriosis is induced by prostaglandins released from the endometrial lining of the uterus. By blocking prostaglandin production, women who use NSAIDS will experience relief from dysmenorrhea.

Since NSAIDs block production of pain-causing prostaglandins, they must be taken before these chemicals are produced in order for these medications to be most effective. NSAIDs will not work if taken while you are experiencing pain because the pain-producing prostaglandins have already been released into your body. To be effective, NSAIDs must be taken at least twenty-four hours before the onset of dysmenorrhea and according to your doctor's instructions, usually about every six hours.

Over-the-counter NSAIDS are available in lower doses than prescription NSAIDS. You will have to work with your doctor to find the right type of NSAID and the dose that is more effective for your endometriosis pain. A wide variety of over-the-counter and prescription NSAIDs are available to endometriosis patients. The most commonly prescribed NSAID in gynecology are ibuprofen and naproxen. These are effective in the relief of dysmenorrhea and pelvic pain but may differ in cost and dosage. The brands in these two categories include:

- *Ibuprofen:* Motrin, Motrin IB, Motrin Migraine Pain, Advil, Advil Migraine Liqui-Gels, Ibu-Tab 200, Medipren, Cap-Profen, Tab-Profen, Profen, Ibuprohm, Vicoprofen, Combunox
- *Naproxen:* Aleve, Naprosyn, Anaprox, Anaprox DS, EC-Naproxyn, Naprelan, Naprapac

Cyclooxygenase has two forms: COX-1, which produces prostaglandins beneficial to the body; and COX-2, which produces prostaglandins that cause inflammation and pain. Part of COX-1 prostaglandins' actions is to maintain the lining of the stomach. In addition to blocking COX-2 prostaglandins, NSAIDs also inhibit production of COX-1 prostaglandins, especially suppressing those that protect the stomach lining. This allows for gastric acid to erode the lining of the stomach and causes pelvic ulcers, bleeding, and other gastric irritations. Other side effects include:

- Nausea
- Vomiting
- Diarrhea
- Pain or discomfort
- Dizziness
- Drowsiness or light-headedness
- Mild to moderate headaches
- Heartburn
- Indigestion

It is recommended that you take NSAIDs with food to reduce stomach irritations.

Selective COX-2 Inhibitors—A New Generation of NSAIDs

Recognizing the serious gastric effects of NSAIDS, scientists have come up with a new generation of NSAIDs called selective COX-2 inhibitors. These directly inhibit the production of COX-2 prostaglandins, effectively relieving pain and significantly reducing the risk of developing gastric problems.

Vioxx, Celebrex, and Bextra were released as the medications under this new generation of NSAIDs. However, follow-up studies conducted by the U.S. Food and Drug Administration (FDA) found that selective COX-2 inhibitors are associated with increased risk of heart attacks, strokes, serious allergic reactions, kidney problems, and liver problems. On April 7, 2005, the FDA requested that Pfizer, Inc., manufacturers of Bextra, voluntarily remove the drug from the market because of the unfavorable overall risk versus benefit profile of the drug. Additionally, the FDA has requested that Pfizer place a boxed warning on the label for Celebrex to highlight the potential for increased risk of developing cardiovascular conditions and gastrointestinal bleeding with its use. Merck voluntarily withdrew Vioxx from the market in September 2004. Celebrex is now the only COX-2 inhibitor NSAID on the market.

The FDA has advised OTC NSAID manufacturers to revise their labels and include more specific information about all the potential cardiovascular and gastrointestinal risks associated with these medications to assist consumers in the safer use of these drugs.

Acetaminophen

Whereas NSAIDS work by blocking production of prostaglandins and reducing inflammation, acetaminophens work on the part of the brain that receives "pain messages," essentially blocking pain receptors in the brain. These drugs can be purchased as an OTC in low doses, or your doctor may prescribe higher doses. Additionally, acetaminophens, once taken according to the instructions of your doctor or those on the product label, do not cause gastrointestinal side effects as with NSAIDs.

Common acetaminophen brands currently on the U.S. market include:

- Aceta, Actamin, Aminofen, Apacet, Anacin
- Banesin, Bayer
- Dapa, Datril
- Genapap, Genebs
- Neopap
- Oraphen-PD

- Panadol, Phenaphen Caplets
- Redutemp
- Snaplets-FR, Suppap
- Tapanol, Tempra, Tempra DS, Tylenol
- Valorin, Valorin Extra

Side effects associated with acetaminophens are rare, as long as the medications are taken according to your doctor's instructions or those on the product label. However, if you overdose or take the medication for longer periods than is necessary, side effects will include:

- Diarrhea
- Profuse sweating
- Loss of appetite
- Nausea or vomiting
- Stomach cramps or pain
- Swellings
- Upper abdominal pain or tenderness or pain in the stomach area

Check with your doctor as soon as possible if you experience any of the above symptoms.

If you take more of the drug than is recommended, you risk damaging your liver and kidneys. Additionally, you should not take acetaminophens with other medicines that contain acetaminophens or with alcohol; this will increase the risk of damage to your liver and kidneys. Rare side effects of acetaminophen use associated with liver and kidney damage include:

- Blood in stool
- Blood in urine or cloudy urine
- Severe and/or sharp pains in lower back and/or side

- Pinpoint red spots on skin
- Skin rash, hives, or itching
- Sore throat that was not present before taking the painkiller and is not caused by the condition you are treating
- Unusual bruising or bleeding
- Unusual tiredness or weakness
- Sudden decrease in urine flow

Narcotic/Opioid Analgesics

Narcotic or opioid analgesics are very strong painkillers prescribed for moderate to severe pain. They can be obtained only with a prescription from your doctor. These drugs act directly on the central nervous system (CNS) to relieve pain by reducing the number of pain signals from the CNS and suppressing the brain's reaction to them. This calms your emotional responses to pain due to the inhibited perception of pain from the brain.

Some of the side effects associated with these drugs are directly associated with actions of the medications in the CNS. These include:

- Drowsiness, dizziness, and/or light-headedness
- Fainting
- Nausea and/or vomiting
- Constipation
- Dry mouth
- Sedation
- Confusion
- Difficulty urinating

Symptoms of overdose include:

- Cold/clammy skin
- Confusion
- Seizures

- Severe dizziness
- Severe drowsiness
- Severe nervousness and/or restlessness
- Low blood pressure
- Pinpoint pupils of the eyes
- Slow heartbeat
- Slow or labored breathing
- Severe weakness

Narcotic analgesics can be addictive; however, the risk of addiction is reduced if the medications are taken properly, according to your doctor's instructions, and if you do not have a history of substance abuse. Some common narcotic analgesics include:

- Anileridine
- Buprenorphine, Butorphanol
- Codeine
- Demerol
- Hydrocodone, Hydromorphone
- Levorphanol
- Meperidine, Morphine
- Nalbuphine
- Oxycodone, Oxymorphone
- Pentazocine, Propoxyphene

Your doctor may prescribe a combination pain treatment containing narcotic analgesics and acetaminophen. In some cases, this combination may provide better pain relief, at lower doses, than either medicine used alone. Examples of these combinations include:

- Allay, Anexsia
- Bancap-HC
- Capital with Codeine, Co-Gesic

- Darvocet, DHCplus, Dolacet, Dolagesic, Duocet
- E-Lor, Endocet
- Hycomed, Hyco-Pap, Hydrocet, Hydrogesic
- Lorcet, Lortab
- Margesic
- Oncet
- Panacet, Panlor, Percocet, Phenaphen with Codeine, Polygesic, Propacet 100, Pyregesic-C
- Roxicet, Roxilox
- Stagesic
- Talacen, T-Gesic, Tylenol with Codeine Elixir, Tylox
- Ugesic
- Vanacet, Vendone, Vicodin
- Wygesic
- Zydone

Whatever pain medications you take, whether OTC or prescription, follow their instructions properly to avoid overdosing and inflicting unnecessary harm to your body.

Topical Analgesics

Topical analgesicis are creams or gels that are applied directly on the skin in the area of discomfort to relieve pain. Endometriosis patients have long used numbing agents to relieve their pain. This type of local anesthetic numbs the tissues in the area applied, thus blocking pain signals. The topical analgesic in this category is called EMLA (a eutectic mixture of local anesthetics—lidocaine and prilocaine). A eutectic is a mixture of two solids that becomes a liquid. The drug is most effective one to two hours after application.

Recently, a new topical analgesic became available to endometriosis patients to relieve their pain. It is Menastil, a combination of natural ingredients available as an analgesic. This topical analgesic was released in October 2001 after undergoing four years of research, testing, and development, including two years of FDA clinical trials with more than 3,000 women worldwide testing the product. These tests found that Menastil is effective in relieving menstrual pain. Over 89 percent of the women in these clinical trials found noticeable to complete relief using Menastil. Further tests involving endometriosis patients showed that Menastil was effective in relieving their pain.

The active ingredient in Menastil is calendula oil, an essential oil extracted from marigold petals. Calendula oil has both anti-inflammatory and analgesic properties. The developers of Menastil found a compound in calendula oil that blocks pain signals to the brain. The compound causes the tentacles between nerve cells to retreat, effectively creating a gap that suppresses pain signals to the brain, resulting in pain relief.

How effective this analgesic is will depend on the severity of your pain and your own personality. Many endometriosis patients have experienced pain relief using this product, while others describe Menastil's effectiveness as "only curbing the pain" or "taking the edge off."

▌ Immunotherapy

Immunotherapy involves targeting the dysfunctions at the immune level and effectively treating them to relieve symptoms. Recognizing the increasing number of endometriosis patients with allergies and asthma—as much as 61 percent according to the 2002 EA survey—physicians are now offering to treat women's immune systems as well as the disease itself.

According to the American Academy of Allergy, Asthma and Immunology (AAAAI), immunotherapy is a form of treatment aimed at decreasing your sensitivity to substances called allergens, which trigger allergy symptoms. This treatment program involves a series of allergy shots, consisting of gradually increasing amounts of that particular allergen, over a period of several months. This is called antigen feeding, neutralization, or desensitization—the immune system gradually becomes less sensitive to that particular allergen. Several endometriosis centers across the United States offer immunotherapy as a standard treatment strategy when treating endometriosis patients.

Testing for Allergies

There are several tests available to check for allergies in endometriosis patients. First, there are blood tests to check for autoantibodies and to determine the level of function of certain organs such as the thyroid, liver, adrenals, and kidneys. Then there are hormone sensitivity tests. Many women are allergic to their own hormones. Standard allergy tests are used to check for allergic reactions to estrogen, progesterone, testosterone, and one of the regulating hormones, luteinizing hormone (LH).

One such test is the prick technique. This involves pricking the skin and introducing a small amount of the allergen. If you are allergic to any of the hormones, then it will cause a chain reaction in your body. Another test is the intradermal test. This one involves injecting a small amount of the allergen under the skin.

If you are found to be allergic to any of the above hormones, then allergy desensitization will be administered until the allergic reaction in the immune system stops. This is very much like a vaccination from which your body acquires/builds up an immunity against the allergy.

You may also be tested for environmental allergies such as allergies to mold, trees, dust mites, weed pollen, and so forth, which can contribute to the weakening of your immune system and to the overall disease process.

In a study conducted to test hormone sensitivity in forty-seven endometriosis patients and eighteen asymptomatic controls, Dr. Deborah Metzger, medical director of Helena Women's Health Center in California, found that:

- 85 percent of endometriosis patients were sensitive to estrogen compared to 16.7 percent of the controls.
- 68.1 percent were sensitive to progesterone versus 33.3 percent of the controls.
- 91.5 percent were sensitive to luteinizing hormone (LH) versus 33.3 percent of controls.

Fifty percent received neutralization allergy drops every three months for twelve months. Patients reported a significant reduction in pain, irritable bowel symptoms, and PMS symptoms. Dr. Metzger therefore concludes that women with endometriosis may become hypersensitive to the above hormones, and therapy should also include neutralizing these antibodies for overall treatment of endometriosis.

▌Immunomodulators

Recognizing the immune system's response to the presence of ectopic endometrial cells, scientists are investigating medications to modulate/normalize the hyperstimulated immune response in women with endometriosis. One such immunomodulator is pentoxifylline (Trental).

Pentoxifylline (Trental)

Pentoxifylline (Trental) specifically targets the immune system's inflammatory cells and normalizes their function. The immune system cells involved in the inflammatory process are macrophages, neutrophils (a type of white blood cell that ingests and kills bacteria and provides a defense against infection), T cell lymphocytes, and natural killer (NK) cells. Scientists have found that Trental directly acts on these inflammatory agents and normalizes their function.

The Sher Institutes of Reproductive Medicine (SIRM) administers 400 milligrams of Trental four times daily to patients as a vaginal suppository, localizing treatment where it is needed most. This also reduces the number of side effects elsewhere in the body. Common side effects of Trental include dizziness, headaches, mild stomach upset, diarrhea, nausea, vomiting, drowsiness, and agitation/nervousness. Trental is not a widely used medication for endometriosis-related immune problems. It is also being investigated as a treatment for immune-related infertility in endometriosis patients.

▌ Transcutaneous Electrical Nerve Stimulation (TENS)

Endometriosis patients who have tried this form of treatment report some pain relief. Transcutaneous electrical nerve stimulation (TENS) involves the use of low-voltage electrical current transmitted to the site of pain through electrodes pasted on the skin. The current is delivered from a battery-powered generator. The theory behind this treatment suggests that TENS may affect the pain nerves, interfering with nerve pathways, and may alter the natural chemicals that affect the way pain is perceived and transmitted.

There are three basic types of TENS:

- *Conventional TENS:* Electrical current is transmitted near the site of pain.
- *Acupuncture-like TENS:* Current is transmitted at specific trigger points.
- *Auricular TENS:* Current is applied to the ear.

▌ Pain Clinics and Specialists

Many endometriosis patients are turning to pain specialists and clinics to help manage their endometriosis-associated pain. While many find pain medications and hormonal treatments sufficient to deal with their pain, other women have to seek the help of pain specialists who will not only treat their pain but also its secondary symptoms such as anxiety, depression, quality of sleep, and so on for better outcomes.

A pain specialist is normally affiliated with a pain clinic or center, each with its own mode of pain treatment. One clinic may focus on only one mode of pain treatment or on only one particular type of pain while another will have more variety in terms of treatment. Pain clinics attached to universities or medical schools usually offer more variety in terms of specialists and treatment methods.

The following are some tips on finding a pain specialist:

- Get a referral from your doctor to a reputable pain specialist or clinic. Some clinics/specialists require a referral from your doctor and also a copy of your medical records.
- You can also contact the American Pain Society or the American Academy of Pain Medicine to find pain clinics or specialists in your area.

Once you have found a specialist, determine whether she/he is right for you. The National Pain Foundation (NPF) suggests the following questions you can ask to help in making your decision:

1. How many cases of my type of pain have you treated?
2. What are your special qualifications to treat my pain condition?
3. Have you participated in any special training about pain management techniques? (Pain specialists are certified by the American Board of Anesthesiology and the American Board of Pain Medicine.)
4. What is your philosophy of management of my pain condition in terms of medications and alternative therapies?
5. What types of medications do you usually prescribe?

6. What types of nonmedication therapies do you use? (Pain specialists utilize a variety of therapies to treat varied types of pain. These include injected medications, biofeedback, or transcutaneous electrical nerve stimulation [TENS].)
7. Where do you refer patients who need additional treatments?
8. Is your clinic listed with any professional societies?
9. Are you, or is someone in the clinic, available twenty-four hours a day if I need help?

Another factor to take into consideration is cost. Ensure that you know the overall cost of treatments for your entire program. Also check with your insurance company on what expenses they cover.

▋ Heat Therapy

Heat has long been a close companion to any woman in pain during her menses. This is especially so for women with endometriosis. Heat, when applied to the area from which pain emanates (the abdomen), has a soothing effect that gives temporary relief from pain. When heat penetrates deep below the surface of the skin, it relaxes the muscles and increases blood flow to the tissues. The tissues are washed by the blood, which, in the process, sweeps away the substance that causes pain, resulting in temporary relief. Heat therapy can range from taking a hot bath to using portable microwavable or plug-in heating pads.

Studies have proven the positive effects of heat in the treatment of dysmenorrhea. In one such study, eighty-four participants were placed into four groups: one group received 400 milligrams of ibuprofen and a heated pad; another given 400 milligrams of ibuprofen and an unheated pad; a third received a placebo and a heated pad; and the fourth received a placebo and an unheated pad. The participants were treated for two days and wore the heated or unheated pads for twelve hours and took ibuprofen or placebo every six hours, three times per day. The women recorded their pain levels during the treatment period. At the end of the period, participants in the two heated pad groups reported greater pain relief than those in the unheated pad and placebo groups. The women assigned heated pads reported overall pain relief equivalent to that provided by ibuprofen.

Procter & Gamble later marketed these heat pads as ThermaCare Menstrual HeatPatches, available in packs of three. These patches can be purchased at pharmacies throughout the United States. These portable heat patches are worn under your clothing, attached to your underwear, and are designed to conform to your lower abdomen. The patches warm up when exposed to oxygen in the air and provide consistent heat for up to eight hours. Women with endometriosis who have used ThermaCare Menstrual HeatPatches describe their effect as "a life saver," or "sometimes it is the only thing that takes my pain away."

▌ Advances/Future Directions in Medical Therapy

The negative side effects of current medical treatment options for endometriosis have propelled medical scientists to investigate new types of medications to treat the disease. Many of these new developments are still in their initial stages and not yet available to the public. However, they hold much promise to endometriosis patients.

Gonadotropin-Releasing Hormone (GnRH) Antagonists

Unlike agonists, antagonists block hormonal receptors. Gonadotropin-releasing hormone (GnRH) antagonists block the pituitary gland from releasing the follicle-stimulating hormone (FSH) and luteinizing hormone (LH) needed to begin the ovulatory cycle.

The end result is the same as with GnRH agonists—decreased estrogen production, endometriotic implant reduction, and symptom relief—but with an added benefit. GnRH antagonists do not stimulate an initial flare of FSH and LH as with the first phase of GnRH agonist treatment. GnRH antagonists directly inhibit FSH and LH secretions, resulting in quicker symptom relief and none of GnRH agonists' hypoestrogenic side effects.

The GnRH antagonists currently under study are mainly short-acting treatments, less than ideal for long-term use in the case of the endometriosis patient. These require frequent subcutaneous (under the skin) injections and thus are very expensive. One promising long-acting GnRH antagonist—Abarelix—was recently discovered, and it's currently in clinical trials all over the United States. This drug holds much promise as a long-term antagonist treatment for endometriosis.

Aromatase Inhibitors

Medical scientists have firmly established that endometriotic implants produce their own estrogen as a result of the enzyme aromatase P450 arom. Implants contain high levels of aromatase P450, which leads to the local production of estrogen. This may explain disease symptom recurrence in up to 75 percent of women treated with gonadotropin-releasing hormone (GnRH) agonists, and disease recurrence after hysterectomy and bilateral salpingoooophorectomy in some women. Dr. Serdar Bulun therefore suggests that a larger number of patients may experience longer symptom relief by blocking aromatase activity in endometrial implants.

One promising aromatase inhibitor is letrozole. In a study conducted by Dr. Bulun and colleagues from the University of Illinois, ten women diagnosed with endometriosis and chronic pelvic pain were treated with 2.5 milligrams of oral letrozole plus a progestin as an add-back therapy. All ten patients responded well to the treatment, with no evidence of endometriosis in any of the patients at a second-look laparoscopy. More studies are being done; however, aromatase inhibitors may offer patients a more effective way of suppressing endometriosis.

Selective Estrogen Receptor Modulators (SERMs)

Selective estrogen receptor modulators or SERMs are also referred to as designer estrogens. These designer estrogens mimic the action of estrogen where it is needed, such as the cardiovascular and skeletal systems, and block the effects of estrogen in others, such as in the breasts and uterine tissues. In the case of endometriosis, SERMs would act by depriving ectopic endometrium of the estrogen it needs to grow and develop into active disease. SERMs have been shown to prevent bone loss and do not promote a hypoestrogenic state as with gonadotropin-releasing hormone (GnRH) agonists. However, SERMs such as raloxifene do not share estrogen's ability to reduce hot flashes. These designer estrogens are still being investigated as treatments for endometriosis.

Extracellular Matrix Modulators (EMMs)

Endometriotic implants produce matrix metalloproteinase (MMP), an enzyme that plays an important role in tissue remodeling. This enzyme has been found to be an integral factor in endometriotic tissue implantation and development at ectopic locations throughout the body. Armed with this knowledge, scientists are now investigating the possibility of creating extracellular matrix modulators (EMMs) that, like selective estrogen receptor modulators (SERMs), would block, isolate, and destroy MMPs. Further studies are being conducted.

RU-486 (Mifepristone)

RU-486 is controversially known as the abortion pill. It has been used to terminate pregnancies and looks promising as a medical treatment for endometriosis. RU-486 is an anti-progestin (an antagonist); this means that its main action is to block progesterone activity as in the case of gonadotropin-releasing hormone (GnRH) antagonists. It binds itself to progesterone receptors on the wall of the uterus, inhibiting progesterone buildup and maintenance of the uterine lining (endometrium) for possible pregnancy. This inhibition triggers the shedding of the endometrial lining, as in the case of a normal menses. RU-486 is also an anti-estrogenic compound, which blocks estrogen to implants.

Studies have shown that treatments of RU-486, with doses from 50 to 100 milligrams daily, decrease ovulation, induce amenorrhea, and improve overall endometriosis symptoms in patients. Further studies on the effectiveness of RU-486 as a treatment for endometriosis are being conducted.

Mesoprogestins

There are progestins (an agonist—medroxyprogesterone acetate), anti-progestins (an antagonist—RU-486), and now scientists have discovered a third category: mesoprogestins. This form of progestin lies between the former two progestin extremes but exhibits both agonist and antagonist actions on progesterone receptors. In other words, mesoprogestins both mimic *and* block progesterone activities. Scientists found that in the absence of other progestins such as medroxyprogesterone acetate, mesoprogestins act as agonists. In the presence of other progestins, they act as antagonists. In the case of the endometriosis patient, mesoprogestins have the ability to allow ovulation but block menstruation.

A small number of women and animals treated with the mesoprogestin Asoprisnil in clinical and animal studies showed signs of inhibited ovulatory cycles. But in all studies mesoprogestins suppressed menstruation. Mesoprogestins therefore antagonize the proliferative effect of estrogen, showing a preferential effect on endometrium. The endometrial lining does not develop, menstruation does not occur and, it is expected, ectopic endometrial tissue will not experience cyclic growth and shedding. The result is less inflammation to the surrounding peritoneal tissues, fewer adhesions, and less pain. In effect, symptoms improve. Further studies will be conducted on Asoprisnil, which was well tolerated by participants in early clinical studies, as a new treatment for endometriosis.

Angiostatic Therapy (Inhibition of Development of New Blood Vessels)

Scientists have found that angiogenesis, the natural process of the formation of new blood vessels, is a major factor in the development of endometriosis. Endometrial implants recruit new blood vessels to continue developing. Researchers therefore suggest that angiostatic therapy (treatment that inhibits the development of new blood vessels) may prevent new endometriotic lesions from growing and may also block already-existing implants from recruiting blood to maintain growth. Research from the Netherlands used four angiostatic compounds on human endometrium transplanted into forty-nine mice and allowed to grow into endometriotic lesions. The researchers found that the compounds inhibited the number of newly developed blood vessels around implants. However, mature vessels surrounded by smooth muscle cells were not affected. These findings suggest that angiostatic therapy may prevent recurrence of endometriosis after surgical or hormonal therapy.

In research from the United States, mouse endometrium was treated with endostatin, an angiostatic treatment. The study found that the growth and numbers of endometrial implants were reduced by as much as a half. Endostatin was also found to be the most effective of all four angiostatic compounds in the Netherlands study.

▮ ▮ ▮ Endometriosis ▮ ▮ ▮
The Four Pillars of Healing

By Deborah A. Metzger, MD, PhD, Medical Director,
Helena Women's Health Center

(Reprinted with permission from Dr. Deborah A. Metzger)

Treatment options for women with endometriosis are quite limited and generally directed at eradicating or suppressing the implants. Recurrence of symptoms following treatment is common, implying that these treatments fail to address the systemic manifestations of the disease. One of the challenges to health care providers is to provide patients with optimal management of the common symptoms of endometriosis: pelvic pain, dysmenorrhea, and fatigue. Over the past eleven years, my practice has consisted predominantly of caring for women with endometriosis, particularly those who have not had success with the standard treatments for endometriosis. As a result of their suggestions and willingness to try new approaches, I have developed an approach that I call the "Four Pillars of Healing"[1]. The following four approaches form the foundation for the science and art of the treatment of endometriosis: (1) accurate diagnosis, (2) thorough excision of implants, (3) hormonal therapy, and (4) immunotherapy.

Accurate Diagnosis

The most common tool for the diagnosis of chronic pelvic pain is a diagnostic laparoscopy under the assumption that whatever is causing the pain will be visible. Endometriosis implants are usually visible, but other, more subtle appearances of the disease can be missed, particularly in young women. Once the diagnosis of endometriosis is made, all of the patient's pain symptoms are often attributed to endometriosis, even though other sources of pain are commonly found in association with endometriosis such as interstitial cystitis, occult inguinal hernias[2], abdominal wall trigger points, vulvodynia, ovarian vein syndrome[3], ovarian remnant syndrome, and pelvic floor tension myalgia[4]. Screening for these sources of pain should be a routine part of the assessment of any woman with chronic pelvic pain[5]. Optimal resolution of pelvic pain will depend on treatment directed toward all of the causes of chronic pelvic pain.

Thorough Excision of Implants

For superficial implants, ablation of the implants is sufficient. However, for implants that demonstrate scarring, retraction, immobility of the peritoneum, or nodularity, wide local excision is necessary to remove the entire implant. Failure to excise deep-seated implants in the cul-de-sac, particularly where there is complete or partial obliteration of the cul-de-sac, may be responsible for rapid recurrence of symptoms following surgery or hormonal suppression. Bowel resection may be necessary in some cases. Endometriomas respond poorly to hormonal suppression and recurrence is common following surgical drainage. The endometrioma capsule must be removed in order to minimize recurrence. Selected patients may benefit from adjunctive pain-relieving measures such as presacral neurectomy, uterosacral nerve transection, or uterine suspension[6].

Although effective in relieving pain, surgery removes the implants but leaves the systemic disease intact, which may explain the recurrence of symptoms in 12 to 54 percent of all women within a year of surgery[7]. Thus, surgery should not be viewed as curative, but merely a way of debulking disease to improve response to the other three pillars of treatment.

Hormonal Therapy

Given the clear association between estrogen exposure development and progression of endometriosis, medical therapy for patients with endometriosis is most frequently based on the need to produce a hypoestrogenic environment that can be achieved using gonadotropin-releasing hormone analogues, high-dose progestins, Danocrine, or continuous oral contraceptives. Controlled studies show a high degree of efficacy of hormonal therapy when relief of pain and dysmenorrhea are used as endpoints. However, dysmenorrhea invariably returns with the resumption of cyclic menses and approximately 25 to 30 percent report recurrence of pelvic pain symptoms within six months of treatment[8].

Women who are more likely to have recurrences include those with severe disease, deep fibrotic disease, or large endometriomas which are better managed surgically. Continuous oral contraceptives (OCPs) may be used to continue the hormonal suppression and symptom improvement initially achieved with GnRH agonists or other hormonal therapy. Unlike surgical treatment, hormonal therapy appears to have beneficial effects on the immune system[9].

Immunotherapy

In spite of the overwhelming evidence suggesting an immune imbalance in women with endometriosis, little attention has been paid to treating the immune system. In treating women with endometriosis, I have been impressed by the large proportion of these women who continue to complain of fatigue in spite of relief of their pain, implying that the systemic part of the disease has not been addressed. Because fatigue can result from a variety of conditions, I routinely perform a fatigue screening workshop that includes the following tests: Zung depression questionnaire, complete blood count with differential, sedimentation rate, liver functions, antinuclear antibody, free T4, TSH, magnesium, calcium, creatinine, BUN, Lyme screen with confirmatory Western blot, AM/PM cortisol, glycosylated hemoglobin, rheumatoid factor, and HIV. In a series of forty consecutive endometriosis patients with fatigue, but no pain, eleven patients had mild to moderate depression while on antidepressant therapy, one patient was found to have adrenal insufficiency, four had mild hypothyroidism, four had mild anemia, and two had Lyme disease[10]. Almost without exception, fatigue persisted in spite of correction of these abnormalities.

An often-overlooked cause of fatigue is allergy to environmental (pollen, dust mites, molds, cold, heat) or endogenous (foods, drugs, Candida, hormones) allergens. Any of these substances can trigger an immediate or delayed hypersensitivity reaction that is manifested as nasal congestion, asthma, diarrhea/constipation, skin rashes, fever, fatigue, muscle pain, and/or joint pain. Often the responsible allergen(s) is something that a person comes in contact with on a regular basis. In the previously described series of forty patients with fatigue, 67.5 percent (twenty-seven) had allergic symptoms and were positive IgE and/or IgG mediated allergies[11]. Identification of and desensitization to the offending allergen(s) has alleviated fatigue in about one-third of patients with endometriosis.

Increasingly there are reports of an association between endometriosis and opportunistic infections, specifically with Candida albicans[12]. Half of the women in our fatigue study had an overgrowth of Candida species on stool culture[13]. Moreover, a high proportion of women with endometriosis have antibodies to Candida[14]. It is not known if *C. albicans* is a primary pathogen or an opportunist and marker for other underlying problems, or both. *C. albicans* is a potent antigen that induces production of interleukin-1[15], tumor necrosis factor[16], and interleukin-6[17]. It activates macrophages[18] and at the same time can inhibit phagocytosis[19]. Women with recurrent Candidal vaginitis have peripheral monocytes that are defective in their ability to proliferate in response to Candidal antigens and have elevated antibody titers to *C. albicans* in their serum and vaginal washings. Although there is an extensive European literature regarding the association between endometriosis and Candida, the lack of published research in Western peer-reviewed journals has inhibited pursuit of this association[20]. My patients have reported that treatment of Candida is as important as surgery and hormonal therapy in contributing to their return to health[21].

Desensitization, neutralization, and tolerization are treatments commonly used to treat allergic symptoms that are not responsive to medications. Three-year follow-up of oral tolerization with dilute solutions of Candida has been proven beneficial in women with Candida allergies[22]. Moreover, Kresch[23] has also shown that 87 percent of women with endometriosis have allergies to estradiol, progesterone, or LH compared to 22 percent of control women. The results of neutralization treatment during a three-year follow-up reveals significant improvement in symptoms in the majority of patients.

Other nonspecific treatments directed toward decreasing stress and improving immune function have also been utilized with success in the overall management of fatigue associated with endometriosis. A low refined carbohydrate diet consisting of no caffeine, no sugar, and no preservatives/additives has been helpful along with the addition of a multivitamin with minerals. Physical activity, such as walking or swimming, has been helpful in reducing pain. Attention to reduction of emotional stress through meditation, counseling, antidepressants, and stress management can contribute greatly to the overall success of an endometriosis program.

The rationale behind the treatment of endometriosis is based on the factors thought to be involved in its pathogenesis: retrograde menstruation, implants, estrogen, and the immune system. One of the reasons that recurrence of symptoms is common among women with endometriosis may be that only one or two of the pillars of healing has been utilized. We may be able to achieve more long-term successes by routinely employing all four of the pillars of healing for endometriosis.

References

1. Leo Galland. *The Four Pillars of Healing*. Random House, New York, 1997.
2. D A Metzger, I Daoud. Occult hernias in women with chronic pelvic pain. International Cognress of Gynecologic Endoscopy AAGL 26th Annual Meeting, September 23–28, 1997, Seattle, WA (plenary abstract).
3. D A Metzger, N Epstein. Conservative management of chronic pelvic pain associates with ovarian vein varicosities. International Congress of Synecologic Endoscopy AAGL 26th Annual Meeting, September 23–28, 1997, Seattle, WA.
4. D A Metzger. Additional sources of pain in women with treatment resistant or recurrent endometriosis. International Congress of Gynecologic Endoscopy AAGL 27th Annual Meeting, Nov. 10–15, 1998, Atlanta, GA.
5. D A Metzger, I Daoud, P Bosco, J Peters-Gee. A systematic approach to the diagnosis and management of chronic pelvic pain. International Congress of Gynecologic Endoscopy AAGL 27th Annual Meeting, Nov. 10–15, 1998, Atlanta, GA (plenary abstract).
6. D A Metzger. An integrated approach to endometriosis. In *Chronic Pelvic Pain: An Integrated Approach* (Steege JA, Metzger DA, Levy B, eds) WB Saunders Co, Philadelphia, 1998.
7. G B Candiani, L Fedele, P Vercellini, S Bianchi, G DiNola. Repetitive conservative surgery for recurrence of endometriosis. *Obstet Gynecol* 1991; 77:421–424
8. A M Dlugi, J D Miller, K Knittle. Lupron depot (leuprolide acetate for depot suspension) in the treatment of endometriosis: a randomized, placebo-controlled, double blind study. *Fertil Steril* 54:419–27, 1990; Fedele L, Parazzi F, Bianchi S, et al (1990). Stage and localization of pelvic endometriosis and pain. *Fertil Steril* 53:155–158; Waller K G, Shaw R W. Gonadotropin-releasing hormone analogue for endometriosis recurrence after treatment. *Br J Obstet Gynaecol* 100:177, 1993.

9. W P Dmowski, D P Braun (1997). Immunologic aspects of endometriosis. In *Endometrium & Endometriosis* (Diamond MP, Osteen KG, eds) Blackwell Science, Malden MA, 174–181.

10. D A Metzger, J Santilli. Fatigue associates with endometriosis. VI World Congress on Endometriosis, June 30–July 4, 1998, Quebec.

11. Ibid.

12. K Lamb, T R Nichols (1986). Endometriosis: a comparison of associates disease histories. *Am J Prev Med* 2:324–329.

13. Metzger and Santilli.

14. A J Kresch. Combining new immune therapies with traditional endometriosis treatment. Presented as an abstract at the 25th Annual Meeting of the AAGL, Chicago, IL, Sept. 24–29, 1996.

15. C M Ausiello, F Urbani, S Gessani, et al (1993). Cytokine gene expression in human peripheral blood mononuclear cells stimulated by mannoprotein constituents from C. *albicans. Infect Immun* 61:4105–4111.

16. E Blasi, L Pitzurra, M Pulita, et al (1992). C. *albicans* hyphal form enhances tumor necrosis factor mRNA levels and protein secretion in murine ANA-1 macrophages. *Cell Immunol* 142:137–144.

17. M C Ghezzi, G Raponi, F Filadoro, et al (1994). The release of TNF-a and IL-6 from human monocytes stimulated by filtrates of C. *albicans* after treatment with amphotericin B. *J Antomierob Chemother* 33:1039–1043.

18. N Vasquez, H R Buckley, D M Mosser, et al (1995). Activation of murine resident peritoneal macrophages by a cell wall extract of C. *albicans. J Med Vet Mycol* 33:385–393.

19. I Szabo, L Guan, T J Rogers (1995). Modulation of macrophage phagocyctic activity by cell wall components of C. *albicans. Cell Immunol* 164:182–188.

20. C R Mabray (1997). The allergy-endocrine-endometriosis connection. In *Endometrium & Endometriosis* (Diamond MP, Osteen KG, eds) Blackwell Science, 342–346.

21. D A Metzger. Efficacy of conventional and alternative treatments for endometriosis. VI World Congress on Endometriosis, June 30–July 4, 1998, Quebec.

22. Kresch.

23. Ibid.

8

Treating Endometriosis-
Associated Infertility

Infertility occurs in one in three women or between 30 to 50 percent of women diagnosed with endometriosis. The condition occurs in all four stages of the disease; however, the causal relationship between stages I and II disease and infertility is problematic. Extensive scarring and blocking of the reproductive tract as a result of adhesions and obstructive implants in stages III and IV disease can easily account for infertility. However, other mechanisms may account for infertility in all stages of the disease. Failure to recognize the role of these other mechanisms will only delay a patient's chances of conceiving.

▌The Endometriosis-Infertility Connection

Medical scientists have found several different mechanisms through which endometriosis can affect your fertility.

Anatomic Distortions

Extensive scarring from adhesions and bleeding from old lesions that causes further adhesions can interfere with the normal anatomy of the reproductive tract. Adhesions have been found to freeze the reproductive organs in place and prevent the transfer of an egg to the fallopian tube. Adhesions create abnormal connections between normally separate parts. Thus, adhesions may cause the fallopian tubes and ovaries to adhere to the lining of the pelvis and to each other, restricting their movement. Additionally, endometriosis can obstruct the inside of the fallopian tubes, impeding the path of the egg to the uterus.

Peritoneal Fluid Effects

Abnormalities in the peritoneal fluid of women with endometriosis may account for endometriosis-associated infertility.

Effects on Sperm Motility

Recently, researchers have found evidence that the epithelium of the isthmic (narrow) region of the fallopian tube, thought to play an important part in sperm transportation to the site of fertilization, may be disrupted in women with endometriosis. The findings of this study, reported in the March 2005 issue of the *Journal of Human Reproduction,* suggest that the sperm-binding properties of the epithelium in women with endometriosis may be disrupted, trapping more sperm than in normal uterine epithelium. More sperm bound per unit area to the epithelium of the fallopian tubes taken from women with endometriosis than in women without the disease. This has the potential to interfere with the motility of select sperm with the right physiological status to take part in the fertilization process.

Researchers have also observed inflammation in the peritoneal fluid surrounding the uterus, characterized by an increase in the number and activity of macrophages and cytokines. Their increased presence creates a hostile environment that may adversely affect sperm motility and survival. One laboratory test noted slower sperm motility in peritoneal fluid taken from women with moderate or severe endometriosis but not from women with mild endometriosis.

Missing Proteins

Dr. Bruce A. Lessey, associate professor of obstetrics and gynecology at the University of North Carolina at Chapel Hill School of Medicine, discovered that infertility in women with mild endometriosis may be caused by a lack of certain proteins in the peritoneal fluid. In his study, peritoneal fluid from women with and without minimal endometriosis was injected into recently mated mice around the time of embryo implantation. The mice given peritoneal fluid from infertile women with mild endometriosis had fewer implantations than did mice receiving fluid from fertile women without minimal endometriosis. Protein levels were also reduced among mice given peritoneal fluid from infertile women with mild endometriosis. These mice were missing the cellular proteins $alpha_v beta_3$ and had reduced levels of leukemia inhibitory factor (LIF). These are present in uterine cells around day twenty of the normal twenty-eight-day menstrual cycle and may play an important role in the embryo's subsequent attachment to the uterine lining. The findings of the study, published in the July 2000 issue of *Fertility and Sterility,* suggests that $alpha_v beta_3$ and LIF reduction in women with endometriosis may interfere with embryo implantation in the uterine lining.

Reduced Ciliary Beat Frequency

Research conducted by the London School of Medicine provides preliminary evidence to suggest that peritoneal fluid in women with endometriosis significantly reduces ciliary beat frequency that would negatively impact transport of the egg. Cilia are the tiny hairs in the fallopian tubes that help the movement of the egg toward sperm. In this study, sections of fallopian tubes from seventeen women who had undergone hysterectomies were exposed to peritoneal fluid. Six sections were exposed to fluid from women with early-stage endometriosis and another six exposed to fluid from women without. Ciliary beat frequency was reduced by about a quarter in those sections exposed to peritoneal fluid from women with endometriosis.

Genetic Defects

A research team from Stanford University in California found that genetic defects may hinder embryo implantation in the uterine wall and can partly explain the association between endometriosis and infertility. The team collected samples of endometrial tissue from eight women with endometriosis and seven without during the "window of implantation" of the menstrual cycle. During this period the uterus becomes most receptive to the embryo. Microarray analysis, a high throughput gene test technique, was then used to assess the expression of 12,686 genes found in the samples. The scientists found 91 genes expressed more than twice as much in the women with endometriosis compared to those without, while 115 genes were expressed less than half as much in the women with endometriosis than those without.

Within this latter set of genes, the team found the gene responsible for mediating adhesion between embryos and endometrium expressed significantly lower in the samples collected from women with endometriosis compared to those without. The researchers conclude that these findings support the theory that the presence of certain genes in the incorrect amount and/or expressed abnormally, contributes to the development of endometriosis. This in turn creates an inhospitable environment for embryo implantation.

Hormonal Effects

Elevated levels of prostaglandin hormones, secreted by active endometrial implants, may induce muscular contractions or spasms. These may hinder the ability of the fallopian tube to transport the egg, resulting in an unsuccessful implantation.

Immune System Factors

The altered immune response in a woman with endometriosis may also affect her fertility. Several dysfunctions have been noticed at the immune system level in women with endometriosis-associated infertility.

Antibodies Formed Against the Embryo

Although the exact mechanisms are unclear, researchers suggest that antibodies formed against ectopic endometrial tissue may also attack the uterine lining and cause spontaneous abortion in women with endometriosis. Spontaneous abortions are up to three times the normal rate in women with endometriosis compared to the general female population. If consistently attacked by antibodies over a period of time, the fallopian tubes may become inflamed and severely blocked by adhesions. The tubes will no longer be able to provide safe passage for egg, sperm, and embryo, increasing the likelihood of ectopic pregnancies, up to sixteen times more likely (16 percent) in women with endometriosis than the general female population (1 percent).

Antiphospholipid Antibodies (APA)

Scientists have found a link between the incidence of miscarriages in women with endometriosis and the formation of antiphospholipid antibodies (APA). These antibodies are formed against phospholipids that make up part of the membrane in the cells of the body. The immune system detects phospholipids as foreign matter and creates antibodies (autoantibodies) against them. These antibodies can be detected by blood tests. In women with endometriosis, the APAs may arise from the general immune response to rid the body of ectopic endometrial cells.

APAs have been found in 66 percent of women with endometriosis. The experts found that APAs can bind to human trophoblast (the tissue that forms the wall of the embryo in its early stages). This inhibits the implantation of the embryo into the uterine wall, resulting in a miscarriage.

Abnormal Natural Killer (NK) Cell Activity

Abnormal natural killer (NK) cell activity and number may also affect your fertility. Research has shown that NK cells play an important role in early pregnancy. NK cells produce growth factors that stimulate the development of placenta. The NK cells also monitor placental development to restrict excessive placental invasion into the uterine wall.

In women with endometriosis, abnormal numbers and activity in NK cells affects the proper implantation of the embryo. These NK cells attack the implanting embryo, resulting in miscarriages and infertility. Approximately 30 percent of women with endometriosis-associated infertility have abnormal NK cell activity.

Lack of Attachment Molecules (Integrins)

The embryo's ability to attach to the uterine wall is facilitated by proteins called integrins, also called cell-to-cell adhesion molecules. Integrins bind with complementary molecules on the surface of the uterine lining. Like a key in a lock, once the adhesion molecules come into contact with its complementary molecules, they interlock and initiate the attachment of the embryo to the uterine wall. Scientists have found that up to 50 percent of women who suffer from endometriosis-associated infertility do not develop cell-to-cell adhesion molecules.

Luteinized Unruptured Follicle Syndrome (LUF)

The inability of the mature follicle to release an egg has been referred to as luteinized unruptured follicle syndrome (LUF). In this case, the patient will ovulate, but an egg is not released, instead becoming trapped in the ovary. This condition is seen in 63 percent of women diagnosed with endometriosis. Ovulation dysfunction accounts for 25 to 30 percent of infertility cases in women with endometriosis.

Luteal Phase Defect

The corpus luteum, in the second half (last two weeks) of the menstrual cycle, produces large amounts of progesterone. This hormone plays a very critical role in the proper implantation of a fertilized egg by preparing the endometrial lining of the uterus (endometrium) for pregnancy. Studies indicate that women with endometriosis are deficient in progesterone during this luteal phase—luteal phase defect—resulting in the inability to properly implant the fertilized egg.

Whatever may be the causes of endometriosis-associated infertility, the thought of not being able to have children can be psychologically traumatic. Andrea describes her situation:

I'd never really thought about having children, although I knew I'd always wanted them. Now that I had been told I couldn't have children, my need for them was great. I became very depressed. I found myself looking at babies in the street as I passed by, cringing as a diaper ad came on the TV. All of a sudden everywhere I went there were babies.

Then my younger sister found out she was pregnant. I was so devastated that I ran to my grandma's and broke down in tears. She knew what it was about; she always did. I never had to explain anything to her . . . she knew me best.

I found myself keeping clear of the sister I once was very

*close to. She knew and was upset that I felt this way. She
needed support, and I couldn't give her any. I hated her. How
could she do this?*

■ Surgical Treatment of Endometriosis-Associated Infertility

Laparoscopic Surgery

Conservative laparoscopic surgery has become a standard and effective approach in the treatment of endometriosis-associated infertility. A randomized controlled trial done by Dr. Sylvie Marcoux and colleagues from the Canadian Collaborative Group on Endometriosis in 1997 demonstrated that laparoscopic resection or ablation of minimal and mild endometriosis enhances fertility in infertile women. In this study, 341 infertile women with stage I or II endometriosis were randomly chosen to have a diagnostic laparoscopy or a diagnostic laparoscopy combined with surgical resection or ablation of endometriostic lesions. The researchers found that resection or ablation of minimal and mild endometriosis, compared to diagnostic laparoscopy alone, increased the likelihood of pregnancy in infertile women. Of 172 women who had resection or ablation of endometriosis, 50 became pregnant. Their pregnancies continued for twenty weeks or longer. Of 169 women who had diagnostic laparoscopy, 29 became pregnant. Fetal losses occurred in approximately 20 percent of the recognized pregnancies, irrespective of the study group.

On the other hand, the Gruppo Italiano per lo Studio dell'Endometriosi conducted a randomized clinical trial in 1999 to analyze the effectiveness of resection/ablation of minimal/mild endometriotic lesions for improving fertility. The women chosen for this trial were a maximum of thirty-six years of age, trying to conceive, and had been diagnosed via laparoscopy of minimal/mild endometriosis (stage I or II), yet experienced infertility. In this study, 51 women were randomly assigned to resection or ablation of visible endometriosis and 45 to diagnostic laparoscopy only. After laparoscopy, the women tried to conceive spontaneously for one year. There were 12 (24 percent) in the resection/ablation group and 13 (29 percent) in the no-treatment group who conceived. Two spontaneous abortions were observed in the resection/ablation group and three in the no-treatment one. The researchers concluded that the results do not confirm that ablation of endometriotic lesions in an early stage markedly improves fertility rates compared with no treatment.

Overall, however, surgery has been found to be very instrumental in improving fertility once endometriotic lesions have been removed, adhesions cut out, and normal anatomical relations restored and maintained to the reproductive tract.

∎ Surgical Treatment of Ovarian Endometriomas

Removal of ovarian endometriomas also improves fecundity rates in women with endometriosis. Surgeons traditionally take two approaches to remove endometriomas. In the first approach, they made an abdominal incision to access the endometrioma and then aspirated (drained) the cyst of its contents. This was not an effective method since the cyst wall was left behind with viable endometrial cells that go on to bleed and reaccumulate within months, requiring further surgeries.

A newer generation of endometrioma surgical techniques involves laparoscopic drainage of the contents of the cyst, followed by removal of the cyst wall. This approach is generally associated with lower disease recurrence rates and improved pregnancy rates. A 2002 study of thirty-nine women—twenty-eight with stage IV disease— who were treated laparoscopically for ovarian endometriomas reported pregnancies occurring within nine months of the surgery. The cumulative pregnancy rate after surgery was 39.5 percent.

However, in many cases, normal ovarian tissue is inadvertently removed along with the cyst wall. This harms the follicular reserve in the ovaries, interrupts estradiol production (which may induce menopausal symptoms such as hot flashes) and causes adverse changes in blood flow to the ovaries. Additionally, there is increased risk of adhesions forming at the site of cyst removal, further affecting fertility.

Today, surgeons are employing a new type of surgical technique, called sclerotherapy, to effectively remove ovarian endometriomas and reduce the complications and risks of the two techniques described above. While new to endometrioma treatment, sclerotherapy is not new to the general field of surgery. Sclerotherapy has long been used to treat varicose veins.

In the treatment of ovarian endometriomas, the patient is given a general anesthetic, and a pelvic ultrasound machine is used to show the ovaries and other pelvic organs and the cyst to be treated. Next, using the ultrasound as a guide, the surgeon inserts a fine needle through the back of the vagina into the cyst. The surgeon aspirates the cyst until it collapses. The cyst cavity is then washed out with a sterile saline solution. Afterward, a solution of tetracycline is inserted into the cyst cavity. The tetracycline irritates the walls of the cyst and replaces the cells of the cyst with fibrous tissue. Essentially, all viable endometrial cells are destroyed, preventing the risk of recurrence.

In the March 2005 issue of *Fertility and Sterility,* Jeffrey D. Fisch and Geoffrey Sher reported complete resolution of endometriomas in twenty-four (75 percent) out of thirty-two patients after sclerotherapy surgery. Only one patient did not respond to the surgery. In twenty-eight patients who subsequently underwent in vitro fertilization (IVF), sixteen (57 percent) had ongoing pregnancies.

▌Expectant Fertility Management

Women with less severe forms of the disease may have more time as well as more treatment options available to them to aid conception. One such method is expectant fertility management, or becoming more aware of your fertility through natural family-planning techniques. By becoming more aware of your body's changes during the menstrual cycle, you will be better able to determine when ovulation occurs. Additionally, if no other problems are apparent that may reduce your chances of becoming pregnant, expectant management techniques will be beneficial.

Fertility awareness techniques include:

Calendar (Rhythm) Method

This method requires vigilant tracking of your menstrual cycle to estimate your most fertile days. This method relies on a regular menstrual cycle and ovulation to occur on a certain day each month. However, as you learned in chapter 3, very few women with endometriosis have regular menstrual cycles, making this a very unreliable method.

Basal Body Temperature (BBT) Method

Basal body temperature (BBT) is the lowest temperature that a healthy person experiences on any given day. The hormonal changes women experience during the menstrual cycle lowers their BBT. This drop occurs one or two days before ovulation and increases one or two days after ovulation. You will have to monitor your body's temperature before getting out of bed every morning, to estimate when you are ovulating. Ovulation increases your BBT by 0.4° F (0.2° C) and keeps it high for over a week. However, many women do not exhibit this drop in BBT, making this an unreliable method for them. Pages 186 to 187 show an example of a BBT chart you can use when charting your BBT.

Cervical Mucus (Billings) Method

This involves observing and recording the appearance of your cervical mucus over several menstrual cycles to estimate when you are ovulating. Cervical mucus is stretchy and becomes clear and slippery just before ovulation.

Ovulation Prediction Kits

Home ovulation prediction kits can be purchased at any pharmacy without a prescription. These kits help identify your most fertile days during a menstrual cycle by testing the luteinizing hormone (LH) levels in your urine. High LH levels mean you are most fertile.

Combined Method

This essentially involves monitoring your body's changes for optimal fertility days by combining all the methods above and making special note of your body's signs of ovulation. You will measure your BBT, observe the changes in your cervical mucus, use home ovulation prediction kits to monitor the luteinizing hormone (LH) levels in your body, and record symptoms such as breast tenderness, abdominal bloating/pain, and mood changes, among others that are specific to you. This combined method is more effective in predicting ovulation than any one of the above methods.

■ Medical Treatments for Endometriosis-Associated Infertility

Medical suppressive therapy has no place in the treatment of endometriosis-associated infertility. Progestins, estrogen-progestogen combinations, synthetic androgens, gonadotropin-releasing hormone (GnRH) agonists, and GnRH antagonists work effectively in depriving the disease of the estrogen it needs to grow by inducing a pseudopregnant or pseudomenopausal state. The results are chronic

Basal Body Temperature (BBT) Chart

Day of Cycle	1	2	3	4	5	6	7	8	9	10	11	12	13	14	15	16	17	18	19	20	21	22	23	24	25	26	27	28	29	30	31
Day of Month																															
Month																															
99.0																															
98.9																															
.8																															
.7																															
.6																															
.5																															
.4																															
.3																															
.2																															
.1																															

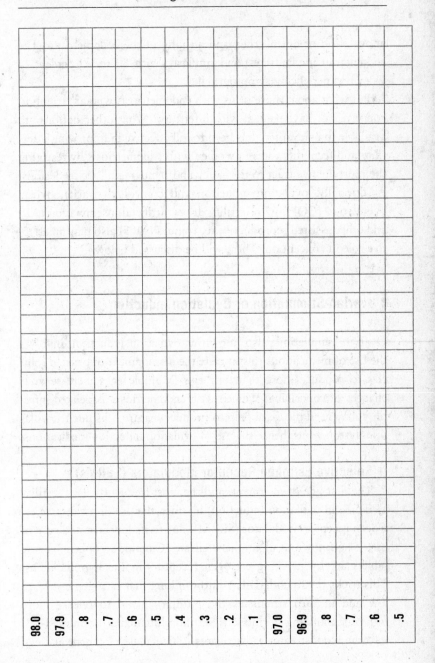

98.0	97.9	.8	.7	.6	.5	.4	.3	.2	.1	97.0	96.9	.8	.7	.6	.5

anovulation or amenorrhea and atrophy of the endometrium. The endometrial implants respond similarly, with 80 to 90 percent of women experiencing symptom relief.

But what about those of us with endometriosis who are trying to conceive but have to deal with infertility? What other options are available to us? Surgery has been found effective in improving infertility and fecundity rates in women with endometriosis by restoring the reproductive tract to normalcy and removing all visible lesions. Additionally, ovulation induction and controlled ovarian hyperstimulation (COH) with fertility drugs, artificial insemination (AI), and other assisted reproductive techniques (ART) also play an effective role in conception. These will be discussed below.

▌ Ovarian Stimulation or Ovulation Induction

Ovarian stimulation, also known as ovulation induction, involves the use of medications to stimulate the development of ovarian follicles to produce more than one egg. Multiple eggs increase your chances of conceiving. Women with endometriosis-associated infertility may need the extra help to produce mature eggs due to ovulation dysfunctions, hence the use of ovulation induction medications.

Selective Estrogen Receptor Modulators (SERMs)

The first line of treatment, and the most frequently used fertility medicine in ovulation induction, involves the use of a selective estrogen receptor modulator (SERM), due to its low cost and ease of use. Also known as clomiphene citrate (Clomid, Serophene), these tablets act by blocking estrogen receptors in the hypothalamus. This tricks the hypothalamus into thinking that estrogen levels are low and in turn stimulates the pituitary gland to release more follicle-stimulating hormone (FSH) and luteinizing hormone (LH) into the bloodstream. This triggers follicular development and egg maturation in the ovaries. As the follicles mature, estrogen is released into the bloodstream as in the normal menstrual cycle.

A week after taking the last clomiphene tablet, your hypothalamus becomes unblocked and, sensing the elevated estradiol levels, stimulates the pituitary gland to release a large amount of LH that triggers ovulation. If the expected ovulation does not take place, the doctor may increase your dosage of clomiphene citrate or add human chorionic gonadotropin (hCG) if this increased dosage does not work. hCG mimics the natural LH surge, triggers the release of the egg from the mature follicle, and encourages the ovary to produce progesterone. Brand names of this drug are A.P.L., Pregnyl, Profasi, and Novarel. Side effects associated with its use include headaches, pain at the injection site, depression, restlessness, irritability, fatigue, and fluid retention.

The clomiphene citrate treatment cycle may be as long as thirty-five days. Some doctors also rely on the patient's menstrual cycle, charted basal body temperature (BBT), LH levels determined from the use of home ovulation prediction kits and/or serum progesterone levels to monitor her response to the treatment.

The side effects of clomiphene citrate treatment include hot flashes, breast tenderness, mood changes, headaches, blurred vision, nausea, vomiting, thick/dry cervical mucus, increased risk of developing ovarian cysts, abdominal discomfort, depression, and increased nervousness. There is also the risk of developing multiple gestations, approximately 10 percent for twins and 1 percent for triplets.

Brandilyn describes some of the side effects she experienced with Clomid:

The side effects from Clomid that I had noticed were mood swings the week I was on the pills (days five to nine of my cycle), frequent headaches, hot flashes, and an increased appetite. I lived through those. I did ovulate, according to the ovulation predictor kit. I had done everything the doctor had requested me to do on the Clomid series, and we didn't conceive. So I refilled my prescription and here's round two! Same side effects, but this time I experienced vaginal dryness during intercourse, which made things difficult, when in order to conceive you have to have sexual intercourse. At the end of this round, I experienced something entirely different. Sure I ovulated and always felt the ovaries pound during that time of the month, but this feeling kept in the same spot for three weeks. By end of week one, I was tired of that feeling and notified [the] doctor's office. She did a vaginal exam, and didn't find anything, sent me home, and I called the same day in severe pain from the pounding of the lower abdominal area. It really felt like my uterus was going to fall straight out of my body! She wanted me in the next day to do another vaginal ultrasound as apparently Clomid has a history of causing cysts and ulcers. Nothing showed up on the ultrasound, and she stated that it's just the Clomid overstimulating the ovaries and recommended I rest one month before going back on Clomid.

▌Controlled Ovarian Hyperstimulation (COH)

This is similar to ovulation induction; however, with controlled ovarian hyperstimulation (COH) more potent fertility drugs are administered for more intensive ovulation induction. The doctor also has more control over ovulation during COH.

Three main categories of ovarian induction medications are used during COH.

Human Menopausal Gonadotropins (hMGs)

Gonadotropin therapy is prescribed if clomiphene citrate treatment failed or if you are about to undergo in vitro fertilization (IVF) therapy. Gonadotropins are very potent fertility drugs that act directly on the ovaries and stimulate follicular maturation and development of multiple eggs. There are three main brands of human menopausal gonadotropins (hMGs): Pergonal, Repronex, and Humegon. These injectable medications contain equal parts of follicle-stimulating hormone (FSH) and luteinizing hormone (LH) derived from the urine of postmenopausal women.

Treatment usually begins on the second or third day of the menstrual cycle for a period of seven to twelve days. Patients are closely monitored during treatment, through regular ultrasounds and blood tests, to monitor the response and number of follicles developing and to ascertain if the appropriate hormone levels have been reached. If the tests reveal that the ovaries are not responding, your doctor may increase the dose. When the follicles are mature and the right hormone levels are reached, hCG is administered to trigger release of the eggs. It is expected that ovulation will occur in thirty-six hours after hCG is given.

There is a high risk of developing multiple pregnancies, approximately 25 percent, with two-thirds developing twins and one-third developing triplets or more. There is also the risk of premature deliveries due to the greater number of fetuses in the uterus. Other side effects include the formation of ovarian cysts, enlargement of the ovaries, abdominal pain, nausea, vomiting, diarrhea, abdominal bloating, irritation at the injection site, dizziness, and the formation of body rashes.

Follitropins (Follicle-Stimulating Hormones [FSH])

These are also injectable forms of gonadotropins that contain only follicle-stimulating hormone (FSH). They mimic the body's own production of FSH and stimulate follicular maturation. Brand names of follitropins are Fertinex, Bravelle, Gonal-F, and Follistim. Fertinex and Bravelle are derived from the urine of postmenopausal women, while Gonal-F and Follistim are purified synthetic FSH. All three medications are administered subcutaneously (injected directly under the skin). Side effects are similar to those of hMG treatments.

Gonadotropin-Releasing Hormone (GnRH) Agonists and Antagonists

Gonadotropin-releasing hormone (GnRH) agonists and antagonists are prescribed during gonadotropin therapy to prevent premature ovulation. Both types of medications are injected subcutaneously. GnRH agonists include leuprolide acetate (injected—Lupron), nafarelin acetate (nasal spray—Synarel) and goserelin acetate (implant—Zoladex). GnRH antagonists include ganirelix acetate (Antagon) and cetrorelix acetate (Cetrotide).

As described in chapter 7, GnRH agonists act by first overloading the pituitary gland with chemical messages to secrete more follicle-stimulating hormone (FSH) and luteinizing hormone (LH) into the bloodstream. This in turn leads the ovaries to produce more estradiol, creating a hypoestrogenic state. After this initial flare, continued administration of GnRH agonists induces a down regulation of hormone receptors in the pituitary gland. This stops FSH and LH to the ovaries, leading to reduced ovarian function and decreased estradiol production. GnRH antagonists have the same effect but without the initial flare/hypoestrogenic state. By suppressing the ovaries, GnRH agonists gives the physician greater control over ovulation induction with hMG injections. These injections will be the only source of follicle stimulation. The side effects are the same as those discussed in chapter 7.

Progesterone

Progesterone supplementation is sometimes used with clomiphene citrate and/or gonadotropin treatment but almost always used with gonadotropin-releasing hormone (GnRH) agonists to mimic a regular menstrual cycle. The fertility drugs clomiphene citrate, human menopausal gonadotropins (hMG), and GnRH agonists and antagonists trigger ovulation in the body and allow fertilization to take place. Combined with progesterone supplementation, the uterine lining is also prepared, increasing your chance of a successful pregnancy.

Progesterone supplements come in the form of an intravaginal gel (Crinone) and an oral capsule (Prometrium). Your pharmacist can also compound progesterone into intramuscular injections, vaginal suppositories, or oral troches. Troches dissolve slowly in your mouth. The dose is dependent on the individual and her needs, and the specific form of the progesterone to be taken.

Side effects associated with progesterone use include nausea, constipation, breast enlargement and tenderness, headaches, drowsiness, vaginal discharge, joint discomfort, fluid retention, and depression.

■ Ovarian Hyperstimulation Syndrome (OHSS)

Ovarian hyperstimulation syndrome (OHSS) is a complication that occurs in 1 percent of women undergoing controlled ovarian hyperstimulation (COH). This occurs when the ovaries overrespond to the medical stimulation. Many eggs are produced in the ovaries, causing them to swell, enlarge, and become very painful. This results in a chemical imbalance in the body, and fluid may accumulate in the abdomen and the lungs.

OHSS occurs more frequently with gonadotropin treatment than with clomiphene citrate treatment. Hospitalization may be required;

severe OHSS can be fatal due to extensive accumulation of abdominal fluid, changes in blood clotting, and dehydration that can lead to kidney and heart failure. Women undergoing gonadotropin treatment have to be especially monitored to reduce their risk of developing OHSS.

▌ Infertility Drug Treatment Chart

The opposite chart summarizes information on all the above fertility drug treatments for your easy access.

▌ Assisted Reproductive Technologies (ART)

Aside from ovulation induction, women with endometriosis-associated infertility have the option of assisted reproductive techniques (ART) to help them conceive.

Intrauterine Insemination (IUI)

Intrauterine insemination (IUI) is a form of artificial insemination (AI) that involves the placement of healthy sperm directly inside the uterine cavity around the time of ovulation to increase the chances that one of those sperms will fertilize an egg. There are several types of artificial insemination techniques available to women; however, IUI has been found more effective than the others to achieve conception.

Other types of AI include:

▌ Intravaginal insemination (IVI): sperm is collected from the male partner and directly inserted in the vagina using a self-insemination syringe (women can inject the sperm into their vagina themselves).

Generic Name	Trade Name	Form	Actions	Side Effects
Clomiphene citrate	Clomid Serophene	Oral tablets	Blocks estrogen receptors in the hypothalamus. This tricks the hypothalamus that estrogen levels are low and in turn stimulates the pituitary gland to release more FSH and LH into the bloodstream. This triggers follicular development and egg maturation in the ovaries. A week after taking the last clomiphene tablet, the hypothalamus becomes unblocked and, sensing the elevated estradiol levels, stimulates the pituitary gland to release a large amount of LH that triggers ovulation.	Hot flashes; breast tenderness; mood changes; headaches; blurred vision; nausea; vomiting; thick/dry cervical mucus; ovarian cysts; abdominal discomfort; depression; increased nervousness; multiple pregnancies
Human chorionic gonadotropin (hCG)	A.P.L. Pregnyl Profasi Novarel	Intramuscular injections	Mimics the natural LH surge, triggers the release of the egg from the mature follicle and encourages the ovary to produce progesterone.	Headaches; pain at the injection site; depression; restlessness; irritability; fatigue; fluid retention
Human menopausal gonadotropins (hMG)	Pergonal Repronex Humegon	Intramuscular injections	Gonadotropins act directly on the ovaries, stimulating follicular maturation and development of multiple eggs.	Multiple pregnancies; ovarian cysts; enlargement of the ovaries; abdominal pain; nausea; vomiting; diarrhea; abdominal bloating; irritation at injection site; dizziness; body rashes
Follitropins (FSH)	Fertinex Bravelle Gonal-F Follistim	Subcutaneous injections	Mimic the body's own production of FSH and stimulates follicular maturation.	Multiple pregnancies; ovarian cysts; enlargement of the ovaries; abdominal pain; nausea; vomiting; diarrhea; abdominal bloating; irritation at

Generic Name	Trade Name	Form	Actions	Side Effects
				injection site; dizziness; body rashes
GnRH agonists	Lupron Synarel Zoladex	Intra-muscular injection Nasal spray Monthly implant	Prevents premature ovulation.	Hot flashes; sleep disturbances; vaginal dryness; joint pain; breakthrough bleeding; headaches; mood changes; bone loss; reduced sex drive; mild breast swelling or tenderness; fatigue; decreased HDL; increased LDL
GnRH antagonists	Antagon Cetrotide	Intra-muscular injection	Prevents premature ovulation.	Hot flashes; sleep disturbances; vaginal dryness; joint pain; breakthrough bleeding; headaches; mood changes; bone loss; reduced sex drive; mild breast swelling or tenderness; fatigue; decreased HDL; increased LDL
Progesterone	Crinone Prometrium	Intra-vaginal gel Oral capsule	Mimics the functions of the body's own progesterone hormone and prepares the endometrial lining for a possible pregnancy.	Nausea; constipation; breast enlargement and tenderness; headaches; drowsiness; vaginal discharge; joint discomfort; fluid retention; depression

▪ Intracervical insemination (ICI): a nurse or a doctor uses a catheter to directly insert the sperm into the woman's cervical canal.

▪ Intrafollicular insemination (IFI): washed sperm is inserted directly into an ovarian follicle.

▪ Intrafallopian insemination (IFI): washed sperm is inserted directly into a fallopian tube using a special plastic catheter.

IUI is a relatively easy procedure that can be done in an office setting. The procedure involves inserting a sterilized sperm-filled catheter directly through the cervical canal and into the uterine cavity. The sperm are then injected directly into the uterus. Patients are required to remain lying down with their hips elevated for up to forty-five minutes to reduce the risk of sperm exiting the body. Once the fallopian tubes are functioning properly and there is no significant problem with the semen, then IUI may be offered as a first-line assisted reproductive technique for infertile endometriosis patients. While they may conceive with IUI treatment, their chances of conceiving are significantly lower than women without endometriosis.

Controlled Ovarian Hyperstimulation with Intrauterine Insemination (COH-IUI)

Pregnancy rates improve when women are administered controlled ovarian hyperstimulation with intrauterine insemination (COH-IUI). This combined method increases the chance of pregnancy, as the inseminated sperm will have more than one opportunity. Since COH usually results in the release of more than one mature egg, it is hoped that there will be a greater chance of pregnancy occurring.

Studies have found that women treated with COH-IUI have a higher fecundity rate than women who use expectant management techniques to conceive. In one study, an 11 percent pregnancy rate was reported during COH-IUI treatment cycles among women with endometriosis. Based on these and other findings, the experts suggest that COH-IUI should be recommended as the first line of treatment for women with stages I and II endometriosis as long as there are no other infertility problems. If COH-IUI is unsuccessful, then patients should try in vitro fertilization (IVF).

▌ In Vitro Fertilization (IVF)

If intrauterine insemination (IUI) and/or controlled ovarian hyperstimulation with intrauterine insemination (COH-IUI) fail to produce a pregnancy, then the next treatment option available is in vitro fertilization (IVF). The experts theorize that IVF in women with endometriosis should increase the chance of a successful pregnancy because the actual fertilization occurs in a laboratory. IVF significantly reduces interaction between egg and sperm with the hostile peritoneal fluid environment of the pelvic cavity and bypasses the distorted fallopian tubes associated with endometriosis.

There are four steps involved in the standard IVF procedure.

Step One—Ovarian Hyperstimulation

The first step in this procedure is ovarian hyperstimulation. Over a period of time, the doctor induces ovarian hyperstimulation to stimulate production of several viable eggs in the ovaries, using any of the fertility drugs discussed above. A woman is also administered a gonadotropin-releasing hormone (GnRH) agonist to prevent premature ovulation. The most common GnRH agonist used in IVF treatments is Lupron. The patient is carefully monitored during this hyperstimulation period with ultrasounds and blood tests. Ultrasounds are done to check on the development, number, and size of the maturing follicles. Blood tests, normally done every other day, monitor estradiol levels in the blood to indicate to the doctor when to administer human chorionic gonadotropin (hCG) to stimulate final maturation of the follicles.

Step Two—Egg Retrieval

In step two of IVF the eggs are harvested before they are naturally released from the mature follicles. Egg retrieval can be done either through a laparoscopy or an ultrasound-guided aspiration. During the laparoscopy, an aspiration device attached to the laparoscope uses light suction to retrieve the eggs. The ultrasound-guided aspiration technique, done vaginally, is used more often than the laparoscopy. It is less invasive, does not require general anesthesia, and does not leave a scar. A probe is used to guide a needle into the ovaries and, guided by the images on the monitor, more accurate aspiration of the eggs is accomplished. Harvested eggs are then transferred to a sterile container to be fertilized in the laboratory.

Step Three—Fertilization

Two hours before the eggs are harvested, semen from the male partner is collected and washed (sperm washing) to select the most viable, active sperm for the fertilization process. Mature, healthy eggs are then combined with the washed sperm in a petri dish and incubated at the same temperature as that in a woman's body. Fertilization normally takes place within forty-eight to seventy-two hours.

Step Four—Embryo Implantation

The successfully fertilized eggs (embryos) are then reimplanted into the woman's uterus several days later. The embryos are placed in a catheter, which is then inserted through the vagina and cervix and into the uterus. The number of embryos to be inserted into the woman's uterus will be determined by the doctor and the woman/couple. Any remaining fertilized eggs will be cryopreserved (frozen) for future IVF treatments.

Efficacy of In Vitro Fertilization (IVF)

Studies have shown that in vitro fertilization (IVF) pregnancy rates in women with endometriosis are about the same as those in women without the disease. Prolonged use of gonadotropin-releasing hormone (GnRH) agonists prior to IVF treatment seem to have a beneficial effect on the outcome of treatment, especially in women with stage III and IV disease. Ovarian endometriomas may have an adverse effect on the outcome of IVF treatments. Studies have reported decreased ovarian response to IVF treatments in the presence of endometriomas. This requires the use of higher doses of gonadotropins to trigger ovarian hyperstimulation.

The effect of surgical removal of endometriomas on IVF treatments has also been studied, but the findings have been inconclusive. Some studies have found no effect on IVF treatments. Others report reduced follicular response after surgical resection of endometriomas in natural fertilization and clomiphene-stimulated ovarian hyperstimulation cycles but no effect on ovarian response after gonadotropin stimulation. On the other hand, favorable responses have been found in women treated via sclerotherapy for ovarian endometriomas.

Variations of In Vitro Fertilization (IVF)

There are four variations of the standard in vitro fertilization (IVF):

Gamete Intrafallopian Transfer (GIFT)

In this procedure fertilization takes place in the fallopian tube. Eggs are produced and harvested as in the standard IVF procedure. They are mixed with the sperm in a petri dish and immediately injected back into the woman's uterus, in the exact place they would be in natural fertilization.

Zygote Intrafallopian Transfer (ZIFT)

This procedure is a combination of IVF and GIFT. Eggs are produced and harvested as in the standard IVF procedure. They are then mixed with the sperm and fertilized in the laboratory. As in GIFT, the fertilized eggs are implanted in the uterus.

In Vitro Fertilization with Intracytoplasmic Injection (ICSI)

This is a highly sophisticated technique referred to as micromanipulation (using micro instruments to achieve/manipulate fertilization). Eggs are produced and harvested as in the standard in vitro fertilization (IVF) technique. Microscopic instruments are then used to inject a single sperm into the center of an egg to obtain fertilization. Once this happens, the fertilized egg is then transferred to the woman's uterus and a blood test administered two weeks later to confirm pregnancy.

Blastocyst Transfer

Blastocysts are five-day old embryos. In standard in vitro fertilization (IVF) treatments, two- to three-day-old embryos are inserted into the uterus. Only the strongest eggs make it to the blastocyst stage, resulting in a better chance for embryo implantation once the eggs are reintroduced to the uterus. The procedure also reduces the incidence of multiple births, as fewer eggs would be transferred than in standard IVF.

Julie relays her experience with IVF:

After the laparoscopy, I started ovulation induction with Fertinex. When I went in for the first ultrasound of my ovaries, they found that I was producing way too many eggs. I would have to finish the cycle with in vitro instead because they didn't want to risk my having higher order multiples.

Even though I had eleven eggs and eight embryos during the first in vitro cycle, I didn't get pregnant. The second in vitro cycle, I had even more eggs and embryos, but I didn't get pregnant. The third cycle, we told the doctors that I wanted to wait until the embryos were five days old, and then transfer them into me. I had thirty eggs and twenty-four embryos. Only two lived until the day five transfer. However, this time, it worked. I got pregnant with twins.

▌ Selective Immunotherapy

Recognizing the immunological dysfunctions apparent in women with endometriosis and women with unexplained infertility, reproductive specialists are treating these dysfunctions to increase the woman's chances of conceiving and carrying out a full pregnancy

▌▌▌ Infertility and Endometriosis ▌▌▌
By Ellen T. Johnson

(Reprinted with permission from Ellen T. Johnson and http://www.endometriosis.org).

I've often wondered exactly how the mere presence of endometriosis can cause so many of us to have difficulty conceiving and carrying a pregnancy to term. Is it a direct cause and effect? Theories have been discussed and proposed, but so far, no one knows for certain.

Maybe it happens on a biochemical or genetic level. Perhaps endometriosis affects egg quality and ovulation. Perhaps it creates a hostile and inflammatory environment for the sperm or embryos. Possibly it affects hormone levels during the luteal phase of our cycles. Or maybe it causes multiple changes in the way our reproductive organs function. Whatever this disease is doing to our reproductive health and the way it's doing it, I know one thing for certain: infertility is very real and very painful for many of us.

I know because I went through it. Believe me, it's not an easy thing to endure. First they tried medication. Followed by surgery. When that failed, fertility drugs and high-tech fertility procedures. When that didn't work, more surgery. Then a heart-wrenching miscarriage. Finally, after a near total depletion of physical, mental, and financial resources, it was time to stop pursuing infertility treatment and accept the cards I'd been dealt.

Those were difficult times. But over the years, the longing and sorrow gradually departed and acceptance took their place. My child-free life—though not what I envisioned for myself—is nevertheless full, interesting, and rewarding. It's not how I thought things would turn out, but life doesn't always turn out the way you thought it would. That's one of the major lessons that infertility (and endometriosis for that matter) teaches you.

I've often wondered what I'd tell a woman in her twenties or thirties who has endometriosis and wonders if this disease will affect her own ability to bear children. From my vantage point, these are some of the things we might talk about:

- *I would tell her to be hopeful.* She should understand that infertility doesn't touch every single one of us. It does affect many of us, but not all. And for those who have difficulty conceiving, there are new fertility methods that can help—and more are being discovered every day. There are also alternative methods for becoming a family (such as adoption) that can be considered.
- *I would tell her to make haste.* If she knows she wants to be a mother, she shouldn't delay. I realize that sounds

strange in our modern world. Encouraging a woman to have children sooner rather than later seems so "last century." What about her career? What if she's not ready? What if her mate's not ready? I know, I know. Those are all things she should take into consideration. But she must also realize that age plays a huge role in fertility. Her ability to conceive will begin declining in her early thirties and will get progressively worse thereafter. That's because women are born with all the eggs they'll ever have—and when they're gone, they're gone. That's for all women, not just those with endometriosis. If you throw endometriosis into the equation, there's even more of a reason not to delay.

▪ *I would tell her to be aggressive.* She should try on her own for six months. And by "trying," I mean working it like a second job. That includes charting her temperature and using an ovulation predictor kit and having intercourse on a regular basis. If there's no pregnancy within six months, she should see a real reproductive specialist. And by "real reproductive specialist," I mean someone who has the training, experience, and expertise to do all the fancy whiz-bang procedures—not a doctor with a mere "interest" in infertility who decides to hang out a shingle.

▪ *And finally, I would tell her to listen to her heart.* As she makes decisions about her reproductive health, she will hear many voices and many opinions. Some are well intentioned, some are not. I would remind her that this is her body and her choice. Only she can decide what is right for her.

For more information about infertility, http://www.obgyn.net/infertility/infertility.asp.

with in vitro fertilization (IVF) treatments. This immunologically based treatment, called selective immunotherapy, targets natural killer (NK) cells to bring their activities back to normal levels, and antiphospholipid autoantibodies (APAs), to suppress their binding actions on attachment molecules (integrins).

Intravenous Immunoglobulin (IVIg) Therapy

This is a standard immunotherapy treatment that involves normalizing NK cell activity. The procedure involves using intravenous immunoglobulin (IVIg), a sterile protein derived from human blood. IVIg works by suppressing NK cell activity and inhibits the effects of APAs, thus protecting the embryo and increasing the chances of embryo implantation to the uterine wall. Dr. Geoffrey Sher from the Sher Institute for Reproductive Medicine (SIRM) found that 63 percent of women who had repeat IVF failures and a positive NK cell activity test got pregnant after being treated with IVIg therapy.

However, one key concern with this treatment has to do with the safety of the blood and the question of transmission of viral infections, especially the human immunodeficiency virus (HIV). To significantly reduce this risk, IVIg is specially treated to kill viruses. There have been no reports of viral infections transmitted through IVIg therapy in the United States.

Side effects of this treatment includes headaches, lower-back aches, fever, joint pains, increase in heart rate (tachycardia), and muscle pains (myalgia).

Heparin

For women undergoing IVF who test negative for abnormal NK cell activity but test positive for APAs, low doses of heparin, an anticoagulant medication, may help. Scientists theorize that heparin acts by repelling APAs from attaching to the phospholipid outer surface of the trophoblast, increasing the chances of a successful embryo implantation.

PART THREE

Think Holistically

9

Herbs and Supplements for Healing

Conventional treatment options for endometriosis—medicine and surgery—have a number of side effects and negative drawbacks, leaving many endometriosis patients dissatisfied. Faced with continuing/worsening symptoms, many are turning to complementary and alternative medicines (CAM) to relieve their symptoms, especially pain.

One such CAM category that many are turning to is supplementation with herbs, vitamins, and minerals. When combined with other lifestyle and dietary changes, supplements can make significant differences to daily life with endometriosis. For me, the daily multivitamin combined with exercise and other stress relievers, as well as attempts at a healthy diet (which I struggled with for years), helped significantly with my attempts to manage this disease, especially its psychological effects, and also my kidney issues.

Endometriosis patients are turning to these herbs and supplements to *complement* their conventional treatment strategies, *not* to replace them. For many, this gives them a sense of control over the disease and empowers them to work even harder to create a treatment program that is unique to them.

Elisabet felt that sense of control when she decided to complement her conventional treatment program with alternative medicine:

Alternative treatments are a way for me to cope both physically and mentally. I need to have the feeling of control. Life gets too scary otherwise. Alternative treatments give me that sense of empowerment and control back. So instead of turning to the doctors for a pill that will cure me, I started looking into alternative coping strategies. . . . I just don't think I can expect to eat awful food, not exercise, and then hope a doctor will give me a quick fix. So I read and learned as much as I could about general healthy living. To begin with, I started exercising regularly, doing yoga. After I learned the impact of nutrition on endometriosis . . . I changed what I ate.

There is a lot of prejudice against alternative treatments, and most people seem to forget that alternative treatments most likely function as a complement to Western treatments. Why choose, if there can be a benefit from both? I still to this day have never met anyone who strictly stuck to alternative treatments, without even the yearly traditional checkup.

However, a word of caution. While scientists have studied some popular herbs such as black cohosh, evening primrose oil, and milk thistle extensively, many others have not gone under vigorous scientific investigation to verify their healing properties. Additionally, herbs are classified as dietary supplements in the United States and, as such, are not regulated as medicines. Instead, manufacturers of dietary supplements are responsible for ensuring that their products are safe and meet the standards set forth in the 1994 Dietary Supplement and Health Education Act (DSHEA).

You can reduce the risk of self-administering incorrect herbs and supplements or incorrect doses of a particular herb/supplement by first consulting with your doctor and getting his/her advice about the types of herbs and supplements you can take in conjunction with your conventional treatments. It is often thought that because a product is "natural," that means it is "safe" to use. This is far from the case. Many herbs contain active ingredients that can harm you if taken with certain prescription or over-the-counter (OTC) medications.

Educate yourself thoroughly about any herbs and/or supplements you are interested in including in your treatment regime. Find out about their actions, properties, and side effects. Also look for any clinical studies conducted by the National Center for Complementary and Alternative Medicine (NCCAM), http://nccam.nih.gov. Carefully read the labels on the containers and look for the U.S. Pharmacopoeia's "USP Dietary Supplement Verified" seal, which indicates that the supplement's manufacturer met certain manufacturing standards before releasing the product on the market. The Good Housekeeping Institute, affiliated with *Good Housekeeping* magazine, also certifies some herbal supplements. To be certified, manufacturers have to make sure their products are tested for uniformity, cleanliness, and freedom from environmental pollutants such as lead, mercury, or drugs.

The following discussion will focus on herbs and vitamin and mineral supplements that can help relieve endometriosis-associated pain and other symptoms. Again, this is for educational purposes only and cannot replace advice from your doctor. Additionally, you may require the services of a practitioner—a trained herbalist—who will take into account your medical history, lifestyle, and diet, as well as your particular disease symptoms, to prescribe the correct herbs to deal with your situation. Such professional practitioners include naturopaths and homeopaths.

▌Herbs

Certain herbs beneficial to endometriosis patients have two main actions. First, there are herbs that can help balance the body's hormones and lower excessive estrogen levels to relieve symptoms. As we all know endometriosis is an estrogen-dependent disease and anything we can do to remove excess estrogen will help to relieve symptoms and allow for better management of the disease. Second, there are those herbs that have anti-inflammatory properties that relieve endometriosis pain such as menstrual cramps and dysmenorrhea. Each category of herb will be reviewed in turn.

Hormone-Balancing Herbs

Black Cohosh (Actaea racemosa and Cimicifuga racemosa)

Black cohosh, a perennial plant native to North America, is a member of the buttercup family. Its roots and underground stems (rhizomes) are used to make preparations that are marketed in tablet or liquid form. Remifemin is one marketed tablet brand of black cohosh. Black cohosh has long been known for its effect in balancing a woman's hormones as she approaches menopause and relieving her menopausal symptoms.

As a woman enters menopause, she experiences a gradual hormonal shift due to changes in her menstrual cycle. The ovaries cease to produce an egg, and the pituitary gland and the ovaries gradually stop communicating with each other. This leads to drastically reduced estradiol levels in the body. Sensing this low estrogen level, the pituitary gland secretes more and more luteinizing hormone (LH) into the bloodstream to stimulate the ovaries to produce the required amounts of estradiol to balance the hormone levels.

Menopausal women thus have low estrogen levels and higher levels of LH, resulting in common menopausal symptoms: hot flashes, vaginal dryness, and mood changes, among others.

This hormonal imbalance also occurs in premenopausal women who had a hysterectomy or those endometriosis patients who are treated with the gonadotropin-releasing hormone (GnRH) agonists Lupron, Lupron Depot, Synarel, and Zoladex.

It is not quite known exactly how black cohosh works, but scientists theorize that it decreases secretions of LH into the bloodstream. An excessive level of LH in the bloodstream has been found to be the cause of hot flashes in pre- and menopausal women. The rhizome also contains powerful plant compounds called phytoestrogens that bind to the body's estrogen receptors, such as the uterus and breasts, and mimic the effects of estrogen. Black cohosh thus offsets the decline in estrogen and reduces menopausal symptoms.

The most recent study on black cohosh's hormone-balancing properties comes from Germany. In the study, 304 women with various menopausal symptoms were administered 40 milligrams of Remifemin or a placebo per day for twelve weeks. At the end of the twelve weeks, Remifemin was found significantly more effective in relieving symptoms than the placebo. These findings were published in the May 2005 issue of *Obstetrics and Gynecology*.

Some uncommon side effects include stomach discomfort, weight gain, and dizziness. Large amounts (above your doctor's prescribed dose) of black cohosh may cause abdominal pain, nausea, vomiting, headaches, diarrhea, dizziness, joint pains, and a lowered heart rate. The experts recommend 250 milligrams of black cohosh extract in the pill form or thirty drops of the liquid to be taken three times daily. Look for tablets that contain 5 percent deoxyactein, one of the active components in black cohosh. Some precautions:

■ Do not take black cohosh for more than six months.
■ Do not take black cohosh with oral contraceptives; this will interfere with your body's hormone production.

Chasteberry (Vitex agnus-castus)

Chasteberry comes from the chaste tree, a shrub found in subtropical climates. It has long been used to relieve menstrual complaints. Like black cohosh, chasteberry has hormone-balancing properties. It has been found that chasteberry stimulates the pituitary gland to secrete more luteinizing hormone (LH) to the ovaries. This stimulates the ovaries to produce more progesterone. Additionally, chasteberry also inhibits the secretion of follicle-stimulating hormone (FSH) to the ovaries, reducing the production of estrogen. Thus, hormone levels are balanced, relieving painful endometriosis symptoms.

Chasteberry also helps relieve premenstrual symptoms (PMS). These symptoms, such as irritability, depression, and abdominal bloating, usually occur because of insufficient production of progesterone in the two weeks before menstruation, resulting in high levels of estrogen in the body. By stimulating the ovaries to produce more progesterone, chasteberry balances the hormone levels and provides relief from PMS symptoms.

Chasteberry also lowers prolactin levels to promote ovulation. Prolactin is the hormone that stimulates the corpus luteum in the ovary to produce progesterone and also stimulates breast milk production after childbirth. In some women, however, prolactin levels are very high, with too little progesterone to promote proper ovulation. Chasteberry has been found to lower prolactin levels and raise ovarian production of progesterone. In one study forty-eight women with infertility and luteal phase defect were given chasteberry extract every day for three months. Of the forty-five who completed the study, seven conceived during the study. Progesterone levels normalized in twenty-five women.

Alone or combined with black cohosh or dong quai, the herb is also effective in normalizing the hormonal imbalances in pre-menopausal women with endometriosis who suffer from meno-pausal symptoms due to gonadotropin-releasing hormone (GnRH) agonist use. Chasteberry may increase menstrual flow and may rarely cause an itchy skin rash or stomach discomfort. The recommended dosage for women with endometriosis is 400 to 500 milligrams of the crushed fruit or standardized extract that contains 0.5 percent agnuside, the active ingredient in chasteberry, or one-half teaspoon of the liquid extract three times daily. Take the tablet or capsule form before meals for optimum absorption. Do not take chaste-berry with oral contraceptives; this will interfere with hormone production. If taken on an empty stomach, the liquid form of chasteberry will irritate your stomach because of the herb's alcohol content. Dilute the liquid in a glass of water to prevent this from happening.

Dong Quai (Angelica sinensis)

Dong quai, also known as Chinese angelica, is an herb that has been used in Asia for years as a remedy for dysmenorrhea, amenor-rhea, metrorrhagia (bleeding from the uterus other than a normal menses), and menopausal symptoms. It is also referred to as the "empress of herbs" or "female ginseng," in recognition of its unique ability to relieve women's menstrual problems and promote uterine health.

Dong quai has several properties that make it a unique herbal supplement specifically for women:

- It contains high amounts of vitamins A, B_{12}, C, and E, as well as high amounts of iron, cobalt, niacin, magnesium, and potas-sium.
- It also contains phytochemicals such as coumarins that relax the uterus's smooth muscles and relieve menstrual pain, and

phytoestrogens that bind to estrogen receptors and reduce the negative effects of a woman's own low estrogen levels.

It is theorized that dong quai's phytoestrogenic ability may help to reduce high estrogen levels in women with endometriosis, resulting in relief of symptoms. It works well in combination with chasteberry to induce hormonal balance. This action is also helpful to relieve menopausal symptoms associated with gonadotropin-releasing hormone (GnRH) agonist use, natural menopause, and surgical menopause induced after a hysterectomy. In this instance, dong quai's phytoestrogenic compounds compensate for the dramatic drop in estrogen levels in the body. However, studies have not found much benefit from dong quai in relieving menstrual symptoms compared to a placebo.

Studies have found that dong quai possesses analgesic properties and can also relieve pain associated with endometriosis. The recommended dosage for women with endometriosis is 200 milligrams of standardized extract, taken three times daily, or one-half teaspoon of liquid extract three times per day. Look for extracts with standardized 0.8 percent to 1.1 percent of ligustilide, the active ingredient in dong quai. Do not take dong quai with NSAIDs.

Dong quai may have a laxative effect and may increase menstrual bleeding. Stop taking dong quai if you develop a skin rash or develop photosensitivity (an abnormal reaction to sunlight that may result in severe sunburns or skin rashes). You may have to limit your exposure to sunlight while taking dong quai. This herb contains chemicals called psoralens that can react with sunlight to cause severe skin rashes or sunburns.

Milk Thistle (Silybum marianum)

The milk thistle plant is recognized for its ability to treat liver disorders and help the liver in its normal functions, such as the removal of toxins and excess estrogen from the body. Milk thistle has also been found to be a powerful antioxidant by specifically protecting the cells of the liver, stomach, and intestines from the damaging effects of free radicals, unstable oxygen molecules that can damage cells.

As we learned in chapter 4, liver dysfunctions may inhibit the removal of toxins and excess estrogen from the body, increasing your risk of developing endometriosis or increasing the severity of the disease. Scientists theorize that milk thistle promotes the growth of new liver cells and prevents toxins from invading healthy liver cells by binding itself to liver cell membranes. The active ingredient in milk thistle that does all this is silymarin. This complex of substances protects the liver from damage from toxins and also regenerates damaged liver tissue, restoring the liver to normalcy.

The recommended dosage is 400 to 600 milligrams three times daily, containing 70 percent to 80 percent of silymarin, at least thirty minutes before meals for maximum effectiveness. You may experience mild diarrhea while taking milk thistle.

Lipotropic Combinations (with Milk Thistle)

The experts suggest trying a lipotropic combination that typically contains milk thistle along with choline, inositol, and methionine (amino acids), vitamins B_{12} and folic acid, and other herbs such as dandelion and turmeric. This lipotropic combination helps the liver process excess estrogen and thus helps relieve your symptoms of endometriosis. Lipotropic combinations enhance the liver's functions, in essence speeding up the removal of excess estrogen from the body. Choline, inositol, and methionine help to maintain the liver's cell membranes. Dandelion helps maintain the liver's function, while turmeric is a powerful antioxidant, like milk thistle, that protects the liver's cells from the damaging effects of free radicals. The recommended dose for endometriosis patients is one or two pills two or three times per day.

Pain-Relieving Herbs

Evening Primrose (Oenothera biennis)

Evening primrose is a wildflower found throughout North America, Europe, and Asia. The active ingredient in this plant is an essential fatty acid (EFA) called gamma-linolenic acid (GLA), extracted from its flowers and seeds. The body converts GLA into anti-inflammatory prostaglandins that help regulate various body functions such as maintaining the structural integrity of the stomach wall. In women with endometriosis, GLA inhibits the production of inflammatory prostaglandins released during menstruation from the endometrium, thus relieving dysmenorrhea and relieving the inflammatory effect of the disease.

GLA is also found in black currant seed oil, flaxseed oil, and borage seed oil. Evening primrose oil may cause headaches, nausea, loose stools, and stomach pain. The recommended dose is 1,000 milligrams two times per day. Take evening primrose oil with food to ensure maximum absorption in the body.

Wild Yam (Dioscorea villosa)

Wild yam can reduce inflammation and soothe the uterine muscles, reducing pain. This is in part the action of substances in wild yams called alkaloids. Wild yam extract (a liquid) should be taken with food to reduce the risk of irritating the stomach. High dosage can result in nausea and diarrhea. The recommended dose for women with endometriosis is one-half teaspoon or 500 milligrams of liquid extract two times per day.

Cramp Bark (Viburnum opulus)

Cramp bark is a deciduous tree or shrub native to Europe and the eastern United States. It is especially known for its antispasmodic (relieves muscle spasms) properties beneficial to endometriosis patients.

As an antispasmodic agent it helps relieve the pain of dysmenorrhea by soothing the uterine muscles. The experts recommend taking cramp bark a day before the estimated start of menstruation to effectively treat dysmenorrhea. Black haw (*Viburnum prunifolium*) is a close relative of cramp bark with the same properties.

White Willow Bark (Salix alba)

The bark of the white willow tree is popularly referred to as "herbal aspirin" because of its unique analgesic and anti-inflammatory effects. It is known to relieve acute and chronic pain, including menstrual cramps, and may be helpful to endometriosis patients. The active ingredient in the bark is salicin, which the body coverts into salicylic acid. Salicylic acid works by reducing the levels of inflammatory prostaglandins in the body, resulting in pain relief. Unlike NSAIDs such as aspirin, white willow bark does not affect the stomach lining. The recommended dose for women with endometriosis is 40 to 80 milligrams of salicin three times per day or one-half teaspoon of liquid extract three times per day. Do not take white willow bark with NSAIDs such as ibuprofen; this can increase the risk of damage to the stomach. High doses may result in stomach discomfort, nausea, or ringing in the ears (tinnitus). Avoid taking white willow bark if you are sensitive to aspirin or already experiencing tinnitus.

Feverfew (Chrysanthemum parthenium)

This herb has become a popular remedy for migraine headaches. The active ingredient in feverfew is parthenolides, which acts by inhibiting the release of serotonin and histamine, substances that are responsible for dilating blood vessels and that also act on pain receptors, causing pain. Feverfew also prevents spasms in blood vessels that trigger migraines. Feverfew may also be beneficial to endometriosis patients by reducing the production of inflammatory prostaglandins during menstruation, thus relieving pain. Feverfew is much more effective if taken *before* the start of your menses, which allows it to limit the production of inflammatory prostaglandins. For migraines take 250 to 400 milligrams of feverfew, with a maximum of 0.4 percent parthenolides, every morning. For menstrual cramps take two capsules two or three times on the day before the start of your menses.

As a preventative measure, feverfew can also reduce the intensity of a migraine and lessen a migraine's associated symptoms such as nausea and vomiting but does not have any effect on a migraine already in progress. Do not take feverfew in combination with NSAIDs. You may experience some stomach discomfort while taking feverfew.

Paivi decided to try herbs, vitamins, and mineral supplementation instead of hormone treatments. This is her experience:

During my post-op appointment, the gyno explained what he found and how he treated it. The lesions were attached to my uterus, ovaries, and tubes. He said there were some hidden in cracks and nooks that were very hard to get to, but he thought he'd cut away most of it. He suggested several post-op treatment plans, one of which was hormone treatment. I researched my options and didn't like the side effects of the hormones, so I opted for vitamin/mineral/herb therapy.

I bought a book (a thick one) on every known vitamin/mineral/herb, explaining what each one's properties were and how each one affected the body. I chose every one that had anything to do with blood, the reproductive system, pelvic pain, hormones, and anything else that had anything to do with menses or women in particular. I paid close attention to the dosage, how each one affected the other, and their side ef-

fects. From this, I chose a treatment plan for myself. I was taking about twelve to fifteen pills three times a day. I did this for about a year after my surgery. I decided to listen and pay attention to what my body was telling me. When I felt nauseous or got a headache from my concoction, it was time to cut something back or change the dosage. My body was telling me it had reached its optimum level of something. I would alter my concoction, and if it felt better, then I knew I was on the right track.

After about a year, I no longer needed to take the highest dose of these natural medicines. I cut back to just bare necessary daily vitamins. I can say with great joy that my menstrual symptoms are now bearable. Once in a while, very rarely, I get cramps that I need to take painkillers for. Most of the time, though, I can get through the days without missing work or soiling my clothes.

I'm not sure if my success story is the result of the doctor doing a very good cleanup job, if it was the home therapy, just a positive attitude, or a combination of all three. I am now forty and, for the last two years, have not had to count days on the calendar, planning my life around my monthly menses, but rather have been able to enjoy activities and life.

▌ Vitamins and Mineral Supplements

Strong scientific evidence links the persistent development of endometriosis to a weakened immune system. While medical scientists are still investigating medications directly aimed at improving the immune system, there are several vitamins and mineral supplements that can help to bolster your immune system to improve overall health and reduce endometriosis symptoms. In fact, once used correctly and taken regularly, vitamins and mineral supplements can help balance your hormones and reduce estrogen levels. Vitamin and mineral supplements can be purchased at your pharmacy or local health food store.

Vitamins

Vitamins are substances that are needed by the body in small amounts to support most of its functions. There are thirteen such vitamins, and they are broken into two groups:

- *Water-soluble vitamins:* Members of this group are the B vitamins (thiamin [B_1], riboflavin [B_2], niacin [B_3], pantothenic acid [B_5], pyridoxine [B_6], cobalamin [B_{12}], folic acid [B complex], and biotin [B complex]); and vitamin C (ascorbic acid). These vitamins support the enzyme systems in the body and have other specific functions.
- *Fat-soluble vitamins:* These include vitamin A (retinal and beta-carotene); vitamin D (ergocalciferol); vitamin E (D-alpha tocopherol), and vitamin K (phylloquinone). Each has a specific function. Vitamin A supports the eyes, especially night vision, and keeps the skin healthy. Vitamin D enhances the body's ability to absorb calcium to promote healthy bones. Vitamin E is an antioxidant that keeps red blood cells and the body's tissues healthy. Vitamin K controls the clotting of blood and may help keep bones healthy.

The Food and Nutrition Board of the Institute of Medicine (National Academy of Sciences—NAS) established the Recommended Daily Allowance (RDA) for vitamins, to guide the amount needed in each person's diet for maximum effect. However, some experts, like Dr. Susan M. Lark, author of *Fibroid Tumors & Endometriosis Self Help Book,* recommends that women with endometriosis take more than the RDA of such vitamins as the B complex.

B Vitamins

Because endometriosis is an estrogen-dependent disease, getting rid of excess estrogen and normalizing the hormone levels in the body will result in gradual symptom relief. This is where the B complex vitamins come in. The B complex vitamins are essential to the normal functioning of the liver to degrade excess estradiol into the less powerful estriol.

B complex vitamins are also required to convert gamma-linolenic acid (GLA) into anti-inflammatory prostaglandins. B complex vitamins are required to work with the liver enzymes to convert GLA into a form that can be used by the body to make these anti-inflammatory prostaglandins. Without this conversion, the body would produce more of the inflammatory prostaglandins, which would increase endometriosis-associated pain.

By complementing your treatment regime with a daily intake of B complex vitamins, you will reduce endometriosis-associated pain by balancing the hormones estrogen and progesterone and maintain the function of the liver to remove excess estrogen from the body. Dr. Susan M. Lark recommends taking 50 to 100 milligrams of B complex vitamins daily.

The following table gives the RDA and safe upper limit for each B vitamin, as recommended by the Food and Nutrition Board, as well as some good food sources for each:

Vitamin	Recommended Dietary Allowance (RDA) in milligrams (mg) or micrograms (mcg)	Safe Upper Limit (UL)* in milligrams (mg) or micrograms (mcg)	Some Good Food Sources
Thiamin (B$_1$)	1.1 mg	—	Pork, liver, lamb, chicken, peas, beans, lentils, potatoes, tomatoes, lettuce, enriched cereals
Riboflavin (B$_2$)	1.1 mg	—	Liver, milk, cheese, green leafy vegetables, fish, eggs, tomatoes, beans
Niacin (B$_3$)	14 mg	35 mg	Pork, fish, eggs, peas, beans, lentils, peanuts, yeast, potatoes, enriched cereals, tomatoes
Pantothenic acid (B$_5$)	5 mg		Egg yolk, fish, whole-grain cereals, green leafy vegetables, cabbage, beans, peas, strawberries, nuts
Pyridoxine (B$_6$)	1.3 mg	100 mg	Tuna, turkey, chicken, liver and other organ meats, egg yolk, bananas, cauliflower, carrots, beans, peas, potatoes, almonds
Cobalamin (B$_{12}$)	2.4 mcg		Liver and other organ meats, beef, pork, shrimp, milk and milk products, chicken, eggs
Folic acid (B complex)	400 mcg	1,000 mcg	Fresh green leafy vegetables, carrots, tomatoes, broccoli, liver and other organ meats, peanuts, peas, beans, lentils, pastas, oranges, grapefruit
Biotin (B complex)	30 mcg		Eggs, rice, tomatoes, almonds, chicken, lamb, liver, kidneys, egg yolk, fish, cauliflower, peas, beans, lentils, peanuts

*UL: This is the daily nutrient intake that the Food and Nutrition Board thinks poses no risk of adverse effects.

Vitamin C

Vitamin C (ascorbic acid) is needed to strengthen the immune system. It has several properties. It is an antibacterial (fights infection), antiviral (fights viruses like the flu virus), and also an antioxidant (reduces cell and tissue damage caused by free radicals). The immune system thus needs vitamin C to enhance its infection- and bacterial-fighting mechanisms, which include the efficient removal of ectopic endometrial cells.

Vitamin C is also a natural antihistamine. It is capable of blocking the inflammatory response to allergens like pollen, pet dander, and dust, and it may even reduce the inflammation characteristic in the peritoneal fluid of women with endometriosis. A recent small study showed that vitamins C and E were effective in improving endometriosis-associated pain and reducing inflammation. In this study, fifty-nine women with endometriosis-associated pain and/or infertility received either a combination of vitamins E and C (forty-six) or a placebo (thirteen) for two months. At the end of the two months, inflammatory markers in the supplemented group were significantly lower than in the placebo group. Of the women in the supplemented group, 43 percent reported an improvement in everyday pain while none in the placebo group experienced pain relief. In the supplemented group as well, 24 percent reported an improvement in dyspareunia compared with none from the placebo group. The research findings suggest an important role for vitamins C and E in improving pain associated with endometriosis.

Some good sources of vitamin C include oranges, cherries, grapefruit, strawberries, green leafy vegetables, tomatoes, and potatoes. The Food and Nutrition Board recommends 75 milligrams per day; the safe upper limit is 2,000 milligrams per day. Dr. Lark recommends 1,000 to 5,000 milligrams of vitamin C per day for endometriosis patients.

Vitamin E

Vitamin E is a powerful antioxidant. Like vitamin C, it helps to reduce the cellular wear and tear caused by the actions of free radicals in the body. Vitamin E also plays a role in the immune function because it is needed for antibody production. It is often combined with its sister antioxidant, vitamin C, which increases its effectiveness for endometriosis sufferers, as indicated in the study described above.

Vitamin E by itself may also be effective in relieving primary dysmenorrhea in women with endometriosis. Researchers from Iran have found that the twice daily intake of vitamin E during menstruation may represent a safe and effective treatment for dysmenorrhea. In the study, reported in the April 2005 *British Journal of Obstetrics and Gynaecology,* 278 girls, ages fifteen to seventeen years, were randomly assigned 200 IU of vitamin E or a placebo, to be taken twice daily for five days at the beginning of menstruation for four months. At the end of the four months, those who took the vitamin E supplements experienced significant pain relief during their menses as well as reduced blood loss compared to the placebo group. It is suggested that vitamin E inhibits the release of arachidonic acid and its conversion to inflammatory prostaglandins. This is an essential fatty acid that, when stimulated by the cyclooxygenase (COX) enzyme, is converted to inflammatory prostaglandins.

Good sources of vitamin E include eggs, fish, whole-grain cereals, vegetable oils, margarine, egg yolk, sunflower seeds, green leafy vegetables, tuna, bananas, brown rice, wheat germ, oatmeal, and avocados. The Food and Nutrition Board recommends 15 milligrams per day; the safe upper limit is 1,000 milligrams per day. Dr. Lark recommends 400 to 800 IU of vitamin E per day for endometriosis patients.

Minerals

Like vitamins, minerals are micronutrients that are needed by the body for its various functions. The minerals required by the body in large amounts are magnesium, calcium, phosphorous, sodium, potassium, chloride, and sulphur. Minerals needed in smaller amounts are iron, copper, iodine, selenium, fluorine, zinc, chromium, manganese, and molybdenum. The body cannot produce any minerals on its own but gets them from the various foods we eat such as fruits, vegetables, grains, beans, and low-fat dairy products.

The minerals that have been found very beneficial to endometriosis patients are calcium, magnesium, iron, zinc, and selenium.

Calcium

Calcium is needed to maintain strong healthy bones, teeth, nails, and muscle tissue. About 99 percent of calcium is stored in the bones and teeth while the remaining 1 percent is shared among the blood, fluid between the cells, and the muscles. Most important for endometriosis patients is calcium's benefit to the body's muscles. Calcium maintains normal muscle tone, which reduces cramping. If there is a deficiency in calcium, muscles will tend to be hyperactive and result in muscle spasms/increased spasms, causing pain for women with endometriosis. Studies have shown that calcium intake relieves premenstrual symptoms (PMS).

Calcium is normally combined with magnesium for maximum symptom relief. The RDA is 1,000 milligrams per day and the safe upper limit is 2,500 milligrams per day. Dr. Lark recommends 800 to 1,500 milligrams per day for women with endometriosis. Some good food sources of calcium include skim milk, plain or low-fat yogurt, eggs, raw broccoli, green leafy vegetables, cheese, calcium-fortified orange juice, and kale.

Magnesium

Magnesium, like calcium, contributes to strong teeth and bones, maintains smooth muscle, and supports a healthy immune system and normal blood pressure, among other functions. For endometriosis patients, magnesium optimizes the absorption of calcium into the body. Magnesium is also a natural muscle relaxant, thus relieving uterine cramps in women with endometriosis.

The RDA for magnesium is 320 milligrams per day and the safe upper limit is 350 milligrams per day. Dr. Lark recommends women with endometriosis take half as much magnesium as calcium or approximately 400 to 750 milligrams per day. Some good food sources of magnesium include green leafy vegetables, whole grains, brown rice, peas, beans, lentils, peanuts, peanut butter, plain yogurt, oatmeal, cashews, and almonds.

Iron

Women with endometriosis usually experience longer durations of menstrual flow, which will increase the risk of iron deficiency. Iron is needed in the formation of healthy red blood cells and in the prevention of anemia. Iron is also needed to help transport oxygen to cells throughout the body and is needed by the immune system to produce antibodies to fight infections. Iron intake will reduce the effects of excessive blood loss during menstruation and replace what is lost during heavy menses. Dr. Lark advises that iron should be taken with vitamin C, which helps with absorption.

The RDA for iron is 18 milligrams per day and the safe upper limit is 45 milligrams per day. Dr. Lark recommends women with endometriosis take 25 milligrams along with 30 milligrams of vitamin C per day. Some good sources of iron include kidneys, beans, lentils, oatmeal, soybeans, spinach, whole-wheat bread, tuna, beef, and turkey.

Zinc

Zinc is found in every cell in the body. It is essential for enzyme activity and works with over 200 enzymes in the body. Zinc supports the functions of the immune system such as the activities of antibodies. Zinc is also known for its action on the hypothalamus by stimulating the production of the gonadotropin-releasing hormones (GnRH) that promotes ovulation. Zinc deficiency can affect your fertility and lower your immune response to infections. This can increase your risk of worsening endometriosis.

The RDA for zinc is 8 milligrams per day and the safe upper limit is 40 milligrams per day. Some good food sources for zinc include oysters, shrimp, turnips, parsley, walnuts, sardines, olive oil, fortified cereals, peanuts, carrots, lettuce, and cucumber.

Selenium

Selenium is a trace mineral that is needed for general good health. It acts to promote a healthy immune system, has anti-inflammatory effects, and also has a protective effect on the liver. Selenium enhances the production of anti-inflammatory prostaglandins to enhance the body's functions while reducing the negative effects of inflammatory prostaglandins. This can have a positive impact on endometriosis patients since prostaglandins released from the endometrial lining can cause severe pain/dysmenorrhea.

Selenium is also a powerful antioxidant like vitamin C and E that can enhance your body's immunity. The RDA for selenium is 55 micrograms per day and the safe upper limit is 400 micrograms per day. Good food sources of selenium include tuna, beef, almonds, Brazil nuts, apple cider, vinegar, walnuts, and a variety of other plants, depending on the soil content of the area from which the plants come from.

▮ Natural Progesterone Cream

Endometriosis is an estrogen-dependent disease. As such, the aim of hormonal and complementary medicine is to remove excessive amounts of the female sex hormone. At the same time, these treatment regimes aim to create a balance between estrogen and progesterone, the other female sex hormone. Why? This has to do with the effects of these hormones. For instance, while progesterone can help use fat as a source of energy, restore a woman's libido, and act as a natural antidepressant, estrogen increases body fat, decreases a woman's sex drive, and causes headaches and depression.

It would then seem beneficial for the endometriosis patient to try to increase her progesterone levels to reduce the negative effects of excessive estrogen. In response to this reality of the endometriosis patient, Dr. John Lee, author of *What Your Doctor May Not Tell You About Premenopause,* treated a number of his patients with natural progesterone cream to block monthly estrogen stimulus to the implants. Natural progesterone cream, like progestins, induces a pseudopregnant state, resulting in increased progesterone levels, that signals to the ovaries to stop producing estrogen. The U.S. Food and Drug Administration (FDA) later approved the use of natural progesterone to relieve endometriosis-associated symptoms.

Natural progesterone cream is bioidentical to the body's own progesterone hormone, thus has fewer side effects than the chemically derived progestins. Natural progesterone is a topical analgesic. The effect is not immediate. Patients who use natural progesterone creams may have to wait four to six months before the full effect of the cream is felt. However, the monthly pains gradually subside.

10

Diet, Body, Mind, and Lifestyle

Lifestyle changes are essential to living well with endometriosis, an important lesson I learned while adjusting to my new life with this disease. The following are some suggestions from Ellen T. Johnson on how to incorporate certain lifestyle changes to live well with endometriosis in her article "Be Good to Yourself."

▌Diet

Apart from adding supplements to your treatment program, experts like clinical nutritionist Dian Shepperson Mills are advocating women with endometriosis to pay closer attention to their diets and overall nutrition to aid symptom relief. What dietary modifications should you take into consideration to enhance your body's immune system and relieve symptoms and overall health?

Remove Wheat

Wheat has been found to have a negative effect on many women with endometriosis. It is supposed that wheat may contain hormones that have estrogenic effects when introduced into the body. Many endometriosis patients have developed an intolerance to wheat and wheat-based products. Ms. Shepperson Mills has found that in her own practice, when wheat is taken out of women's diets, pain subsides in 80 percent of patients. Additionally, when wheat is reintroduced into their diets, the pain returns.

Examples of wheat-based products include pastas, breads, cakes, pizza, muffins, and pastries, to name a few. You can purchase wheat-free products such as cakes, breads, and muffins at your neighborhood health food store.

Reduce Red Meat and Ham Intake

A recent study conducted by Dr. Fabio Parazzini and colleagues from the University of Milan has found that eating red meat and ham may increase your risk of developing endometriosis. The scientists surveyed 504 women admitted for laparoscopically confirmed endometriosis and 504 women admitted for acute nongynecological, nonhormonal conditions. The participants were asked about their diet in the year prior to the interview. The study found that the women who had a high consumption of red meat and ham were associated with an 80 to 100 percent increase in the incidence of endometriosis.

This may occur as a result of several reasons. Red meat and ham, unless they were organically produced, will be full of hormones and unwanted chemicals that can adversely affect the hormonal balance, increasing the body's estrogen level and stimulating the development of the disease. Animal fats also absorb the environmental pollutant TCCD or dioxin that has been found to increase the risk of developing endometriosis and increasing the severity of the disease.

Additionally, meats contain saturated fats that, when introduced into the body, put stress on the liver to remove the excess fats. The stressed liver may lose some of its ability to remove excess estrogen from the body, thus increasing the severity of the disease. Saturated fats from animal protein also enhance the production of inflammatory prostaglandins, which contribute to worsening endometriosis-associated pain.

Eat Fresh Fruits and Vegetables

The same study conducted by Dr. Parazzini also found that consumption of lots of fruits and vegetables may lower a woman's chances of developing the disease. But the study found that a high consumption of fresh fruits and green vegetables from commercial suppliers resulted in increased risk for endometriosis developing as these would be sprayed with pesticides, exposing them to dioxins. Try to eat organic fruits and vegetables, which are now available at most local grocers.

Reduce Coffee and Alcohol Intake

A 2001 study found that drinking more than two cups of coffee daily will increase estrogen levels in your body and stimulate the continued development of the disease. The study found that women who consumed more than one cup of coffee daily had significantly higher levels of estrogen levels, or 70 percent more estrogen during the follicular phase of their menstrual cycle than women who drank no more than 100 milligrams daily.

Additionally, coffee reduces the body's store of B complex vitamins and also negatively affects the liver's functions. Alcohol also negatively affects the function of the liver, which will adversely affect the process of getting rid of excess estrogen. The liver also overstresses when eliminating alcohol from the body, which again adversely affects its ability to eliminate excess estrogen from the body. Caffeine—in the form of coffee and black tea—and alcoholic beverages should be avoided entirely.

Cut Out Dairy Products

Dairy products, like animal proteins, contain saturated fats that put stress on the liver, which can lead to excess estrogen in the body. And, like animal proteins, dairy products can increase your risk of producing more inflammatory prostaglandins, which will worsen endometriosis-associated pain.

Eat More Fish or Supplement with Omega-3

Omega-3 is a form of polyunsaturated fatty acid that comes from the fat in fish. The two forms of omega-3 are eicosapentaenoate (EPA) and docosahexaenoic acid (DHA), which can be found in cold-water fish such as salmon, tuna, and trout. Another type of omega-3 is alpha-linolenic acid (ALA), which comes from evening primrose oil and flaxseed oil.

Omega-3 plays several key roles in the body, including reducing the risk of heart disease and acting as a general anti-inflammatory agent—good news for endometriosis patients. You can purchase omega-3 supplements at the pharmacy or local health food store. Or you can include more fish in your diet and get the omega-3 fatty acids straight from the source.

Two animal studies have found omega-3 fatty acids effective in reducing dysmenorrhea, due to their anti-inflammatory properties, in women with endometriosis. Omega-3 fatty acids are needed by the body to produce the anti-inflammatory prostaglandins for their various functions. By increasing your intake of omega-3 you will reduce the production of inflammatory prostaglandins and reduce pain symptoms.

Carefully watching your diet and removing the foods that can enhance your symptoms are instrumental to dealing with endometriosis. Errikka found that out when she systematically evaluated her own diet:

I began looking for alternative ways to manage my pain. I found that changing my diet helped me tremendously. I kept a journal of my meals, snacks, and pain, and tried to identify any patterns. I eliminated several foods that seemed to either trigger the pain or increase it. I was able to determine which foods were aggravating the endo. I ended up with a very strict diet. I eliminated caffeine, acidic foods, gassy foods, oily and greasy foods, and decreased my dairy intake. Since I love to eat, this was a very difficult challenge for me, but the results were dramatic, so I stuck with the diet, and to this day I think it is the best thing I've done to minimize the pain.

Others, however, while possessing good intentions, find it hard to stick to such a routine. Take Melissa, for instance:

It . . . seemed like a good idea to the painless me to try eating very healthy (no salt, no caffeine, no dairy, no alcohol, no red meat—these aggravate pain symptoms, say some). However, when in pain I feel rather self-destructive and sometimes develop cravings for salt, coffee, chocolate, greasy food, cigarettes, and wine. I don't even smoke. Salt and coffee are the strongest cravings, and they actually do make me feel better after having them. Is it all in my head? Does that matter when you're in this much goddamn pain? Pass the Hershey's!

▌The Mind-Body Approach

Within the parameters of complementary and alternative medicine (CAM) is a category called mind-body medicine. This CAM focuses on using the mind to affect the body's functions. In essence, mind-body medicine focuses on intervention strategies, such as meditation, yoga, biofeedback, tai chi, and others, to promote overall health.

Endometriosis patients have tried some of these techniques and, while not showing any impact on the disease itself, they have helped in their overall outlook on their health and life with endometriosis.

The following are reviews of some of the common forms of mind-body strategies that are available to you and that some women with endometriosis have tried.

Biofeedback

Biofeedback involves the use of a special monitoring machine to teach individuals how to control certain bodily functions to improve their overall health and well-being. In essence, you are taught to will certain physical ailments to disappear. During a biofeedback session, a therapist will apply electrical sensors to different parts of your body. These sensors relay your reactions to stress, such as the muscular contractions caused by tension in your shoulders or neck, in a beeping sound or flashing light. You will begin to associate your body's response to certain physical functions; in this case, pain as a result of muscular tension.

Once you recognize that the pain in your neck or shoulder is a result of tense muscles, your next step would be to learn techniques to relax the specific muscles to achieve pain relief.

While no studies have been conducted on the effect of biofeedback on endometriosis or its associated symptoms, this technique may help relieve the migraine headaches to which we are often prone. Biofeedback has been found helpful in treating about 150 medical conditions, including headaches, incontinence, irritable bowel syndrome (IBS), hot flashes, high blood pressure, irregular heartbeats, asthma, Reynaud's disease, and nausea and vomiting associated with chemotherapy.

Consult with a qualified biofeedback therapist to ensure proper treatment. The Biofeedback Certification Institute of America

(BCIA) certifies biofeedback therapists. Therapists must also be licensed in another area of health care; thus, they are usually physicians or clinical psychologists who have taken special training in this technique. Check with the BCIA for a listing of biofeedback practitioners in your area, or ask your doctor for recommendations.

Guided Imagery (Healing Visualizations)

Guided imagery involves using the mind to visualize your body in the process of healing. People use their imaginations all the time—they dream about winning the lottery or starting their own business. Guided imagery goes one step further. A trained therapist can teach you to use your mental powers to invoke healthy changes in your body.

The process is simple. A trained practitioner (oftentimes a psychiatrist or psychologist) may use an interactive or objective approach to encourage patients to visualize their picture of optimal health. For instance, Dr. Carl Simonton developed a technique in the 1970s—later called the Simonton method—that utilized guided imagery to treat cancer patients. The patients visualized their cancer cells being attacked by white blood cells, much like in a Pac-Man game. The more graphic the scenes the patients created, the more effective the process. Some patients visualized their cancer cells as tiny fish being attacked by sharks.

Many endometriosis patients have created their own images of the disease and its main symptom: pain. The figure on the following page is Deborah Ann's mental image of herself with the disease.

Using this image, the next step for Deborah Ann, according to Dr. Simonton in his book *Getting Well Again*, would be to visualize any treatment she is receiving eliminating the source of the disease, or strengthening her body against its symptoms. Deborah Ann should also visualize her own body defending itself against the disease and imagine herself free from the pain of the disease.

You can also create your own image of the disease and visualize

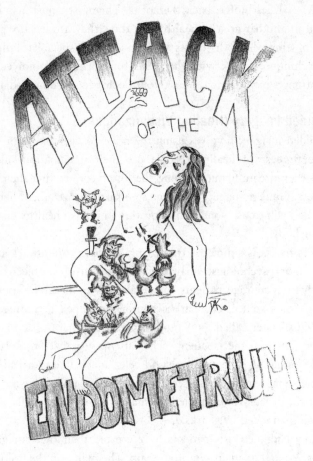

your treatments and/or your body eliminating its presence in your body. There are tapes that you can purchase to guide you in the process, or you can consult with a trained practitioner. There are no certification boards for practitioners of guided imagery.

Meditation

Meditation is a very common mind-body technique that has been practiced for thousands of years. The process involves strengthening the communication between your mind and body during quiet alone periods to reduce stress and even pain. There are three main types of meditation techniques practiced in the United States:

- Transcendental meditation (TM) involves repeating a word or sound (called a mantra) to focus thinking and help achieve calm.
- Breath meditation involves focusing on the breathing process—inhaling and exhaling—to clear the mind.
- Mindfulness meditation involves focusing on the present moment, for example, keeping your awareness on a specific physical sensation.

The aim of meditation is to induce a relaxed state to better deal with the emotional aspects of illnesses, to better cope with stress, and to induce a sense of well-being. A 2002 study involving magnetic resonance imaging (MRI) has shown that meditation significantly increases left-sided brain activity. This activity is associated with positive emotional states. There also seems to be a beneficial effect on the immune system. The same study found that meditation resulted in increased antibody production against the flu.

Tai Chi

Tai chi is sometimes described as "mediation in motion." This is a gentle form of exercise that aims to improve mental and physical health while promoting balance, flexibility, strength, and posture. Tai chi involves a series of slow, deliberate, but graceful movements while standing. The technique has been found to have both physical and mental benefits, including:

- Reduced stress
- Sharpened reflexes
- Increased flexibility
- Improved balance and coordination
- Increased energy and stamina
- Increased bone mineral density after menopause
- Reduced anxiety and depression
- Reduced blood pressure

While tai chi may not relieve your worst physical symptoms of endometriosis, it may help with the mental and psychological stress of endometriosis you experience on a daily basis. Jennifer found just that:

> By the time it came back, I had learned tai chi and was prepared to meditate my way through the pain. Stress seemed to trigger a lot of the pain, so I tried to keep stress at bay as much as possible.

Yoga

Yoga, like tai chi, aims to improve mental as well as physical health through exercises that improve flexibility, muscle tone, and balance. Many endometriosis patients are not able to do intense physical workouts due to their debilitating pain levels. Yoga and tai chi may offer gentler alternatives to relieve some of the physical and emotional stresses of the disease. Exercise releases endorphins, naturally occurring chemicals in the brain that have pain-relieving properties similar to opiates—ideal for endometriosis patients.

Research from the Fred Hutchinson Cancer Research Center in Seattle found that high-intensity workouts such as jogging, bicycling, and/or doing aerobics could reduce your risk of endometriosis by two thirds. However, it has been shown that endometriosis-associated pain may hinder exercise programs, even if the patient was active before being diagnosed. The experts therefore suggest light to moderate exercises such as walking, yoga, and tai chi.

Laughter

Researchers are discovering that laughter does have some physical as well as psychological effects on patients. People generally feel good after a really good laugh. This can momentarily reduce the sensation of pain. Dr. Donald Black, professor of psychiatry at the University of Iowa College of Medicine, suggests that laughter triggers the release of hormones from the endocrine system, which sends painkilling chemicals throughout the body. This is similar to the effect of exercise. Dr. Black describes laughter as "internal jogging" that keeps the body and mind fit.

Therapists have used laughter to treat depression and with some effect to heal stroke patients.

In Jamaica, we have a saying: "Tek bad tings mek joke." This basically means to find humor even in the worst of situations. Doing so puts the event into perspective, allowing you to find a solution or to think more clearly about a solution. In the meantime, you also get a good laugh, which helps you to feel good temporarily. Coming from a family of belly laughers myself, this wasn't hard for me to do.

Relaxation

Endometriosis by itself can cause great physical and emotional stress. Added to this are the everyday stresses of work, school, home life, finances, and personal relationships. Dr. Susan M. Lark, author of *Fibroid Tumors & Endometriosis Self Help Book*, has found that stress is a common and significant problem associated with many recurrent and chronic health problems like endometriosis. Research has shown that stress can impair immune function and hormone balance. For women with endometriosis this means upsetting the estrogen and progesterone balance, which can lead to disease and symptom severity.

Endometriosis patients have their own relaxation techniques. For

Cassandra, a show horse trainer who had to give up her career because of endometriosis, it was her horse:

> I got my horse from a friend. A very cute pony, small and Western, when I had mainly ridden English jumping fences, but quiet and safe. That helped my quality of life tremendously. I wasn't able to take lessons or compete but would trail ride as often as I could, and no matter how bad I felt even just going and brushing her helped me more that I can describe. The best antidepressant I have ever been on, in fact.

Other relaxation techniques include relaxed breathing. High stress levels are usually accompanied by rapid, shallow breathing. By controlling and relaxing your breathing, you will be able to reduce the body's responses to stress, such as rapid heart rate and perspiration. The steps are as follows:

1. Close your mouth and inhale slowly through your nostrils. Inhale as deeply as you can to the count of six. Keep your shoulders relaxed.
2. Hold the air in your lungs to the count of four. Count slowly.
3. Slowly release the air through your mouth to the count of six.
4. Repeat the process three to five more times.

▌ Massage Therapy

Massage therapy is a form of complementary and alternative medicine (CAM) within the category of manipulative and body-based practices. These techniques focus on the bones, joints, soft tissues, and circulatory and lymphatic systems to relieve symptoms. These complement your treatment regimes for overall well-being.

Massage therapy involves the manipulation of the soft tissues of the body—muscles, tendons, and skin—using the fingertips, hands, and fists. Massage has several benefits for the endometriosis patient:

- Massage relieves tense muscles, which compress blood vessels and stretch nerves, constricting blood flow and causing pain. As the muscle is massaged, the blood vessels and nerves become loosened, resulting in pain relief.
- Massage also has been shown to increase the body's production of endorphins, resulting in temporary pain relief.

Julie experienced temporary pain relief from both massage and acupressure:

In attempts to feel better, I've tried acupressure and massage, which were absolutely wonderful for temporarily relieving pain. However, this became too expensive as I am staying home to care for our two children. So this became a luxury that we can only afford to do a few times a year.

The National Certification Board for Therapeutic Massage and Bodywork (NCBTMB) certifies massage therapists in the United States. Check with this board about massage therapists in your area, or check on the status of any therapist you are interested in consulting. Also, make sure that she/he is a member of the American Massage Therapy Association (AMTA).

▌ Acupuncture

Acupuncture is a form of traditional Chinese medicine that involves the insertion of stainless-steel needles at different depths at strategic locations on your body. Within complementary and alternative medicine (CAM) this form of treatment is classified as energy medicine.

Within traditional Chinese medicine, illness is seen as caused by imbalances within the energy flow of life called qi or chi. Qi flows through twenty major pathways or meridians in the body, which can be accessed in the body through 400 different acupuncture points. Acupuncture needles are inserted into these acupuncture points in different combinations to rebalance your energy flow and help with the healing process.

Studies have found that acupuncture may help treat a variety of health conditions. The National Institutes of Health (NIH) suggest three explanations for this:

- Acupuncture may stimulate the central nervous system (CNS) to trigger the body's own natural healing properties.
- Acupuncture may release endorphins that relieve pain.
- As changes occur in the CNS, other bodily changes may occur, such as alterations in the regulation of blood pressure, blood flow, and body temperature.

Jude found acupuncture beneficial to her:

At a time when I was in terrible pain I found acupuncture a great relief, and I would have two days a week pain-free after a treatment.

Melissa also found acupuncture helpful:

Though my experience with acupuncture was a good one and I would recommend it to others, I did not find reduced symptoms. I went to acupuncture every week for three months, but none of those appointments happened to coincide with my times of greatest pain. It did not hurt and was actually much less scary than a regular doctor's appointment. The best thing about going to acupuncture was that I felt extremely listened to and respected by the doctors. They gave me the feeling that I was in control, and they were professional yet compassionate. Though my pain was not reduced, it was healing in a different way for me to have a positive connection with a medical professional.

In one study, women diagnosed with dysmenorrhea due to endometriosis were treated with ear acupuncture. (Ear acupuncture involves stimulating along the external ear about 130 acupuncture points that correspond to certain organs in the body.) A total of sixty-seven women were selected, half treated with ear acupuncture and the other half used as a control. The researchers reported that 81 percent of the former group had less painful menses after the acupuncture treatments. The findings were published in the December 2002 issue of the *Journal of Traditional Chinese Medicine*.

If you are considering trying acupuncture, make sure that you consult with a certified acupuncturist. The National Certification Commission for Acupuncture and Oriental Medicine (NCCAOM) certifies all acupuncturists in the United States.

▌ Exercise

I took a water aerobics class. I took it because a neighbor, who had seen me do a little water aerobics routine at our neighborhood pool while I was pregnant the first time, asked me if I would lead a water aerobics class for a small group of women in our neighborhood. At first, I thought this was crazy. How could I lead an aerobics class when I am one of the unhealthiest women on the planet? But she kept asking me to do it, so I finally said okay. I signed up for a water aerobics class at the community pool. I took the class in the morning, and showed our neighbors what I had learned in the evenings.

Within two weeks I noticed a huge difference in how I felt. My joint pain was greatly relieved each time I got in the water, which made sense to me. But never in my wildest imagination did I think that this would help with my endometriosis symptoms. This little bit of exercise (which wasn't hard to do) was very much helping to relieve my pelvic pain. So much so that when the summer was drawing to a close, I started to become really sad, thinking of having to give this up. In fact, I continued to do water aerobics through the beginning of October! When I could no longer be in the pool, I started walking and lifting weights at our community center. At first this was a little harder on my body than being in the water, but I eventually adjusted to it. I am now even able to jog instead of walk.

This is the very best that I have felt in years. My periods are now down to five days instead of ten most of the time. They are still very painful (I have to take Darvocet the first few days of my period), and I've had a few ovarian cysts that have caused pain, but in general my pain seems more manageable than before I started exercising. Being active has been so good for my mind and spirit that I think it is affecting how I feel about and treat my body. Each time I go jogging, I picture the webby mess in my stomach breaking apart. It may sound silly, but this is helping me deal with this disease. Exercising has improved my self-image. I no longer feel like I am just lying around powerless, unable to help myself.

You can almost feel Julie's excitement in her words above. Her experience mirrors that of many endometriosis patients who have begun various exercise routines to try to relieve their symptoms. While many are not able to do intense aerobic exercises, or have had to give up their former intense exercise routines—in my case I had to give up my much-loved martial arts training for a while—light exercises can be just as effective.

Instead of karate, I joined a gym and went two or three days out of each week. My routine consisted of light weight training and aerobic exercises. If the routine became too strenuous, I would concentrate on the treadmill and light aerobics.

I found this routine very helpful in terms of my pain levels. While surgery and my three-month injections of Depo-Provera significantly reduced my pain symptoms each month, the addition of an exercise program made me feel very good and further reduced my already reduced symptoms. I felt so much better, in fact, that I slowly resumed karate training in early 2005.

Why does exercise have this effect on a woman in pain? Exercise helps the body release its natural pain-relieving chemicals, called endorphins, which work by blocking pain signals to your brain. These chemicals are also known to relieve depression and anxiety, an effect that Julie can attest. Exercise can also improve your sleeping habits and give you more energy to deal with your endometriosis-associated pain.

But, as with any other condition with chronic pain, start slowly. Lay out a moderate exercise routine and stick to it, such as walking around the neighborhood park or participating in water aerobics, like Julie. Add variety to the routine as well, so you don't get bored too quickly. You may add yoga or tai chi along with your daily strolls through the park. Alternate these activities. Join a health club if you need more variety.

▊ Stress Management

Women with endometriosis are no strangers to stress. The debilitating nature of the disease brings with it stress as an inevitable side effect. Coupled with everyday stressors from work, family life, and school, you will feel constantly bogged down and at increased risk of worsening health. Take Linda, for example. The stress of endometriosis, the inability to have a child, and demanding work schedules coupled with an abusive marriage took a major toll on her health:

> *I had a complete and total nervous breakdown. The working so much, the abusive marriage, the inability to have a child, the new house, the being sick all the time, everything had become too much. I could not sleep, eat, or function in any way. My family doctor prescribed Prozac and some time off work. After three months I became worse instead of better. I was living in a nightmare marriage and too sick to find the strength to leave. I thought if only we could have a child then things would be better, but this child would never come. In hindsight I know this would not have fixed my marriage. I began seeing a psychiatrist and entered a program as an outpatient at the hospital, which I attended every day. I was diagnosed with severe depression, severe anxiety disorder, agoraphobia, post-traumatic stress disorder, and battered women's syndrome. Years of problems had finally caught up with me.*

Stress can have several physical manifestations. These include:

▊ Depression
▊ Anxiety
▊ Trouble sleeping

- Lack of energy
- Trouble concentrating
- Headaches
- Diarrhea
- High blood pressure
- Tension
- Stomach cramps
- Reduced libido
- Weight gain or loss
- Skin problems/acne/rashes
- Anger
- Constipation

In women with endometriosis these symptoms may be elevated due to the direct effects of the disease or side effects of the medications we are taking to control the disease. It is essential, therefore, to deal with those stressors we can in order to optimize our treatment of the disease. The techniques reviewed in this chapter can help you manage stress and relax.

▌ Writing About It

Many women with endometriosis have found that writing about the disease's myriad effects on their lives can positively impact how they deal with the disease. Studies have shown that writing about traumatic events in our lives has therapeutic value. It can help you to come to terms with your illness, ultimately reducing the impact on your physical health.

Dr. Joshua Smyth and colleagues from the State University of New York at Stony Brook School of Medicine conducted a study on the effect of writing about traumatic life events on asthma and rheumatoid arthritis patients. The patients (fifty-eight asthma patients and forty-nine rheumatoid arthritis patients) were assessed at two weeks, two months, and four months after the writing exercise. The researchers found that asthma patients showed improved lung function from 63.9 percent at the start of the study to 76.3 percent at the four-month assessment. Rheumatoid arthritis patients showed overall improvement in disease severity. Control groups for both conditions showed no change.

Dr. Smyth asserts that writing about traumatic events gives you a sense of control over the event. The exercise of writing allows you to break down the event into small pieces, making it more manageable and giving you a sense of understanding about the situation. This relieves stress and leads to personal growth, as Andrea describes:

> *I started creating a Web site for others to read. My story, my life with endometriosis in hope that it would reach just someone and let them know that they were not alone, that they could overcome this disease too. My site, www.emptyarms .co.uk, became so popular I spent months replying to others who had contacted me, supporting them and giving them the strength to get themselves clued up on the disease so they could demand their own treatment.*

This form of therapy, called writing therapy, comes in various forms. One popular form is journal therapy, in which the patient expresses the emotional impact of problems in a journal. Two other forms are letter therapy and poetry therapy. Letter therapy involves writing very personal letters to people, whether they are alive or dead. The aim is to allow the writer to express her innermost thoughts and feelings about any problems/issue without the stress of a face-to-face contact. These letters are usually never sent, although there are exceptions. Take Antonia, for instance. She found it easier to express herself to her fiancé in a letter. This is what Antonia wrote:

Hi Sweetheart,

As you may have gathered from my earlier e-mail, I am unable to sleep and so I thought I would write to you.

It is nearly 3:00 a.m. and I am wide awake and in pain. I have taken my painkillers and now have a glass of whiskey by my bedside that I am slowly sipping. I am hoping that once this is written the whiskey will be finished and so I will then be able to get some sleep.

I don't really know what it is that I want to write to you about. But I know that I am better at expressing myself in words on paper than in words by mouth.

The other night when you said that you were frustrated, you gave me such a fright. I really thought that you were going to tell me that you had had enough, and that you wanted to end it all. It was the most terrifying feeling that I have had in a long time.

You said that you wanted to know how I feel and what I am thinking. To tell you the truth, I don't honestly know at the moment. I feel as though I am in limbo and that I have no direction in life. I know that one day all of this will seem like a long bad dream, but at the moment I feel that it has well and truly taken over my life. I don't feel that I have a say in my life anymore. I have to live by the rules that are determined by my body, my hormones, and my pain. I can no longer live by my rules, doing what I want to do, when I want to do it.

I don't feel as though I am in charge anymore. I feel as though everyone else has a say in what I do except for me. I know it sounds silly—and to a certain extent I am still in charge. I can still keep an eye on what I am given drug-wise, and if I have to I can persuade the doctors to listen to me. But this isn't the life that I had planned out for me. This is not where I want to be, and I wouldn't wish this kind of life on anyone else. My mother tells me that I should count my *blessings and that I am extremely lucky in many ways. I have a house that is paid for, I have you, and to a certain extent I have my health. I have all my faculties, and I am not dying.*

Great. What about a life? When I look around at you, and all our friends, I see people getting on with their lives. I see people living their lives to the full—doing what they want to do, and achieving things that I should be doing and achieving.

By now I should be in a job where I am happy and fulfilled, going out and enjoying myself, and generally having a laugh. But all of that has had to be put on the back burner while I concentrate on my health.

I am so jealous of all of you. It eats away at me sometimes when I see you all going out and enjoying yourselves. Sometimes when I am in the hospital, and I hear that you have all been out and had a brilliant time, I cry myself to sleep. Other times I get determined that I will be there with you, when I know that it will make me worse—and it always does.

If someone had told me four years ago that I would be living this life, I would have laughed in their face and told them not to be so silly.

When I was diagnosed with endo, no one told me that it would be like this. No one prepared me for this oblivion. Not even when I called the help line was I warned that it could go on and on and on.

Every time the pain went away, it was like a small miracle, and my hopes were raised. Every time my pain went away, the hopes of my family were raised too—and I was "better." Then of course it all started to come back and I was suddenly ill again, but according to everyone else it was all in my head.

It has been so hard to try and get people to understand this disease, and then you come along and take it all on board. You have been amazing. You have accepted me from day one as me. You have stood by me, where other people would have run away. I know that you have found it hard, and I know that you are still finding it hard, but you have a strength in you that no one else has had.

I know that my friends have stood by me—but they have watched me over the years, and gone up and down with me. You—on the other hand—just walked in and took it all in.

When we first met and I told you that I could get ill, you accepted it, but I don't think that you knew how hard it was going to be. I wish that I could have prepared you better, but then I don't think I knew either.

This thing has a habit of creeping up on me slowly, and starts to pull down my defenses and barriers that I have built up during the short time that I have a break from it. It is a bit like a fog that crawls and creeps its way in from the sea, slowly covering every nook and cranny, covering everything that gets in its way. There is no way of stopping it—once it decides that it is going to happen.

The only thing to do is to try to control it as best as I can—and even then that is hard work. The drugs that I have been on have made me worse, the painkillers slow me down, and basically I am a mess at the moment. I don't know how you put up with me, I really don't.

So far the Mirena seems to have made me worse rather than better, but at least there are no horrific side effects, like I had with the Zoladex.

I am bitter about this whole thing, and wish that it had never happened. I am scared that it will last forever and that it will never go away.

I often think, "Why me?" and that I want my life back—I know that it isn't going to kill me, but at the same time, I know that I don't have the energy or the get-up-and-go that I used to have because of it.

I am scared of the future. I am scared that I won't be able to have children, or that if I do I will be in so much pain that I won't be able to care for them.

I am scared that you will get fed up with it all and leave me. I don't think that I will find someone as good and as kind as you. You are a good man. I am so very, very lucky to have met you.

So basically, I have not come to terms with this disease, and I don't know if I ever will. I am fed up with living like this, and of letting everyone down all of the time—especially you.

I know that there is hope on the horizon—the Mirena might work and I will be pain free—but it seems so far away and so much like a dream that I just can't get my hopes up—if I do I know they will be dashed to the ground again. Instead I will just live my life day to day—and take each day as it comes.

I am sorry if this is so depressing, but you wanted to know what is really going on inside my head. I have laid myself bare to you. You now know what I feel—most of the time.

I hope that you will understand me better now—either that, or you won't want to know me anymore.

I love you, and will go on loving you as long as you want me and need me.

—Antonia

For some, another aspect of letter therapy involves writing to the disease itself. Some find this act of discourse quite empowering—looking your enemy squarely in the eyes and properly telling it off—releasing the pent-up anger and refocusing your attention on your main goal: ridding your body of its presence.

Danielle did just that. She wrote a letter to endometriosis during a particularly rough period with the disease. Note her anger but also note the resolve in her words:

Okay you beast! Are you ready for me? The time has come for us to do yet another battle over my life. You have raised the banners of war over my body once again, and I am here to face your challenge. But first you will have to listen to me before I come another step. I hate you! I hate the way you make me feel like I am less of a woman. I hate what you have done to my health. I am a twenty-three-year-old young woman with so many hopes and dreams in my life: dreams of children, grandchildren, dreams of being able to hold down a job, dreams of the day when you are no longer hiding like a coward deep within me. That's right, I called you a coward! You beckon me into a war that leaves me scarred, hurt, and ready to destroy you only to hide behind my womanhood when we come to attack. Well, I'm sick of playing your games if you are going to be a coward every time I allow a doctor to cut me open to find you. Be the beast you claim to be when I'm not lying on the operating table. Show yourself to me and allow me the chance to kill you once and for all!

For almost five years the game you play has controlled my life. I have spent countless days in bed unable to walk, unable to do anything but wither in pain and cry myself to sleep. You know you have stolen the luxury of sleep as well. You have made the pain severe enough to keep me awake for twenty-six hours now and I'm tired of this battle. You know I am coming for you again, don't you? Is this your punishment for the extra herbs and vitamins I've thrown at you lately? Do you always have to fight dirty? Can't you battle like a true warrior, face-to-face with your enemy?

What will be your next punishment? Will I wake up from surgery to find you have stolen my left ovary? You sure seem to like that one. Or will you steal my dreams of being a mother, of feeling my baby grow and kick inside me, the one thing that sustains me? Well, here's your warning, coward! If you take another thing from me, you will pay dearly. I will take no mercy in ridding my body of your diseased being. After all, you have caused so much torment, anger, frustration, and sadness in my life. How much more do you think I will take from you? Yeah, you've had me almost ready to give up and wave the hysterectomy flag a few times, but I am stronger than you. . . . You wait and see, I will win this war over you; you will be defeated.

Writing has always been a great joy and escape for me. I easily turned to the blank pages in the form of poems and unsent letters to loved ones to express my feelings. In fact, I find that I express myself much better in the written word and have used this outlet to pour out my soul about this or any new path in my life. Here is one such poem written during my postdiagnosis/postsurgery period. I marvel at how trapped I felt about this disease:

I know I am strong.
Yet weakness is my friend.
We play together, laugh together.
Strength a façade.

I challenge life's characters and play them one by one.
Laugh in the face of battle.
Smirk at a challenge others might not have done.

Yet at nights the shadows haunt me and beads of sweat soak
*   my ice-cold skin.*
I hate the dark, which hides the secrets.
And cringe with fear as each is revealed.

Oh please let the light shine again!
Take away all the hurt and pain!

Cast away the demons, which battle over my soul
And perish the devils from my whole!

The light is here again and I know I am strong.
The night a forgotten nightmare
The day a long-lost friend.

▌ Prayer/Spirituality

Published evidence has shown that prayer and other forms of religious and spiritual expressions can positively impact your health. The American Academy of Family Physicians defines spirituality as the way you find meaning, hope, comfort, and inner peace in your life. Many find it through religion. Others find it through art, music, or by observing nature.

A national survey on Americans' use of complementary and alternative medicine (CAM) conducted by the National Center for Complementary and Alternative Medicine (NCCAM), released in May 2004, found that when prayer was included in the definition of CAM, 62 percent of respondents declared they had used CAM. The survey also found that:

- 45 percent prayed for health reasons.
- 43 percent prayed for their own health.
- 25 percent had others pray for them.
- 10 percent participated in a prayer group for their health.

Research on spirituality and health has found religious activities such as attending church services, meditation, or prayer result in positive beliefs and better methods of coping with your illness. In fact, studies have shown that spiritual people live on average seven years longer than nonreligious persons.

Jeffrey Levin, a social epidemiologist and author of *God, Faith, and Health: Exploring the Spirituality-Healing Connection*, asserts the following about the benefits of spirituality on health:

▮ Spirituality encourages a healthier lifestyle.
▮ It contributes to a more positive and contented outlook on life that can positively impact health.
▮ Going to church offers times for social interaction and builds supportive relationships.

Danielle knows the positive impact of a spiritual/religious outlook on life. She depends on her spiritual relationship with God to help her get through the toughest periods with endometriosis:

Through hormone therapy and God's grace I lived nearly twelve years pain-free. I felt I'd finally escaped my prison and lived fully. I went back to school, rekindled old friendships, and relearned who I was inside. I built a new foundation for a walk with Christ and focused on a new life with Him. Like everybody else, I have my good days where I'm determined I will not let this disease win my body or my mind, and I have days where I wonder, "Why me, Lord?" It angers me that the medical world will spend millions of dollars on developing Viagra to cure men's impotence, yet so many of us suffer daily in silence. And there are times I wonder who would ever want to marry me, broken as I feel; what man will ever commit to spending forever with me, if I can't promise him children of his own flesh. These days I feel defective and incomplete.

But God doesn't make mistakes, and I try to keep my focus on the reason I feel He gave me this disease: education of others. I try educating those around me about what it means to be an endo sister. . . .

■ ■ ■ Be Good to Yourself ■ ■ ■

By Ellen T. Johnson

(Reprinted with permission from Ellen T. Johnson and
http://www.endometriosis.org)

Women with endometriosis are inundated with so-called
"good advice." We've heard it all—from "just relax" to "just
have a baby and the pain will go away." We're smart enough to
know that most of this well-meaning advice doesn't really
work. We're left wondering if anything can actually help us.

One thing we know for sure is that endometriosis is a very
individualized disease. No woman experiences it exactly the
same way as another. So what works for one person might not
work for another. We also know that this disease can take a toll
on us physically, mentally, and emotionally. It can cause us un-
told stress and the stress often makes our symptoms worse.

So how do we take care of ourselves as individuals while
dealing with this disease? Let's look at a few things that might
actually help.

Some Foods Might Cause More Pain

Try eliminating caffeine, alcohol, sugar, red meat, fried foods,
and wheat from your diet just before and during menstruation.
Add foods high in omega-3 fatty acids (such as salmon,
flaxseeds, and herring). You might have less pain.

Relaxation Isn't Just Good in Theory

Try to carve out a few minutes each day to relax. This can be as
simple as putting on headphones and listening to relaxing music. Breathing exercises also help calm the body.

Sleep, Sleep, Sleep

Studies suggest that sleep deprivation results in hormonal and metabolic changes, inflammation, and increased levels of pain. If you're having trouble sleeping, try homeopathic sleep remedies, a cup of chamomile tea, or a spritz of diluted lavender oil on your pillow. Getting outside during the day can also result in better sleep. If sleep deprivation becomes a problem, see your physician.

Replace Negative Thoughts with Positive Ones

According to Harvard researchers, optimism results in better overall health. Make an effort to turn negative thoughts into positive ones. It will make you feel better if you find ways to be hopeful while facing the day-to-day challenges of endometriosis. Suggested reading: *Learned Optimism: How to Change Your Mind & Your Life,* by Martin E. Seligman.

Move When You Can

Researchers have also found that physical activities can ease tension and release endorphins (your body's natural painkiller). Take advantage of the times when you're able to be physically active. When you don't feel up to brisk activity, try something simpler, such as taking a walk around the block. It might be slow going at first, but you will probably feel better afterward.

Simplify Your Life

Most women are strained with too many commitments and too little time, which takes a toll on us after a while. If you're overburdened, you might consider simplifying your life by asking what tasks or responsibilities can be eliminated or delegated to others. Suggested reading: the Simplify Your Life series of books by Elaine St. James.

Avoid Toxins in Your Environment

Try to eliminate as many toxins in your life as possible, opting instead for natural products.

Join a Support Group

If a support group exists in your area, join. They understand what you're going through when others might not. If no support group exists in your area, try to find at least one supportive person to share your concerns with. Don't keep all your frustrations inside!

PART FOUR

Your Endometriosis Repair Plan

11

Endometriosis Symptoms and Evaluation Toolkit

Before a definite diagnosis of endometriosis can be made, you need to be aware of the range of your symptoms. This chapter provides you with three tools to help you on your path to a proper diagnosis and repairing the damage of endometriosis: a symptoms chart to record a month's worth of daily symptoms; a pain map to pinpoint the precise locations of your pain; and a risk factors and symptoms checklist, which is a listing of all known endometriosis risk factors and symptoms discussed in chapters 4 and 5 that you can fill out and take with you to your next doctor's appointment.

■ Monthly Symptoms Chart

A monthly symptoms chart is used to record the range of your symptoms throughout any month. Place a check mark next to the symptoms you feel within each day of your cycle. Chart your symptoms for three months or more and take it with you to your next doctor's appointment.

Monthly Symptoms Chart

Date:

Day of Cycle

Type of Pain	1	2	3	4	5	6	7	8	9	10	11	12	13	14	15	16	17	18	19	20	21	22	23	24	25	26	27	28	29	30	31
Gynecolocial																															
* Cramps (pelvic)																															
* Cramps (other)																															
* Heavy menses																															
* Heavy clotting																															
* Premenstrual spotting																															
* Painful menses																															
* Pain during sex																															
* Pain after sex																															
* Pain with ovulation																															
* Pelvic pain (right)																															
* Pelvic pain (left)																															
* Pelvic pain (low middle)																															
* Pelvic pain (other)																															
Gastrointestinal																															
* Abdominal bloating																															
* Abdominal pain																															
* Blood in stool																															

Type of Pain	1	2	3	4	5	6	7	8	9	10	11	12	13	14	15	16	17	18	19	20	21	22	23	24	25	26	27	28	29	30	31
Gastrointestinal (cont.)																															
* Cramps																															
* Constipation																															
* Nausea																															
* Pain/bowel movements (before)																															
* Pain/bowel movements (during)																															
* Pain/bowel movements (after)																															
* Pain when passing gas																															
* Rectal bleeding																															
* Rectal pain																															
* Spasms																															
* Tailbone pain																															
* Vomiting																															
Urinary																															
* Blood in urine																															
* Burning/ painful urination																															
* Difficult urination																															
* Flank pain toward groin																															
* Frequent urination																															
* Incontinence																															
* Low back pain																															
* Pain above pelvic bone																															
* Tenderness around kidneys																															

Monthly Symptoms Chart (continued)

Date:

Type of Pain	Day of Cycle																														
	1	2	3	4	5	6	7	8	9	10	11	12	13	14	15	16	17	18	19	20	21	22	23	24	25	26	27	28	29	30	31
Urinary (cont.)																															
* Urgent need to empty bladder																															
* Urine retention																															
Thoracic																															
* Coughing up bloody sputum																															
* Chest pain																															
* Difficulty breathing																															
* Right or left shoulder pain																															
Sciatic																															
* Cramping in left leg																															
* Left foot drop and weakness																															
* Motor deficit																															
* Pain in hip that radiates down leg																															

Type of Pain	1	2	3	4	5	6	7	8	9	10	11	12	13	14	15	16	17	18	19	20	21	22	23	24	25	26	27	28	29	30	31
Mental																															
* Anger																															
* Anxiety																															
* Depression																															
* Irritability																															
Neurological																															
* Dizziness																															
* Fainting																															
* Headaches/migraines																															
Others																															
* Fatigue																															
* Fever																															
* Insomnia																															
* General aches and pains																															
* Light-headedness																															
* Low blood pressure																															
* Pounding heartbeat/ palpitations																															

Description of pain—check all that apply:
Dull ache □   Constricting □   Nagging □   Stabbing □   Throbbing □
Burning □   Pinching □   Itching □   Shooting □   Cramping □

List all medications taken:

▮ Pain Map

Dr. Arnold Kresch developed the pain map and used it extensively with his own patients to pinpoint the precise locations of their pain, with much accuracy. Pain maps are very helpful because they suggest to your doctor that certain areas should be carefully examined for possible endometriosis involvement.

Make a copy of the pain map opposite and place in the boxes 1, 2, 3, and so on up to 10 (10 being the number representing the most severe pain) in the locations where you feel the pain.

▮ Risk Factors and Symptoms Checklist

You can use the risk factors and symptoms checklist to identify your risks for developing endometriosis, and the full range of your symptoms. If you are not already diagnosed, the checklist, along with the monthly symptoms chart and pain map, can help you get a diagnosis. If you are already diagnosed, the checklist can serve as a tool to assess whether new symptoms are developing or the disease is developing in severity.

Make copies of this checklist, check those risk factors and symptoms unique to you, and, at your next appointment, give one copy to your doctor. This will help her/him identify those areas on which to concentrate and repair the damages of endometriosis.

Risk Factors

Menstrual/Reproductive Factors
____ Earlier age of menarche (first menstrual cycle at eleven years or earlier)
____ Heavy menstrual flow (may have to wear both sanitary napkin and tampon for protection)
____ Heavy clotting

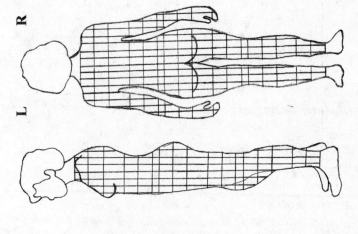

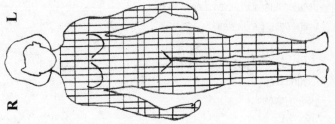

____ Longer duration of menstrual flow (ten days or more)
____ Longer menstrual cycles (thirty-six-day or longer cycles)
____ Shorter menstrual cycles (twenty-seven days or less)
____ Late/no pregnancy
____ Previous intrauterine device (IUD) use
____ Previous oral contraceptive (OC) use

Family History
____ Mother/sister with endometriosis
____ Cousin with endometriosis

Body Characteristics
____ Above average height
____ Above average weight
____ Red hair color

Lifestyle/Environmental Factors
____ Lack of exercise
____ Overconsumption of coffee (more than five cups of coffee daily)
____ Overconsumption of red meat and ham
____ Overexposure to dioxin

Anatomic Abnormalities/Organ Dysfunctions
____ Abnormal cul-de-sac (pouch of Douglas)
____ Kissing ovaries
____ Liver dysfunction

Autoimmune Medical Conditions

It is thought that your risk of developing endometriosis may increase if your immune system is already weakened by autoimmune disorders such as fibromyalgia, chronic fatigue syndrome (CFS), asthma, and allergies.

Symptoms Checklist

Chronic Pain and Aches/Discomfort

___ Abdominal pain, indicative of gastrointestinal tract involvement

___ Abdominal pain that is constant or occurs during the menstrual cycle, indicative of urinary tract involvement

___ Backaches/lower back pains, indicative of pelvic, urinary, and gastrointestinal involvement

___ Chronic/intermittent pelvic pain, one of the key symptoms indicative of reproductive organ involvement

___ Constricting/deep chest pain, indicative of lung and diaphragm involvement

___ Cramping in the left leg when walking for long distances, indicative of sciatic nerve involvement

___ Extremely painful menstruation that occurs before, during, and after menses (dysmenorrhea)

___ Painful bowel movements, indicative of gastrointestinal tract involvement (dyschezia)

___ Pain experienced during sexual intercourse (dyspareunia—especially with deep penetration)

___ Pain with ovulation that worsens over time (*mittelschmerz*)

___ Flank pain that radiates toward the groin, indicative of urinary tract involvement

___ Intestinal cramping, indicative of gastrointestinal tract involvement

___ Left or right shoulder pain associated with menses, indicative of lung and diaphragm involvement

___ Leg pains, indicative of pelvic involvement

___ Lower back discomfort that radiates to the left leg, indicative of sciatic nerve involvement

___ Pain above the pelvic bone (suprapubic), indicative of urinary tract involvement

____ Pain after sexual intercourse, may last for a few hours or a few days with bleeding

____ Pain experienced during internal examination of the vagina, indicative of endometriosis on the reproductive organs

____ Pain during rectal examinations, indicative of gastrointestinal tract involvement

____ Pain in the hip that radiates down the leg, indicative of sciatic nerve involvement

____ Pain that begins just before menstruation and lasts several days after menses, indicative of sciatic nerve involvement

____ Pain when passing gas, indicative of gastrointestinal tract involvement

____ Pain when sitting, indicative of gastrointestinal tract involvement

____ Painful or burning urination, indicative of urinary tract involvement

____ Painful incisional nodules/masses (mass is slow-growing and pain is cyclic, occurring during menses), indicative of incisional scar involvement

____ Painful nodules/swellings along the skin, indicative of skin involvement

____ Rectal pain, indicative of gastrointestinal tract involvement

____ Rectal pain and pressure, indicative of urinary tract and gastrointestinal tract involvement

____ Tailbone pain, indicative of gastrointestinal tract involvement

____ Tenderness around the kidneys, indicative of urinary tract involvement

____ Tenderness of sciatic notch, indicative of sciatic nerve involvement

Sleep Changes

____ Difficulty falling asleep (associated with constant chronic pain)

____ Insomnia (associated with constant chronic pain that disrupts/prevents sleep)

____ Interrupted sleep/frequent waking (associated with chronic pain and urinary symptoms)

Fatigue

____ Fatigue with or after normal activities (includes fatigue with long hours at work, normal exercise routines, shopping, driving, etc.)

____ Unrefreshing sleep (fatigue felt even after ten or more hours of sleep)

____ Fatigue associated with catamenial pneumothorax (CPT—recurrence of air in the lungs during menstruation, which causes them to collapse)

Reproductive/Menstrual/Sexual Problems

____ Ectopic pregnancies (women with endometriosis have a higher than average risk of ectopic/abnormal pregnancies)

____ Heavy menses (often with heavy clotting)

____ Infertility/problems conceiving (occurs in 30 to 50 percent of women with endometriosis)

____ Long duration of menses (more than seven days)

____ Miscarriages (women with endometriosis have a higher than average risk of having miscarriages)

____ Painful intercourse (dyspareunia—especially during deep penetration)

____ Premenstrual spotting (experienced the week before menstruation)

____ Reduced sex drive (often associated with pain that accompanies sexual intercourse)

Neurological Problems

____ Dizziness (symptomatic of increased blood loss/anemia and/or air caught in the lungs during menstruation, that causes the lungs to collapse—called catamenial pneumothorax [CPT])

____ Fainting (symptomatic of increased blood loss/anemia)

____ Headaches/migraines

Urinary Problems

____ Stress incontinence (urine leakage brought on by a sneeze, cough, laugh, or sudden movement)

____ Urge incontinence (urine leakage that occurs when you feel the urge to urinate but may not have enough time to get to the bathroom)

____ Frequent urination (urinating more than fifteen times per day and going to the bathroom very often during the night)

____ Hematuria (blood in the urine—indicative of urinary tract involvement)

____ Urine retention

____ Difficult urination (dysuria)

____ Urinary urgency (urgent need to empty the bladder)

Gastrointestinal/Bowel Problems

____ Nausea

____ Vomiting

____ Abdominal bloating

____ Constipation

____ Alternating between constipation and diarrhea

____ Rectal bleeding that may occur during menses

____ Blood in stool (hematochezia)

____ Spasms

Thoracic/Diaphragmatic Problems

____ Recurrent cough

____ Coughing up blood or bloody sputum, especially during menses (catamenial hemoptysis)

____ Accumulation of air in the pleural cavity that leads to lung collapse (catamenial pneumothorax [CPT])

____ Collection of blood in the pleural cavity (hemothorax)

____ Difficulty breathing/shortness of breath (dyspnea)

____ Water on the lung (pleural effusion)

____ Accumulation of air in the chest cavity (pneumomediastinum)

____ Pulmonary nodules present in the pleural cavity

____ Pleural masses

Sciatic Involvement

____ Motor deficit

____ Left foot drop and weakness

____ Cramping in the left leg when walking for long distances

Psychological Symptoms

____ Anger

____ Anxiety

____ Depression

____ Irritability

____ Stress

Infections/Autoimmune Disorders/Allergies

____ Chronic yeast infections

____ Sinus infections

____ Very frequent allergies

____ Chronic fatigue syndrome (CFS—one hundred times more common among women with endometriosis)

____ Fibromyalgia (twice as common among women with endometriosis)

____ Hypothyroidism (five times more common among women with endometriosis)

____ Systemic lupus erythematosus, rheumatoid arthritis, multiple sclerosis, or Sjögren's syndrome (occur more frequently in women with endometriosis)

____ Allergies (occur in 61 percent of women with endometriosis compared to 18 percent of the general female population)

Other Symptoms

____ Fever

____ High blood pressure (hypertension)

____ Light-headedness

____ Pounding heartbeat/heart palpitations

____ Pale skin

12

Getting Diagnosed

Getting diagnosed is very often a difficult and time-consuming process. A 1998 EA survey found that the average delay in getting a diagnosis is as much as 9.28 years. Approximately 21 percent of patients first experienced dysmenorrhea at age fifteen or younger while 38 percent of patients had their first pelvic pain at age fifteen or younger.

One factor that contributes to this significant delay in diagnosis concerns how seriously patients are taken by their doctors. The EA survey found that 35 percent of patients felt their doctors did not take them seriously, and 38 percent did not find their doctors helpful. Another powerful factor concerns the level of education of the patient about her symptoms. In the survey an overwhelming 58 percent of patients thought their symptoms were normal.

Yet another factor that contributes to delays in getting a diagnosis concerns the symptoms of the disease, which are similar to those of other diseases, such as pelvic inflammatory disease (PID), irritable bowel syndrome (IBS), and interstitial cystitis (IC).

The earlier you get a diagnosis, the better you will be able to deal with the symptoms of the disease. This chapter will discuss what you need to do to ensure an early diagnosis and what is involved in getting a diagnosis of endometriosis. The chapter concludes with a review of the future directions in endometriosis diagnostic techniques.

▌Your Responsibilities

Evaluate Your Symptoms History

One of the first things you need to do before you see a doctor is evaluate the range of your symptoms. The Symptoms Evaluation Toolkit in chapter 11 will help in this process. Make copies of the symptoms chart, and record your daily symptoms for a minimum of three months. On a copy of the pain map, pinpoint the precise locations of your pains with the numbers 1 to 10, signifying pain severity at each location. Fill out a copy of the risk factors and symptoms checklist, recording all the symptoms you had during the three months.

Armed with these tools, your doctor will be better able to assess your symptoms history to make a better and quicker diagnosis. These tools can also be used to assess your symptoms periodically, better treat them, or see if new ones are developing.

Find the Right Doctor

One of the main factors that contribute to delays in getting a proper diagnosis of endometriosis has to do with the type of doctor you are seeing. Many endometriosis patients report seeing doctors who did not take their symptoms seriously and refused to acknowledge their pain.

This is what happened to Gen:

For years I would go see my family doctor to try to get some help controlling the pain I was going through, but the only thing I was told was that it was all in my head. According to him, I could not possibly be in so much pain. So I was told to bear it and that it was normal and every woman had painful periods. He told me I would just have to get used to it.

To avoid delays, make sure that the doctor you are seeing believes you and makes a concerted effort to relieve your pain and find the exact cause of your many symptoms. If you find yourself with a doctor like Gen's, do not waste precious time. Find another doctor who believes you and takes your symptoms seriously. Chapter 13 goes into more details about finding a doctor to treat your endometriosis once you are diagnosed.

∎ The Endometriosis Diagnosis

A positive diagnosis of endometriosis today can be obtained only through a surgical procedure called a laparoscopy. A doctor may suspect a woman has endometriosis based on her symptoms history, pelvic exam, and transvaginal ultrasound, but these have their own shortcomings. Symptoms such as menstrual pain may not be indicative of endometriosis only, and most women with endometriosis have normal ultrasound results. Pelvic exams may indicate the presence of masses or growths, but these may not necessarily be indicative of endometriosis. A definitive diagnosis therefore requires laparoscopic surgery.

The Laparoscopy

A laparoscopy, or lap as members of the endometriosis community call it, is a minimally invasive outpatient procedure. During the laparoscopy, the surgeon looks via a laparoscope inside the abdominal/pelvic cavity through a small incision, about 1 centimeter wide, made through or near the belly button. This is a thin, lighted instrument that is fitted with a telescopic lens. A video camera is also attached to allow the surgeon to see areas in the abdominal cavity she/he cannot see with her/his own eyes. Additional incisions of the same size are also made in the pubic hairline through which other surgical instruments are introduced to treat the condition.

Through the main incision, the surgeon inserts a needle and injects the patient with carbon dioxide (CO_2), which expands the abdominal cavity and lifts and separates the organs to allow for easier insertion of the laparoscope. Through the laparoscope the surgeon is able to view and manipulate the organs, make diagnoses, take biopsies, and remove diseased tissues wherever they may be found.

Once the surgeon is satisfied that the surgery was successful, all instruments are removed, the abdomen is deflated, and the incisions closed with a few dissolvable stitches, then covered by bandages. Scarring is minimal, and discomfort is expected during the two days postsurgery. The patient's recovery depends on the extent of the work done during the laparoscopy, but it generally varies from patient to patient. It may take up to two weeks to recover. On rare occasions, some patients have reported one to two months needed for recovery.

In the past some surgeons would do a laparoscopy only as a diagnostic tool. The patient would then be scheduled for another surgery to remove any endometriosis found during the laparoscopy, a very inefficient system that was also very taxing on the patient. Now it is rare for a surgeon to perform a "diagnostic laparoscopy" and not to treat any disease found during the laparoscopy if she/he can.

Other Names for Laparoscopy

- *Bandage surgery:* Incisions made during surgery are so small that they can be easily covered with a bandage.
- *Belly button surgery:* The laparoscope is often inserted through a small incision near the umbilicus or navel (belly button).

How does it feel to be diagnosed? Relieved, depressed, angry? Or all of the above and more? For many, diagnosis is certainly a relief and a confirmation of years of pain. Says Melissa:

> *They indeed found a moderate amount of endometriosis, and vaporized it with a laser. I was strangely relieved that I had not gone through all of this just to be told that I had been complaining about normal menstrual pain for years.*

Amira also felt relieved by her diagnosis:

> *When I was coming to from surgery, my doctor told me I had endometriosis. I cried and was still crying when they allowed my husband to finally see me. The tears were tears of joy. You wouldn't think I would be so happy to be diagnosed with endometriosis, but after all the suffering and having no answers, it was a welcome relief.*

For many, however, anger is a common reaction to the positive diagnosis. Deborah Ann describes her reaction to the diagnosis:

> *I was diagnosed with recurring ovarian cysts, numerous fibroid tumors, and endometriosis. Doing a little bit of research on my own, I discovered that this diagnosis explained my agonizing cramps, the extremely heavy menstrual flow, the bloating and diarrhea, the terrible leg and lower back pain after and during sex. Violent allergies all year round, and much more. At first I was furious. All those doctors that I had gone to over a span of twenty years let me suffer and think I was crazy! What kind of ignorant, egotistical doctors had I been going to?!*

Advantages and Disadvantages of Laparoscopy

Advantages

- *Reduced post-op pain:* Compared to a laparotomy (traditional open surgery), the overall trauma to the skin and muscles is reduced as a result of a smaller incision. This results in less post-op pain. The patient in turn resumes her normal day-to-day activities more quickly. During a laparotomy, a longer incision is made to gain access to the abdominal cavity. This results in increased postsurgery pain, a longer stay in hospital, and increased risk of developing an infection in the wound.

- *Reduced hospital stay:* A laparoscopy takes between forty-five minutes and five hours, depending on the extent of the individual's case. The hospital stay then is greatly reduced, ranging from half a day to two to three days. Patients go home earlier and return to normal routines much sooner than after an open surgery.

- *Reduced infection:* Laparoscopic surgery also reduces infection, as delicate tissues are not exposed to the air of the operating room over long periods as in a conventional surgery. Further, video magnification offers surgeons a better view of the diseased organs and surrounding vessels and nerves. This significantly reduces the exposure of delicate tissues to the air of the operating room. Delicate maneuvers can be performed to protect these vital structures during the removal of endometrial implants.

- *Less scarring:* The incisions made in the abdomen heal quickly without noticeable scars.

- *Economical:* The amount of medication required by the patient after a laparoscopy is considerably less compared to what's needed following open surgery.

Disadvantages

- *Inability to treat all types of endometriosis:* This is a major disadvantage of laparoscopy. In many cases, the extent of the endometrial implants and their locations do not allow the surgeon to treat the condition during the laparoscopy, and more invasive surgery is required. In these cases, patients then go on to have a laparotomy, a surgical procedure under general anesthesia that requires a wider incision, an extended stay in hospital, and a longer recovery time.

- *Disease recurrence:* Women with severe endometriosis experience recurrence of the disease and require repeat surgeries. Laparoscopic treatment of endometriosis is not a cure for the disease.

- *Complications:* There are also complications associated with laparoscopic treatment of endometriosis. One such complication concerns the use of carbon dioxide (CO_2) gas to expand the abdominal cavity. The CO_2 gas is harsh on tissues, resulting in damage to the peritoneum. Experts suggest that surgeons should warm and humidify the gas as it is injected into the abdominal cavity. This will lessen post-op abdominal discomfort.

- *Unsuitable patients:* Another disadvantage of laparoscopy is that it cannot be performed on all types of patients. For instance, a patient who has had other operations before may have too much scar tissue to allow for a safe procedure.

- *Laparoscopy is surgery:* Laparoscopy is a minimally invasive surgery, but it is still a form of surgery. Needing surgery to diagnose their condition may prevent some patients, especially those without insurance, from pursuing diagnosis and treatment.

▌Other Diagnostic Methods

Transvaginal Laparoscopy

Transvaginal laparoscopy is a minimally invasive diagnostic surgical procedure developed to explore the tubes and ovaries in patients without obvious symptoms. The procedure is done through a needle puncture in the cul-de-sac (pouch of Douglas), using a local anesthetic; it can be done in the doctor's office. Access through the cul-de-sac allows visualization of the posterior wall of the uterus, the ovaries, fallopian tubes, pelvic sidewalls, the uterosacral ligaments, and the cul-de-sac, except for the site of entry. A saline solution is used to keep the organs afloat. This type of solution is very helpful in detecting early endometriotic implants. Minimal endometriosis was found in 30 percent of patients without any complaints of pain using transvaginal laparoscopy. Minimal endometriotic lesions can also be treated during the procedure.

Additionally, transvaginal laparoscopy allows for better inspection of the lower pelvis without manipulation and can test the patency of the fallopian tubes (the state of the tubes, whether they are open or blocked). However, transvaginal laparoscopy cannot replace standard laparoscopy. Although the procedure is less invasive than a standard laparoscopy, the surgeon has the advantage of doing major surgery with a standard laparoscopy, which cannot be done via the transvaginal approach. One major advantage of transvaginal laparoscopy, however, is the ability to detect more adhesions. Examination of the ovaries by transvaginal laparoscopy in patients with mild endometriosis revealed 50 percent more periovarian adhesions compared to standard laparoscopy.

Imaging Techniques

Imaging techniques such as ultrasonography (ultrasound), computerized tomography (CT scans), and magnetic resonance imaging (MRI) have been used as diagnostic tools for endometriosis but with varying success. These techniques offer additional information but may not be useful to make the initial diagnosis.

Ultrasonography (Ultrasound)

Ultrasonography involves the projection of sound waves at a very high frequency, inaudible to the human ear, through a section of a person's body. These sound waves produce images of the interior of that section of the body on a video monitor. This procedure has been used to determine the extent of the disease and involvement of other organs. Ultrasonography has been reported useful only in characterizing masses found in patients already diagnosed with endometriosis by laparoscopy. Additionally, ultrasonography as a diagnostic technique is compromised by a lack of specificity. It does not distinguish endometriotic cysts from ovarian cysts, tumors, or other benign ovarian masses.

Computerized Tomography (CT Scan)

A computerized tomography (CT) scan is a form of X-ray examination in which the CT scanner rotates around the section of the person's body to be scanned. The information gathered is used to produce three-dimensional (3D) computerized images of the scanned sections. As in the case of ultrasounds, CT scans do not specifically distinguish between benign versus malignant masses and are often unable to distinguish between adnexal structures (adjoining parts such as the fallopian tubes and ovaries, which adjoin the uterus) and loops of bowel.

Magnetic Resonance Imaging (MRI)

Magnetic resonance imaging (MRI) is a noninvasive diagnostic technique that involves the analysis of the absorption and transmission of high-frequency radio waves by hydrogen in water molecules and other components of body tissues once placed in a strong magnetic field. In comparison to ultrasonography and computerized tomography (CT) scan, MRI has been found to be more reliable; it can detect the hemorrhagic nature of some endometrial implants. However, MRI cannot detect all types of endometriotic implants, and the procedure does not reveal small adhesions. Therefore, MRI cannot substitute for laparoscopy to definitively diagnose endometriosis.

Serum/Biological Markers

Biological markers have long been investigated by scientists as diagnostic tests for endometriosis. However, these markers are relatively nonspecific, being increased in ovarian cancer, liver disease, colon cancer, pelvic inflammatory disease (PID), and even during menstruation in healthy women.

Serum Cancer Antigen 125 (CA–125)

Serum cancer antigen 125 (CA-125) is an antigen that is found in many normal tissues such as endometrium and peritoneum. This antigen is also found on the surface membranes of endometriotic implants. Studies have reported extremely high levels of CA-125 in women with endometriosis. This may be caused by the endometriosis-associated inflammatory response that increases CA-125 shedding into the peritoneal cavity. High levels of CA-125 have been observed in serum, menstrual effluent, and peritoneal fluid in women with endometriosis. However, CA-125 is more often elevated in advanced stages of the disease—stages III and IV—and less so in stages I and II. This low sensitivity limits the usefulness of the test in diagnosing minimal and mild endometriosis.

Serum Cancer Antigen 19-9 (CA 19-9)

As in the case of serum cancer antigen 125 (CA-125), serum cancer antigen 19-9 (CA 19-9) levels have been found elevated in women with endometriosis and significantly reduced after treatment. CA 19-9 has also been found in the glandular epithelial cells in ovarian endometriomas (chocolate cysts) in many patients. However, the serum's level increases with the severity of the disease, again limiting the usefulness of this serum when screening for minimal and mild endometriosis. CA 19-9 as a diagnostic test is still being studied.

■ Advances/Future Directions

While laparoscopy is considered the gold standard for the diagnosis of endometriosis, the procedure has several shortcomings. Most doctors accept visualization of apparent lesions as sufficient to make a diagnosis. While certain appearances of endometriotic lesions are accepted (chapter 2), to rely on common laparoscopic appearances of lesions to make a diagnosis may lead to inaccurate conclusions. A more definite diagnosis of endometriosis can only be confirmed by a pathology report. Less invasive and noninvasive diagnostic techniques are being investigated to diagnose endometriosis.

Microlaparoscopy

Microlaparoscopy is the newest minimally invasive diagnostic surgical technique. The technique was developed to further reduce surgical trauma, and to allow for a more comfortable recovery and a quicker return to normal activities with reduced socioeconomic costs.

The procedure is the same as a laparoscopy except the instruments are much smaller. A standard laparoscope is 0.39 to 0.5 inch (10 to 12 millimeters) in size while microlaparoscopes are less than 0.12 inch (3 millimeters). Microlaparoscopy involves smaller incisions—the 0.08-inch (2-millimeter) instruments leave a tiny spot with drastically reduced post-op pain. The procedure is often done without orotracheal intubation (tube inserted down throat) and with less anesthesia. There's no accompanying sore throat and a shorter, more comfortable postsurgery recovery.

The benefits to endometriosis patients are tremendous. Patients are more accepting of the procedure because it is minimally invasive, and they return to their normal routines of work, family, or school much faster and with less postsurgery discomfort. Sometimes, however, the surgeon will find a problem that cannot be corrected during the microlaparoscopy, such as significant adhesions, major endometriotic implants, or other abnormalities. In this event, the patient will receive a general anesthetic, and the operation will be completed using standard laparoscopic techniques.

Microlaparoscopy is still in its infancy and is primarily used for diagnostic surgery. However, as newer instruments become available, more uses of microlaparoscopy will be realized.

Immunological Markers

The immune system has been shown to play a major role in the development of endometriosis. For example, studies are under way to determine if cytokines (immunoregulatory proteins) can be used as a screening tool for endometriosis. Peritoneal fluid cytokines such as IL-1, IL-6, IL-8, IL-12, IL-13 and peritoneal fluid tumor necrosis factor-alpha, (TNF-α), are being studied as possible markers for endometriosis. One study found that IL-6 and TNF-α levels were significantly higher in patients with endometriosis and could be used to discriminate between patients with and without endometriosis with a high degree of sensitivity and specificity. In time, these potential immunological markers for endometriosis may allow for a nonsurgical diagnosis of the disease.

Genetic Markers

The fact that endometriosis runs in families and that certain genes are expressed differently in women with endometriosis has led researchers to try to develop a gene-based diagnostic test for endometriosis. Gene-based technologies are currently being investigated with regard to endometriosis, including subtractive cDNA hybridization and microarray techniques. A microarray is also known as a gene chip, and it relies on just a blood test or a biopsy.

Endometrial Aromatase Expression (P450 Arom)

Aromatase P450 is an enzyme present in endometrial implants that can give implants the ability to create their own supply of estrogen, which they need to develop. A recent study found that detection of aromatase P450 in the endometrium of women with endometriosis strongly indicates the presence of endometriosis and may be a potential marker of the disease. More studies are being conducted in this area.

13

Create a Dynamic Treatment Team

There are three aims of any treatment strategy, as we learned in part III: (1) to treat the disease; (2) to treat the disease's associated pain; and (3) to restore the woman's fertility. The therapies advocated for all endometriosis patients include conventional (also known as allopathic) treatments as well as complementary and alternative medicines (CAM)—a multidisciplinary approach to living well with endometriosis.

No one therapeutic approach has been shown to be 100 percent or even 85 percent effective in treating the disease. Treatment failures within medical therapies are common, as many women who undergo gonadotropin-releasing hormone (GnRH) agonist protocols—Lupron, for instance—can attest. As Lone Hummelshøj, editor in chief of www.endometriosis.org, noted in her paper "Meeting Expectations in the Chronically Ill Patient by Extending the Therapeutic Network": "An integrated approach involving a multidisciplinary team is needed, with an open mind to explore combination of therapies, even beyond the medical mainstream, based on patient outcome measures, to improve symptoms, alleviate side effects, and/or to assist recovery after surgery."

A multidisciplinary approach is recommended to treat your disease. This will involve several medical specialists and complementary and alternative medicine practitioners—in essence, a team approach.

This chapter will focus on creating just such a team. While the emphasis is placed on finding and working with an endometriosis specialist, the chapter will first review the types of conventional and complementary and alternative practitioners you may go to for treatment.

▌Family Medicine Practitioners

Often family medicine practitioners are the first point of contact for women who will eventually be diagnosed with endometriosis. Family medicine practitioners can diagnose and treat a variety of conditions and diseases for all age groups and for both sexes. They are trained in several specialties, including gynecology, disease prevention, obstetrics, general surgery, and internal medicine. Their emphasis, as the name suggests, is the care of families, and they will refer patients to specialists for further treatment. The American Board of Family Medicine certifies family medicine practitioners.

▌General Practitioners (GPs)

General practitioners (GPs) are also often the first point of contact for women eventually diagnosed with endometriosis. GPs do not specialize in any one specialty. Instead, they diagnose and treat a variety of conditions and diseases. GPs will refer patients to a specialist such as a gynecologist for further care. There is no board that certifies GPs.

▮ Gynecologists

Gynecologists diagnose and treat disorders and diseases of the female reproductive system. It is the twin specialty to obstetrics, both usually denoted as OB/GYN. Gynecologists focus on women's reproductive health, with many specializing in treating women with endometriosis. They also perform gynecologic surgeries such as laparoscopies to remove endometrial implants. The American Board of Obstetrics and Gynecology (ABOG) certifies gynecologists.

▮ Reproductive Endocrinologists (REs)

Reproductive endocrinology is a subspecialty of obstetrics and gynecology. Reproductive endocrinologists are gynecologists who specialize in infertility—they are concerned with diagnosing and treating the complex problems that may contribute to infertility in women, such as endometriosis. They also diagnose and treat other reproductive and hormonal problems in women.

The American Board of Obstetrics and Gynecology (ABOG) certifies reproductive endocrinologists.

▮ Allergists/Immunologists

Allergists and immunologists diagnose and treat immune-related disorders such as asthma, eczema, food allergies, hormone allergies, and others. Many endometriosis patients also consult with immunologists to treat their various allergy symptoms.

The American Board of Allergy and Immunology (ABAI) certifies immunologists.

▌ Pain Management Specialists

Pain management specialists are medical doctors who have additional training in treating persons with chronic and acute pains. This field is a subspecialty of anesthesiology. The American Board of Anesthesiology (ABA) certifies pain management specialists.

▌ Gastroenterologists

Gastroenterologists diagnose and treat conditions and diseases of the digestive system, including the stomach, gallbladder, liver, and bowels. They also consult with surgeons during abdominal operations. Gastroenterology is a subspecialty of internal medicine, and specialists are certified by the American Board of Internal Medicine (ABIM).

▌ Surgeons

Surgeons are medical doctors who specialize in the treatment of disease through different types of surgeries. These surgeries may be done to diagnose an illness or to treat an illness, as in the case of an endometriosis patient who is treated via a laparoscopy. The American Board of Surgery (ABS) certifies surgeons.

▌ Nutritionists

Nutritionists are becoming important members of endometriosis patients' treatment programs. Recognizing the intrinsic relationship between nutrition and health, women with endometriosis are turning to nutritionists to create individualized nutrition plans.

Nutritionists have extensive education and training in nutrition science. They carry the title of certified nutritionist (CN) or certified clinical nutritionist (CCN). Clinical nutritionists are certified by the Clinical Nutrition Certification Board (CNCB) and certified nutritionists by the National Institute of Nutritional Education (NINE). CCNs and CNs may also be members of the Society of Certified Nutritionists (SCN).

∎ Registered Nurses (RN)

Nurses, often our first contact at hospitals or private medical practices, are an important part of any medical practice and can provide treatment, counseling, and health education. Many endometriosis patients can attest to how essential RNs are, as many nurses educated them about the disease when they were first diagnosed.

∎ Traditional Chinese Medicine (TCM) Practitioners

Many endometriosis patients are turning to traditional Chinese medicine (TCM) practitioners to help relieve their pain and other symptoms. TCM practitioners treat each person individually, creating a treatment approach unique to that person. Treatments include dietary modification, acupuncture, tai chi, and herbal supplements.

Acupuncture is a popularly practiced TCM throughout the United States. Professional acupuncturists are certified by the National Certification Commission for Acupuncture and Oriental Medicine (NCCAOM) and carry the title Licensed Acupuncturist (L.Ac). The American Board of Medical Acupuncture (ABMA) and/or the American Academy of Medical Acupuncture (AAMA) certify physicians trained in acupuncture.

▌ Herbalists

If you choose to add herbal supplements to your treatment strategy, make sure to consult with a professional herbalist. Herbalists may be members of the American Herbalists Guild (AHG), or you may seek the counsel of a licensed naturopathic physician. Make sure that the herbalist you consult has experience treating women with endometriosis.

All these specialists play an important role in your overall treatment program, targeting specific aspects of the disease and its various side effects as well as the whole you. As Hummelshøj asserts, once all these specialties are linked intrinsically to your needs within your own unique therapeutic network, then you should realize long-term and satisfactory outcomes.

▌ Find the Right Endometriosis Specialist

Finding the right endometriosis specialist to treat your endometriosis is a challenge in most cases. Often you will encounter physicians who are not aware of the disease's many symptoms and who are not fully educated about the latest treatment methods. Proper diagnosis can be delayed for years while you undergo numerous unsuccessful treatment regimes for conditions you don't have. Jude advises the following:

> *I choose my specialists based on word of mouth from other people that the work they do is of a high standard. I also think it is important to have a good working relationship with your specialist so you can honestly tell him or her what is happening to you, even the most embarrassing bits.*

I also think trusting your specialist puts you in a good state of mind. However, I also think it is important to listen to your gut feelings. If you have a sense that your specialist is floundering with treatment options, then seek a second opinion. I feel empowered in thinking that I am employing my specialist's services and at the end of the day I call the shots.

Fortunately, there are many doctors in the United States who specialize in treating endometriosis patients. But how do you find them? The following are a few key points to consider when trying to find the right endometriosis specialist for you.

Identify Candidates

Your first priority in the search for an endometriosis specialist is to create a list of several candidates. The best place to begin this search would be with either one or both of the national endometriosis support organizations: the Endometriosis Association (EA) and the Endometriosis Research Center (ERC). They will know which doctors around the country specialize in endometriosis treatment, whether independently or as an affiliate of a hospital or medical center.

Another great tool in this identification process is the opinions of other endometriosis patients. Visit the numerous online endometriosis discussion forums and ask other patients about their experiences with particular endometriosis specialists. Find out who their specialists are, what they think of them, and if they would feel comfortable recommending them to you. Also, search these online message boards for any types of comments about the specialists on your list.

You can also ask for a referral from your family doctor or general practitioner, who may be aware of the leading authorities in endometriosis treatment.

Verify Their Capabilities

You've identified possible candidates and, based on preliminary research, you have two or three possible specialists. It is now time to visit these candidates to further investigate each one's ability to treat your condition. Call their offices and set appointments. Ask each doctor to review your medical records and outline a treatment plan for you. During this consultation the experts suggest you ask the following questions to become better aware of a particular doctor's capabilities in treating you:

1. How much of your practice is dedicated to obstetrics? How much to gynecology? (Heather C. Guidone, program director of the Center for Endometriosis [CEC] and director of operations of the Endometriosis Research Center [ERC], advises that this can be helpful in determining whether your doctor will be called to the delivery ward during an appointment.)

2. How many women have you treated for endometriosis?

3. How many women are you currently treating for endometriosis? (These two questions above will help to determine the experience level of the doctor.)

4. What do you believe to be the proper course of treatment? (Be careful of doctors who immediately recommend pregnancy or hysterectomy as treatments and/or dismiss other treatments. Quickly finish up your consultation, then delete them from your list.)

5. How do you measure the outcome of your treatment? How long do you take to gather that information?

6. Will your treatment be provided at a hospital or clinic where the staff is familiar with the special needs of women with endometriosis?

7. Does your recommended treatment eradicate the disease or temporarily suppress symptoms?

8. If your recommended treatment is unsuccessful, what will be the subsequent course of treatment?

9. What is your treatment philosophy regarding hysterectomy and endometriosis?

10. Have you collected data while treating women with endometriosis and published the results of your work? If so, may I have a list of the articles(s)?

The following questions specifically concern surgery:

1. What method of surgery do you use to remove the implants?

2. Why do you use this method over the others currently available?

3. Will you perform this procedure via a laparoscopy or a laparotomy?

4. Do you remove all the endometriosis?

5. Do you have colleagues consult in the operating room if endometriosis is found in an area outside of your expertise? (Endometriosis found in areas such as the bladder or bowel requires additional surgical experience on the part of the specialist. You will feel much more comfortable knowing that, if implants are found in these delicate areas, the specialist will have the necessary experience to know how to proceed or will call on a colleague to assist in the surgery.)

6. Will the removed tissues be sent to pathology for final identification? (Dr. David Redwine asserts that it is difficult to know for certain if endometriosis is present unless a pathologist examines the removed tissues.)

There are other important factors to take into consideration in order to create an effective patient-physician relationship that will have a positive impact on your treatment.

Selection Criteria

You must decide what other criteria are important to you in selecting a physician. Expertise in treating endometriosis is just one of many other considerations.

Gender

Give some thought as to whether you prefer a male or female physician. This will help you narrow your search and save time. While studies have shown that female patients choose a female doctor more often than male doctors, both male and female patients will choose male doctors. However, a preference for a same-sex doctor becomes much stronger when patients are seeking help for health problems of a more intimate nature such as endometriosis.

A study done in 2003 found that visits to female doctors were associated with greater patient satisfaction. For example, the study found there were important differences in the way female doctors communicated with their patients compared to male doctors. Female doctors were more attentive, emphasizing partnership building in their interactions with their patients. They also shared more information and encouraged their patients to ask questions and to speak freely. Essentially, female doctors' practice style was found to be more patient-centered.

On the other hand, male doctors placed greater emphasis on more technical routines, such as recording the patients medical and family history, doing a physical examination, and performing in-office procedures. The study, however, did not find much difference in the length of time spent on visits between male and female doctors.

Type of Doctor/Practice Style

How you interact with your doctor will affect the outcome of your treatment. Give some thought to the type of doctor you are looking for. Are you looking for a doctor to dictate exactly your course of treatment? Or do you prefer a more involved relationship with your doctor, one in which you are part of the decision-making process—a partner in your own health care?

There are four broad categories of doctor types:

- *Parental/priestly doctor:* This type of doctor acts as the patient's guardian, dictating and implementing treatments that she/he thinks are best. The doctor presents the patient with selected information that will encourage the patient to consent to the treatment the doctor thinks is best.

- *Informative/consumer doctor:* As the name suggests, this type of doctor recognizes the importance of the patient in her own treatment decisions. The doctor provides the patient with all the relevant information so that she can choose the type of treatment she desires.

- *Interpretive doctor:* This type of doctor provides the patient with information about the nature of her condition and advantages of possible treatments. She/he further assists the patient in evaluating her goals in relation to her condition and in determining what treatments are best to realize the specified goals. The interpretive doctor thus acts more as a counselor, engaging the patient in a joint process of understanding who she is in relation to her condition and how the various treatment options bear on her identity.

- *Deliberative doctor:* This type of doctor acts more like a teacher or a friend, someone who engages the patient in dialogue on what course of action is best. A deliberative doctor indicates what the patient *could* do, but, knowing the patient and being aware of her goals in relation to her condition, and wanting to achieve the best outcome, indicates to the patient what she *should* do.

Qualifications and Credentials

Obstetrics and gynecology (OB/GYN) is the discipline that primarily treats endometriosis. Check to make sure that the gynecologist you choose is board certified in this specialty by an accredited specialty board. This means that she/he completed an approved educational training program and passed the accreditation tests to practice in this medical specialty.

Gynecologists are certified by the American Board of Obstetrics and Gynecology (ABOG), a recognized specialty board of the American Board of Medical Specialties (ABMS). Certified specialists are listed in *The Official ABMS Directory of Board Certified Medical Specialists*, published annually. This annual directory can be found in most public hospitals, in university and medical libraries, and is also available on CD-ROM. You can also check on specific physicians through the ABMS Web site at http://www.abms.org via their Who's Certified link. Verification is also available through the ABMS toll-free telephone service by calling 866-ASK-ABMS (275-2267).

You can also check on a physician's credentials by contacting the individual specialty board in the physician's field of practice. In the case of the endometriosis specialist, verification can be obtained from the American College of Obstetricians and Gynecologists (ACOG), which requires doctors to be board certified to become a member. Visit ACOG's online Physician Directory at http://acog.org/member-lookup/disclaimer.cfm to find out more about a particular gynecologist. A doctor who has attained full membership in ACOG is called a Fellow of the society and is entitled to use the society's acronym in all formal communications. In the case of the endometriosis specialist certified by ACOG, she/he will have FACOG (Fellow of the American College of Obstetrics and Gynecology) behind her/his name.

You can also check on a doctor's accreditation through the American Medical Association's Web site at http://www.ama-assn.org.

Hospital Privileges

It is also important to check whether the doctor you've chosen has admitting and surgical privileges at an accredited hospital. A doctor must pass a thorough review of her/his entire training and must demonstrate proficiency in the procedures for which privileges are requested. You can get this information from the medical staff at the hospital where you will have the procedure done. If the doctor does not have privileges there, be suspicious.

Disciplinary and Malpractice History

You will want to know if the doctor has had any disciplinary action or malpractice suits brought against her/him. Contact the applicable state medical board for more information. For a complete listing of state licensing boards, go to the Federation of State Medical Boards' (FSMB) Directory of State Medical Boards link at http://www.fsmb.org/directory_smb.html. FSMB also has a Disciplinary History Report service available at http://www.docinfo.org that provides consumers with paid access to a database of doctors' disciplinary histories.

Good Bedside Manners

A 2001 study titled "The Role of Gender in Determining Strength and Nature of Marketing Relationships" found that while both men and women are concerned about "how" they are treated by their doctor, women care more about having a strong relationship with their doctor. The study concluded that women want to have a sense of control in their doctor-patient relationship and do not want to be talked down to. Men are more interested in treatment.

Female patients therefore expect good bedside manner from their doctors or better communication. As the Third Annual Disease Management Outcomes summit concluded: "Without effective communication, patients and physicians cannot achieve the ideal relationship that leads to the ideal delivery of care." To foster such a relationship, do the following:

- Prepare a list of questions and concerns you wish the physician to address.
- Make the physician aware of these questions and concerns at the beginning of the visit.
- Share your medical history, including symptoms, records, and any treatments with the doctor as completely and accurately as possible.
- Take along with you to the appointment someone who will also make relevant notes of the meeting since you may not catch everything the doctor says.

Also consider the following:

- Did you feel comfortable talking with the doctor?
- Did the doctor answer your questions thoroughly? Did the doctor seem hostile while you asked the questions?
- Did the doctor seem more interested in getting paid than in taking care of you?
- Was any of the doctor's behavior inappropriate?
- Did the doctor dismiss or trivialize any of your symptoms?
- Did the doctor treat you like an intelligent partner in your health care?
- Did the doctor encourage you to communicate freely, or did she/he seem too busy to listen?
- Do you like the doctor? (Follow your own gut feeling about her/him. You will be discussing very intimate details with this person, so how you feel about her/him must be paramount in your evaluation.)
- Did the doctor initially meet you with your clothes on or off? (Ellen T. Johnson advises that the clothes-off position is often

associated with vulnerability, especially since you are meeting with this person for the first time.)

Office Experience

Visits to the doctor's office can significantly impact the quality of your treatment. How the front-desk staff treats or speaks to you or how long you wait to be seen by the doctor will tell you plenty about how you may be treated as a patient. If you call and repeatedly get a busy signal, hear "I'm sorry, Dr. M. is not available right now" again and again, or sit in a waiting room for more than an hour, that's a signal that the doctor is probably too busy and may not be the right one for you.

Get a Referral or a Second Opinion

If after meeting with the doctor, you find that she/he cannot provide the degree of care you need, or you two cannot get along, then ask for a referral to see another specialist. Or if the treatment you receive has not sufficiently accomplished its desired result, then a second opinion may be in order. Second opinions are important; there are different levels of expertise within the endometriosis medical community. The level of expertise of your present doctor may not be sufficient to treat your endometriosis. The September 2004 issue of *Mayo Clinic Women's Health Source* advises a second opinion may be warranted if:

- Your current treatment isn't working.
- Your doctor suggests a procedure that is expensive, risky, or experimental.
- Your health plan will not pay for a certain type of procedure without a second opinion.

The following is a journal entry from Elisabet describing her search for Dr. Right:

Dr. Snake

Today I saw Dr. Snake. . . . Dr. Snake has got a bad vibe around her that I pick up on the minute she enters the room. She seems aggressive, and I feel uncomfortable asking her any questions at all. I'm sure glad that I have my paper with all the questions, or I probably would have left with no info at all. She is visibly upset and comments upon the fact that she knows I'm "looking around for a doctor." But instead of sneering, I think she ought to let me know why I should choose her. She also lets me know that if she were to perform surgery on me, she would have another surgeon there, a real specialist. Basically she admits that she sucks at endo surgery. She gives me two names of specialists and finds it highly amusing that I am unfamiliar with this one medical center in Beverly Hills that apparently is considered a good place. (Yep, she too laughed at me, although she was mostly dry.)

Anyways, her focus is on cancer. She tells me that there is a 1 percent chance of the cysts being malignant. She then reminds me that 1 percent is actually very high. And of course I freak out. She seems so pissed off for some reason. She is looking through my papers and asking me "Who did this ultrasound?" "Where did you get these blood tests?" She is obviously irritated. How dare I use many different doctors? I had no idea that was considered bad in any way.

Needless to say, I felt totally awful after this visit. . . . As I left, I just felt that she's right. I'm screwed. I'm likely to have cancer and I will die alone, a bitter childless person, in real bad pain.

When I went to see Dr. Great later that same day, my hopes were down on zero. I just wanted that article on nutritional approaches that people had told me he had in his possession, but I was actually in for a big surprise.

Dr. Great

Okay, so the conclusion is that two doctors' visits on the same day is just a little more than I can handle. Even without the examination. I started crying after my second sentence in Dr. Great's office. Highly embarrassing. I was sobbing something like, "They tell me I might have cancer and I won't be able to have children." Well, his reaction was big eyes, "Oh really? Cancer?" And then he went to get me some tissues. He is probably very used to this kind of behavior.

Anyway, this doctor's visit was like night and day compared to Dr. Snake. It became very obvious that she was not a specialist in the endo field and that here in front of me was one. On the door to the office it said "Endometriosis Center." It looked promising to me. When I came into the waiting room, I was so glad to see a simple place with no pictures of babies on the walls. It was a relief not to have the walls covered in smiling babies and the waiting room filled with highly pregnant women. It is just not what you need to see when you're in my situation.

I went to sign in and saw a small man who smiled at me and said hi. I was hoping that he would be Dr. Great, and he was. I didn't have to wait a second. I went to the bathroom and they told me to give a urine sample. Then, after my little meltdown cry, Dr. Great told me that I didn't need to worry about not getting pregnant. He had seen so many of his patients get pregnant. He calmly started to slowly, and very carefully, go through the ultrasounds with me. It reminded me of myself the way he checked and compared exactly the increase or decrease in the cysts. Not one of the other doctors had done that. Not one. . . . So it made me feel very good to watch him care, or at least pay attention to detail. That's a good quality in a potential surgeon, I thought.

I still felt stupid for crying, but I started my quiz. He

passed the trick questions easily. No, he certainly did not use medications to clean up. In fact, he didn't use medications at all! Lupron, he said, has no effect. And "there is no scientific evidence that the contraceptive pill has any effect on endometriosis." That's what I like to hear! Not "You'll have to use Lupron and then the contraceptive pill between pregnancies and RU-486 together with the pill and then some Depo-Provera." No "Endo is like a cancer and it has to be treated aggressively." No, no such speeches from Dr. Great. He simply stated that a successful surgery should do the job. There is no need for further medication. He is the first true specialist in the field whom I have met. . . . Don't get me wrong, he is in no way suggesting a cure. He simply is recommending the form of treatment that he has seen in his experience to work the best. I think I should learn my lesson. What I need is an endometriosis specialist. Not infertility doctors or general OB/GYN doctors. This is a specific problem I have; it needs a specific doctor.

I asked for a copy of the nutritional guidelines, and I got what I had originally come for. He then wanted to examine me, but I refused, stating my fear of the exam. He understood, and we decided to make an appointment for a week or two. I would need that anyway to sign consent papers for surgery. Dr. Great didn't laugh at me at any point during our meeting. He took my concerns seriously, and he was friendly. I left the office feeling calm and confident. I said to my partner straightaway when I came out from the office that "I think I have found my surgeon."

But as active partners in our health care, endometriosis patients have their own recommendations for their physicians. Melissa recommends the following:

What doctors may not realize is that when you give a gyne-cological exam to a woman with endometriosis, it can hurt very literally, and it can also bring emotions to the surface in a way that I can't really explain. Plainly, the exam makes me want to cry uncontrollably and I don't completely know why. The obvious thought occurred to me after valiantly or stupidly holding back tears at many appointments, "Maybe you want to cry because she is touching disease." This un-pleasant thought was actually a great relief to me, because I had been asking myself questions like, "Are you embar-rassed by the exam?" "Are you repressing some past abusive experience?" "Why are you so upset?" It is the pronounced emotion and intimacy involved in this disease that make it essential to have a doctor who will listen to you, will trust your interpretations of what is going on in your body, will know that it is sometimes extremely hard to get through an appointment or even to face the fact that there is something wrong inside of you, a doctor who will relate to you as a whole person.

If doctors can find time in their busy day to honor the fact that they are having a very personal interaction with each pa-tient, it can open up a new avenue for healing. I want to honor the fact that doctors possess wonderful knowledge and ability to heal, and I want them to honor the fact that I some-times deal with great pain, and I choose to ask them for help with this very personal issue. I'm not asking for a new friend; I am asking for a genuine interaction.

14

Become an Empowered Patient

Fear is the most common emotion when one has endometriosis. The fear comes from the knowledge that this is a chronic and unpredictable disease. The fear results from the knowledge of the long-term effects that this disease can have on one's ability to have a child, to have long-lasting intimate relationships, and even to function normally on a day-to-day basis. But you can overcome this fear with two very powerful tools: education and support. The following are some tools to help you become more involved in your treatment program and to prepare for your new life with endometriosis so that the fear will no longer be an overriding presence.

■ Become an Educated Patient

Knowledge is power. This holds true if you are diagnosed with a terminal illness or faced with the common cold. Once you are aware of what exactly a disease is, how it progresses, how and what it affects, and how it can be treated, you will be better armed to deal with this invading force in your life. You will make better and more informed decisions about treatments and also create a more effective relationship with your doctor. After all, an educated patient is an empowered patient.

Jude is a strong believer in self-education:

> *I have found it immensely helpful to educate myself about endo. I have read loads of books from the public library and looked at many Internet sites because I think knowing what is happening to my body helps me to cope better. I also think it helps me to communicate with my specialist better because I can ask questions based on a wider knowledge base.*

The importance of self-education in your overall treatment must not be underestimated. Through a consensus process at the Third Annual Disease Management Outcomes summit, under the theme "Defining the Patient-Physician Relationship for the 21st Century," held October 30 to November 2, 2003, in Phoenix, Arizona, more than 200 patients identified seven key components of the doctor-patient relationship, including education. In the document prepared after the summit, education is defined as the "drug of choice" for prevention and treatment of every medical condition. It recommends, among other things, that patients may obtain information from resources other than those offered by their health care provider, including the Internet, newspapers, friends, family, and nonmedically trained sources.

The study shows that once the patient takes the responsibility of education into her own hands, the following will be the possible positive outcomes:

- Improved patient recognition of important symptoms
- More informed decisions by patients
- Positive patient behavior changes
- Patients taking a more active role in their care

- A strong foundation to facilitate self-care
- Improved clinical outcomes

Learn to Read

An empowered patient is more involved in her own health care. This involves searching for as much of the medical and lay literature about endometriosis as possible in order to know exactly what you have. Currently, we are fortunate to have a growing amount of literature about endometriosis ranging from medical journal articles, reports on latest research, books, and very informative Web sites. Appendix A of this book features books and Web sites that provide in-depth information and the latest news about endometriosis.

Your search for literature about endometriosis can begin at any of the two national endometriosis awareness and support organizations, the Endometriosis Research Center (ERC) and the Endometriosis Association (EA). The ERC acts as a resource center for further education about the disease as well as support. It offers literature on endometriosis, fact sheets on many topics pertaining to the disease, and a monthly newsletter. To obtain a copy of the ERC's material request form, which lists all of their available educational materials and their prices, visit their Web site at http://www.endocenter.org or call their offices toll free at 800-239-7280. To receive a free sample copy of the latest edition of their newsletter, send your request, along with a #10 SASE, to 630 Ibis Drive, Delray Beach, FL 33444.

The EA publishes literature on endometriosis and related concerns regularly and also maintains a small library at its headquarters in Milwaukee, Wisconsin. The EA provides educational brochures in twenty-eight languages; a newsletter published four to six times per year that is free with membership; audio- and videotapes; and three books about endometriosis: *Endometriosis: The Complete Reference for Taking Charge of Your Health* (2003), *The Endometriosis Sourcebook* (1995), and *Overcoming Endometriosis* (1987). For a free information packet, call the EA at 800-992-3636.

Whichever method you choose in your search for literature—purchasing books, searching the Internet, contacting the ERC or the EA—reading about the disease should be your first point of attack. For Elisabet:

Reading and learning about endo became my first and most important tool to living with endo. It gave me the knowledge I needed to stick to what I wanted without putting myself at risk.

Join the Endometriosis Research Center (ERC) and/or the Endometriosis Association (EA)

Endometriosis has been described as an enigmatic disease. It is a leading cause of chronic pelvic pain in millions of women and teens; it is a leading cause of female infertility and gynecologic surgery, and it is the second-leading cause of hysterectomies performed annually. However, the disease is still shrouded in mystery, resulting in delayed diagnosis for a majority of women and improper treatments for many who have been diagnosed. How do we uncover the mystery behind endometriosis? This is where the ERC and the EA come in. These two organizations strive to research and understand the disease, promote awareness of the disease's existence and impact on the up to 11 million women and teens diagnosed with endometriosis in the United States, and support the diagnosed and their families.

The ERC is an established 501(c)3 nonprofit organization that was founded by Michelle E. Marvel in 1997, to address the international need for education, research, and support regarding endometriosis. Its six main areas of emphasis:

- To find a cure for endometriosis
- To provide support and help to improve the quality of life for women suffering with endometriosis
- To raise public awareness about the disease

∎ To educate health care providers, patients, policy makers, and the public

∎ To provide an international network for women to exchange information and ideas

∎ To fund further research on all aspects of the disease

Since its beginning in 1997, the ERC has become a recognized figure in efforts to increase recognition of the disease, specifically among policy makers. It has had successes in the legislative arena, raising recognition about issues pertinent to endometriosis education and research among local, state, and federal representatives. It was through its tireless efforts that the first-ever National Endometriosis Awareness Resolution, H. Con. Res. 291, was drafted and unanimously passed by Congress. This resolution recognizes the disease and formally declared March as Endometriosis Awareness month. It has also enjoyed many successes in Florida, California, Pennsylvania, Michigan, Colorado, and New York.

The ERC does not charge members to join the organization or to benefit from its many programs. They offer several in-person support groups throughout the United States, Canada, and the Caribbean as well as the largest online endometriosis support group. To get involved or attend in-person meetings, you can search the listing, which includes complete contact information, at http://www .endocenter.org/supportgroups.htm. The online, moderated discussion group can be found at http://groups.yahoo.com/group/erc. To join, contact:

Endometriosis Research Center

World Headquarters
630 Ibis Drive
Delray Beach, FL 33444
Toll Free: 800-239-7280
Phone: 561-274-7442

Fax: 561-274-0931
URL: http://www.endocenter.org
E-mail: AskERC@aol.com

The EA was the first self-help organization in the world created
for women with endometriosis and has become a recognized au-
thority in the field. Its ultimate goal is to work toward finding a
cure for the disease as well as providing education, support, and
research. The association was founded by Mary Lou Ballweg and
Carolyn Keith in 1980 and has become an international organization with headquarters in Milwaukee, Wisconsin.

Since its beginning, the EA has achieved many goals, including
undertaking mass educational projects, publishing three books, and
leading in research activities. The association currently has a special
program at Dartmouth Medical School and has funded and assisted
a number of researchers from across the world. The association has
recently teamed up with Vanderbilt University School of Medicine
to create a dedicated research facility to address the mechanisms responsible for causing endometriosis.

Other research projects supported by the association include:

■ A study of dioxin-exposed young women in Seveso, Italy
■ Publicity and help obtaining patients and families for a genetic
  study at Oxford University, England
■ Support for research on a noninvasive diagnostic technique by
  a U.S. researcher
■ Small grants and tissue samples for a number of researchers
  studying dioxin and related toxins and endometriosis

The association has a network of chapters and groups in sixty-six
countries and numerous benefits for members. To become a member, you can write to the EA for more information. You will receive
a membership form, which lists the different types of membership

and their corresponding fees. You can also join from their Web site at http://www.endometriosisassn.org/membership_cart.html. To join, contact:

Endometriosis Association

International Headquarters
8585 N. 76th Place
Milwaukee, WI 53223
Toll-free: 800-992-3636
Phone: 414-355-2200
Fax: 414-355-6065
URL: http://www.endometriosisassn.org
E-mail: support@endometriosisassn.org

Become an E-Patient

One very integral tool in the information gathering process is the Internet. According to Roberta Speyer, president of Medispecialty.com and publisher of OBGYN.net, the Internet has become a major educational force and communication tool for many patients. These figures prove it: A Harris poll in 2001 found that 75 percent of all adults nationwide use the Internet to look for health care information. A follow-up Harris poll in 2002 found that the number increased to 110 million adults or 80 percent of all adults online.

A Pew Internet and American Life Project Internet Health Resources survey in 2003 found that 80 percent of adult Internet users, or about 93 million Americans, have searched for at least one of sixteen major health topics online. This makes the act of looking for health or medical information one of the most popular activities online, after sending/receiving e-mail (93 percent) and researching a product or service before buying it (83 percent). The survey found that the most popular health topic search concerns a specific disease or medical problem, with as much as 63 percent of all Internet users seeking information on a particular disease or medical problem.

The study found that, among other things, Internet health seekers go online to:

- Search for health information at any time of the day or night
- Research a diagnosis or prescription
- Prepare for surgery or find out how best to recover from one
- Get tips from other caregivers and e-patients about dealing with a particular symptom
- Give and receive emotional support
- Keep family and friends informed of a loved one's condition
- Find humor and even joy in a bad situation

The study also found that, in general, women are more likely than men to search for health information online, with some 85 percent of women online compared to 75 percent of men. The Internet has now become the number one tool among endometriosis patients to first gather information about what exactly this disease entails.

As Tiffiny explains:

To try and stem my panic and feeling of being totally out of control, I immersed myself into the depth and breadth of the Internet, hungrily looking for anything and everything on endo. In the absence of familiar faces and comfort, I built an armor of knowledge around my fragile body.

The Internet thus empowers you to become an effective advocate in your own health care. As stated by the Pew Internet and American Life Project report: "An educated consumer stands a better chance of getting better treatment, and the Internet can be a significant resource for that health education process."

But how reliable is the information gathered from the Internet? The Internet has become the biggest library in the world, and it has transformed the way many persons seek and find health information.

However, the main drawback of the Internet is the fact that it is un-regulated and the quality of the medical information varies.

The Pew Internet and American Life Project Internet Health Resources report found that "only about one-quarter of health seekers follow the recommended protocol on thoroughly checking the source and timeliness of information and are vigilant about verifying a site's information every time they search for health information." Another quarter of health seekers check a site's information "most of the time," while half of all health seekers "only sometimes," "hardly ever," or "never" check the source or date of the information they read online.

To rule out unreliable information, the Medical Library Association (MLA) recommends the following verification protocols when searching for information on the Internet:

- *Check the health site's sponsor:* Sponsorship is important because it helps establish the site as respected and dependable. The Web address itself can provide additional information about the nature of the site and intent. A .gov, .edu, .org, or .net address represents a government agency, an educational institution such as a university, a professional organization such as a medical association like the American Medical Association (AMA— http://www.ama-assn.org), or a network of similar companies, such as financial institutions. Commercial sites are represented by .com and will most often identify the sponsor as a company.
- *Check the date of the information:* The Web site should be updated frequently and reflect the most current information on the subject. The Web site should also be consistently available, with the date of the latest revision clearly posted, usually at the bottom of the home page.
- *Check the accuracy of the information:* Information should be factual, not opinionated—and capable of being verified from a

primary information source such as a professional journal or
links to other Web pages.

- *Check for the health site's primary audience:* The Web site
should clearly state whether the information is intended for the
consumer or the health professional. On the other hand, many
health information Web sites maintain two different areas—
one for consumers and one for professionals. The design of the
site should make selection of one area over the other clear to
the visitor. For instance, OBGYN.net clearly indicates what is
content for medical professionals and what is intended for
women at the top of the Web site and on every page.

The California Healthcare Foundation also recommends the following:

- Set aside enough time for a health search.
- Visit four to six sites to verify the information you have gathered.
- Discuss the information found on the Internet with a health
care provider before making any treatment decisions.

While the Internet holds great benefit for the information-hungry
endometriosis patient, you need to heed a word of caution. The Internet will never replace an office visit or a personal conversation
with your doctor, but it can be a starting point in taking control
over your endometriosis.

▪ ▪ ▪ How to Become an Empowered Patient ▪ ▪ ▪

By Your Fellow Endo-Sisters

"The more you know, the better you can control the disease."

—Heather C. Guidone

No one understood what I was going through. Sickness is often equated with weakness, and everyone around me thought I was simply weak. Given that endometriosis is a poorly understood disease by society at large, people told me to "just have a hysterectomy and be cured." Frustrated at my inability to get those around me to understand that it's just not that simple, I recognized a new emotion: anger.

The anger saved my life. Anger drove me to learn everything about endometriosis—and to find as many others with the disease as I could. Tapping into the vast resources available on the Internet, I discovered that there were indeed others like me—and they understood, physicians and patients alike. After swimming in a sea of pain, heartbreak, and despair for over a decade, I was a thrown a lifeline.

By the end of 1996, I had become a walking encyclopedia on endometriosis. I knew the proposed etiology of the disease, the vast realm of symptoms, what the best treatment options for this incurable illness were, and how to find others who understood. I found the Endometriosis Research Center and contacted the executive director, expressing to her my interest in wanting to give back some of the support I had received and my desire to learn even more about endometriosis. We began a friendly relationship, unified by the common bond of endometriosis. Later, I was asked to volunteer as a community leader for a prominent women's health network, providing support and education to those interested in learning more about the disease. I felt I had finally found my niche.

The problem that remained, however, was that I was still very, very sick.

Then I hit the Web site of the Center for Endometriosis Care, a specialty surgery center located in Georgia. The surgeons there are among the few in the country who perform excision surgery for endometriosis. The concept is simple: remove all disease from all locations to end the symptoms. It was as if a light went on inside my head: I needed to have surgery with them, and soon. In 1997, I did.

Five weeks later, I was pregnant with my son.

So began my soul-searching process. I knew that I could not continue in my high-stress job and take care of my health—and that of my growing baby's—the way I needed and deserved to. For several weeks, I reflected on how far I had come in my life and thought about where I wanted to go. What would truly make me happy? Then it all became clear. I wanted to work in the endometriosis community.

Since I made the decision to break from mainstream corporate America, I have been volunteering in various medical communities as an endometriosis supporter and educator; working on endometriosis medical sites as content manager, copyeditor, and coordinator; writing (a hidden love of mine since I first had my book of poems published in grade school), and devoting my time to raising my son. I am now with the Endometriosis Research Center full-time, no longer just an occasional volunteer. As an executive board member and the director of operations for the ERC, I have found, aside from being a mom, the most rewarding career I've ever had. Better still, the ERC's executive director and the organization's team members are no longer just mere acquaintances, but closer to me than many of my family members. Many women in the endometriosis community are like sisters to me, separated by distance but bound by our hearts.

Nowadays, aside from being a mom to the son the medical community said I'd never have, I travel on business related to endometriosis, write extensively about the disease for publications and books, speak publicly on endometriosis to women and their families, lobby for more research and funding, and strive every day to raise disease awareness. Best of all, I have made a difference in the lives of others—albeit a small one, but a positive difference nonetheless. Helping others has enabled me to help myself. More important, I have made a difference in my own life. Turning my anger into empowerment and taking back control of my health care enabled me to rise above this disease, much like the proverbial phoenix from the ashes.

Endometriosis does not have to own you. You must be an empowered patient. The more you know, the better you can control the disease. If you had asked me ten years ago where I would be today, I would never have imagined doing any of the things I am today. I am not cured. Some days I am not even well. I am approaching my twentieth year in the battle against endometriosis. I've been on more medications, undergone more surgeries (including a total hysterectomy at age twenty-eight), and spent more time in hospitals than almost anyone I know. I have been subjected to the haughty condescension of doctors and others who told me the pain was all in my head. I have dealt with the suspicion of those around me that I was exaggerating my pain. Relationships in my life have suffered. I have sacrificed a lot to this illness, as most women with endometriosis have.

But at the end of the day I own my disease; it does not own me. Endometriosis has changed me, but in the long run, it has been for the better. I am not a woman defined by my reproductive organs, but by my heart and mind.

If not for endometriosis, I would not have looked long and hard inside myself and decided what was really important in the "big picture" of my life. If not for those in the endometriosis community, I would have not learned until it was too late that there are riches beyond wealth and sometimes, the opportunities of a lifetime are right in front of you.

Take charge and put the control of your health back in your hands. You can live well in spite of endometriosis, and we can beat this disease—one woman at a time.

Some Tips for the Reader

By Moira Allen

1. If you have chronic pain, don't write it off as "normal." Don't assume that it's just something every woman has. Don't let your doctor write it off either. If he (or she) does, find another doctor who will listen and counsel you.
2. Track your pain. Keep a diary of what hurts, and how, and when. Determine when your "worst" pain is—whether it's before, during, or after your period. This can help in diagnosing endometriosis.
3. Don't let a doctor pressure you into a decision you're not prepared to make. When I finally chose to have a hysterectomy, it was MY choice on MY timing. I'd had time to gather information, study (and test) my options, and make an informed decision.
4. If possible, share your situation with your spouse or significant other. It really helps to have an understanding partner who will support you in your decision—and who will actively help out when you're incapacitated.
5. Find a GOOD doctor who will listen to you—not just to your physical complaints, but to how you feel about your body, and about treatment. We all have emotional reactions and responses to our bodies; your doctor needs to be willing to work with you on a treatment

plan that addresses your emotional concerns as well as your physical needs.

6. Don't be afraid to walk away from a doctor who doesn't listen or who gives "orders" rather than "options." Unless you actually have cancer, you don't have to make a decision "today." You've lived with endometriosis for years, and you can live with it for a few more weeks (or months) as you decide the best approach. If you get the impression that you're just another mortgage payment to your doctor (or perhaps a down payment on his yacht), go somewhere else.

7. Believe that things can get better. If you've been living with endometriosis for years, you don't know what "normal life" is either. Instead, you've learned a host of ways to "cope" with a condition that has become so familiar that you scarcely realize how much it is stealing from your life. Fighting endometriosis isn't just about minimizing the pain. It's about getting your life back.

▋ Get Support

Important in your struggle with endometriosis is support. This will be an irreplaceable tool. Knowing that you are not alone will positively impact your treatment. Family members, friends, and in-person and online support groups can make up your support network.

Family Members

They will make up your direct forms of support. These are the persons who see the day-to-day effects of endometriosis on you. Talk to them and explain the extent of your illness. Share with them the lay literature you found on endometriosis and ask for their support in your struggle with this disease. Tell them what you need, do not assume that they will know what you need. The responses you get from them will vary, but you will become aware of those who will be the cornerstone of your support network and those who will not be helpful. Says Jude:

> Telling my family has had mixed reactions from "Endometriosis . . . what's that?" to "You had a hysterectomy and that fixed it." I think it is hard for people to understand that the pain is constant, not just when I'm having my period, and it doesn't just get better on its own (like the flu). I have found it really difficult to get through to some family members that there is no "quick fix" solution and this is a long-term, complex thing. Just because it worked for them does not mean it will work for me.

For Seph the experience was different:

> My family is in the medical profession, with my dad a doctor and my mum a nurse, so I found everyone was supportive from the beginning. I let everyone know what was going on. I think most people thought it explained a lot over the years and that I did have a reason for all my moaning and groaning about being sick all the time.

Still, the task of talking to others about this disease that you have can be a difficult one. So says Amanda:

> It'd be nice to talk about this with my family and friends, but they all are too uncomfortable. They pretend that I do not have endometriosis. They think that I am either a hypochondriac, malingering for attention, or both. If I talk about it,

then I get a strained tone and a quickly changed subject. They have made comments like "That is all over now" or "Why would it come back, don't be silly you had it taken care of." My sister believes me because she has seen the pain, and occasionally she expresses empathy, but she is far away and very distant.

So all I have is my husband. He tries to listen and he tries to understand, and most of the time he does a pretty good job. Sometimes I would like it if he'd speak sharply to our parents and say, "Why are you so unsupportive of your daughter/(in law)? She is suffering a painful disease and having to make choices that normal twenty-four-year-olds do not have to make." I wish he realized how much it hurts me that my family won't acknowledge what I am going through. I do not want their sympathy, but perhaps their interest/caring/empathy and sometimes their ears too. Most of all I want them to realize that I do not want to be this way; I did not choose this disease. I want to be normal.

Spouses and Significant Others

Usually spouses and significant others will find it difficult to understand what endometriosis is all about. Often the male response to a problem is to fix it. Their inability to "fix" endometriosis in their loved ones will make them frustrated. You must make them understand the life-changing effects of this disease. As Ellen T. Johnson says: "The trick in any close relationship is to keep talking, even when you don't feel like it."

Educate them about the disease to ensure the right kind of support from your spouse or significant other when you need it. Instead of fixing, tell them what you need: a backrub, a hot-water bottle, or even their help with cooking dinner. Make them an integral part of your treatment to ensure you get their support in dealing with endometriosis. For Jude:

My husband has found the endometriosis experience very difficult, and I think because we are such good buddies we have stayed together. I think he struggles seeing me in pain because he can't fix it. Whenever I am having surgery, bursts of renovating get done around the house so he can fix something. At times we both ask why our lives are so difficult, with the emotional, financial, and relationship stress that occurs with endometriosis. It is amazing when you get talking to people just how many are affected by endometriosis and the extent to which they and their families suffer.

Nancy Petersen, RN, has this to say about her own experiences as a registered nurse, having to deal with men/husbands whose significant others have endometriosis:

I have sat with hundreds of men while their wives were undergoing surgery for excision of endo. Those who were motivated to travel to a center of excellence in endo excision were also highly supportive of their wives. But they did have a common thread with other men whom I saw throughout the U.S. and Canada when lecturing on endo. They all wanted to FIX IT!!

Men tend to be linear in their thinking, and want it fixed, and it is hard for them to believe that most docs cannot fix it. In many cases it can be fixed for long periods of time and or permanently, but the techniques are spreading slowly, with the big bucks of drug therapy obstructing the process as well as the old tried and supposedly true BUT UNTESTED beliefs of pregnancy, hormonal therapy, laser surgery, and hysterectomy. We now know that endo persisting after all of the above is the norm. An outrageous situation in women's health today when you look at the numbers of women whose lives are severely impacted in adverse ways.

If 5 million men suffered unbearable pain during sex, bowel movements, exercise, pelvic exams (just the thought of this one makes me chuckle), and were offered as treatment pregnancy, feminizing hormones or surgical castration—well you can see where I am going with this—endo would be a national emergency to which we would dedicate the defense budget. These things have been done so long that they are accepted, but in fact excision is the only therapy that has been put to the scientific process and held up.

So, when the docs doubt the patient who has been in pain so long, and nothing works, it tends to seep into the families, parents, siblings, kids, and husbands. It is frustrating but in a way understandable, as they just want life to get better, and to enjoy basic activities such as sex and going places and other fun things. But for women with endo, it is often an insurmountable struggle until they find ways to get their endo out. And until anyone has walked in our shoes . . .

Lorie is sure that she would not have been able to cope with endometriosis without the support of her husband Jimmy:

I have read that endo can be hard on a marriage, and sometimes they will end. I agree that it is very hard at times on a marriage; the mood swings are the worst for my husband and me, but we work really hard to understand that it is my body that makes me moody. The pain and the out-of-wack hormones make me so mean sometimes that I don't think about what I am about to say and the words come out so wrong. I try to let him know that I am having a really bad day and usually I get very quiet because I don't want to say the wrong things. He understands and leaves me alone.

Jimmy is a really great guy, he truly loves me or he wouldn't have stuck by me for the past thirteen years. I thank

God that he gave me a very understanding and caring husband. Without Jimmy's help and support I don't think I could make it as well as I do. He is there for the good times and for the bad. I don't like him to have to see and go through the bad times, but if he weren't here I wouldn't have anyone's shoulder to cry on. Thank you, Jimmy, for all that you do for me. I love you.

Jimmy, Lorie's husband, has some advice for spouses, significant others, and relatives:

I'd . . . like to say a few words to the husbands, boyfriends, or any relative who might be living with a special woman with endo. There may be mood swings, quiet times, and just times that they say (even without speaking a word), "I need my space. I'm not in the mood for intimacy. I don't need the extra pain right now." But be patient. It doesn't mean they have stopped loving you. They may just need time to cope. We all need that from time to time. I know it's hard. But the good times can return. And when they do, make the most of them. Cuddle up on the couch with a good movie. Go out for the night. Whatever you do, make the most of it. It's worth it all just to have a woman who loves you beside you when you fall asleep at night. And if she asks for help, give it to her without question. Chances are that if she could, she would take care of the task herself. She didn't do anything to deserve this and it's our place, as the people who love them, to help them whenever possible. One thing I am trying to learn is not to push her. I just want to make her as comfortable as possible.

There is so much frustration, anger, disappointment, and the list goes on and on. Frustration sets in when the mood swings pop up. I know it isn't her fault, but at those times it seems that I just can't do anything right. And the last thing I want to do is get into an argument. She may kill me for saying this, but at those times I tell her to watch her nagging and go on. Another thing that frustrates me is when she is hurting and I can see it in her face but she won't share it with me. Anger. Now there is a big one. I obviously can't take away the pain for her, but it drives me crazy that we can't seem to find anyone who can.

For now, we will just take it one day at a time and I will continue giving her the same unconditional love that I have been giving her all these years.

Edward shared the following:

My Girlfriend's Pain—My Pain
By Edward Rendini

I am a twenty-three-year-old man who lives with endometriosis every single day. I experience its brutal, relentless nature firsthand, through the ever-present pain and tears welled up in the beautiful eyes of my best friend. I sit by helplessly as it cripples her over and over again. You see, my girlfriend Athina has endometriosis, and much of the time, I feel as if I have it too.

Endometriosis is a horrific, miserable disease that can slowly destroy a relationship. It's evil and I hate it. I hate that my girlfriend suffers because of it. I hate that I have to watch her suffer because of it. I hate that she hasn't had a decent night's sleep in years because of it. I hate that she hasn't had the pleasure of even one pain-free day, in recent memory, because of it. Mostly, though, I hate that there is nothing I can do about it. Nothing I can do to relieve her pain. Nothing I

can do to restore her life. Nothing I can do to make her truly
happy. Nothing.

Without any warning or predictable pattern this disease
steals something very precious to a couple. Time. It rips away
days, then weeks, then months, then years. Time that should
have been spent being happy is instead spent being worried.
Worried about what we can and can't do. Worried about
where we can and can't go. Worried about anything and
everything that might make the pain worse. Endometriosis
controls us. Our plans, our days, our lives.

I have dated Athina for well over three years, and the signs
of her endo were there at the beginning. I hadn't even known
her very long when we had our first trip to the emergency
room because of the pain. They, of course, misdiagnosed her.

She went to other doctors. Doctors whom I found and doctors whom she found. Still she was misdiagnosed over and
over. They actually told her she had a low threshold for pain
and that the problem was simply menstrual cramps combined
with that low threshold.

I knew they were wrong. I knew there was something more
and so did she. I watched her every day keeled over with pain,
in the bed, unable to move, for hours or days on end. Crying
herself to sleep every night. Ice packs, heating pads, pain relievers, prescription drugs; nothing ever helped and nothing
ever worked. She had no relief. I had no relief.

When I was there, I suffered with her. When I wasn't there,
I constantly thought about her suffering. Feeling guilty that I
couldn't do anything to help. Feeling guilty that I couldn't be
there all the time. Feeling guilty that she was in this pain and I
wasn't. Basically just feeling guilty about everything, all the
time.

If I hadn't loved her so much I would have broken up with

her. I know this probably sounds cold, but it's true. It's just too much to go through if you don't love the person. If you're not sure you want to spend the rest of your life with them. If you're not absolutely sure they're the one. It's just too much.

But I do love her that much, and I was always sure. I never doubted it, and so I stayed and helped the best I could and am still helping today. I try to cheer her up. I try to take her mind off the pain. I try to make her happy.

I've been with her through two endo-related operations, countless sleepless nights, depression, mood swings, relationship problems, and much more. Still, she has always made me happy. Being with her makes me happy.

I just wish she could be happier. The pain basically rips away any happiness she manages to muster up. But things are looking up. Her last endo-related procedure was judged a success by both the surgeon and her gynecologist. Although she is still in pain now, it is supposed to slowly subside over the coming months and then, eventually, rear its ugly head only around her time of the month.

I know that may not sound like much. But to me, it's the best news I've ever gotten in my life. The thought of her not being in pain all the time is pure joy.

In my head I know that the endo is a part of her. For good or bad, it comes with the package. In my heart, however, I see it only as a leech that sucks the freedom and happiness out of her life. Something foreign that should not be there. Something that needs to be eliminated.

I feel guilty, almost torn, at times because of how I feel about her disease. It's a part of her that I despise. I hate it. I hate what it puts her through. I hate what it puts us through.

But at the same time I love her. But more importantly, I love her no less than I would if there was no endo.

I never understood how someone could love a person while hating something about them. It never made any sense to me. You either love all of them or none of them. Right?

Wrong.

Now I understand. Now it's the thing about life and relationships that I understand best.

▌▌▌ The Partner's Predicament, ▌▌▌ or What About the Men?

By Robert B. Albee, MD

(Reprinted with permission from Dr. Robert Albee)

Disease and pain cause stress and strain on every relationship. However, they can also offer opportunities for tremendous growth in that relationship. When illness occurs, we naturally focus our attention on the ill person. Because an illness often lessens their coping skills, the sick person's weaknesses may become more noticeable. (For example, a person who is somewhat dependent on others may become increasingly unable to function alone, while a person who is more independent may become increasingly isolated.)

Our natural inclination is to excuse these behaviors because of the illness. This is very easy in short-term illnesses where the diagnosis is straightforward and simple for others to understand. However, when there is trouble getting a diagnosis, or when the diagnosis is difficult to understand, or when the disease seems unending, the behaviors of the sick person can seem unacceptable.

Relationships that are already weak are the most vulnerable to the strains an illness produces. When partners lack communication skills, or don't use them, when they are quick to accuse and slow to forgive, then illness can cause a crippling blow.

Endometriosis is a disease of women. Men do not get endometriosis (they never even experience a normal period, much less the pain of endo). Women with the disease have these questions about their partners:

▪ Why isn't he involved?
▪ Why doesn't he believe I'm in pain?
▪ Why is he so quiet when I'm hurting?
▪ How can I meet his physical needs (and my own) when intercourse is so painful?

Why Isn't He Involved?

This question implies that men should understand your pain and disease. Let's agree that they should *try* to understand. As noted, the entire menstrual cycle is foreign to a man's experience, and endometriosis can be totally confusing. For example, a common question from men is, "If the problem is with the reproductive organs, why does my wife blame her fatigue on endometriosis?"

If men are involved in the entire process of evaluating the problem and seeking a correct diagnosis, they tend to reach a greater level of understanding. Therefore, we in the medical profession need to encourage men to be a co-student in the learning process. More often than not, when I see men with their wives at consultations, pre-op, and post-op visits, I feel I am dealing with a couple who are actively building their relationship, and not allowing it to dissolve.

When I talk to men who are not involved I hear a number of different excuses. Some men say that they think their wives want them not to be present. Some say they are uncomfortable in any medical situation. Lots of men are ill at ease when situations seem out of their control. One man said, "I don't see how we can spend any more money; nothing has worked so far, and we are deep in debt."

To Involve Your Partner:

- Choose a doctor who will educate you and your spouse about endometriosis. Find someone who will take extra time, if needed.
- Know that some doctors are intimidated by certain situations. If bringing your husband to a doctor's appointment makes the doctor obviously uncomfortable, then you need another doctor.
- Communicate! Tell your partner about changes in the way you feel. But try to do it in a way to show him that you are sharing information that can help you both, and not in an angry way, or some other way that could make him feel responsible for your pain.
- Ask him to read informational materials (such as this newsletter) and then tell you what he thinks about things that might relate to your situation.
- If you know another couple dealing with endometriosis, get together to share information and support. It's always easier to cope when we are not alone.
- Offer to set up a personal consultation for him with your doctor (and without you). Attention would be focused on answering his questions and his concerns.
- Reassure him that you want to feel better.
- Don't assume *anything* about his understanding or feelings. Ask him.

Why Doesn't He Believe I'm in Pain?

Endometriosis can't be readily seen or touched. Adequate communication about the disease and the way you feel is essential in helping your partner understand. He can't read your mind: you must tell him how and where you hurt.

Some men are themselves very insensitive to pain, or have never had an experience where pain immobilized them. They do not automatically understand or have sympathy for the variety and intensity of pain that endometriosis can bring.

Sadly, some relationships include routine disbelief between partners. In such situations, communications break down because the truth is *always* questioned.

To Explain the Pain:

- Show him where you hurt, as specifically as you can.
- Don't assume that he knows.
- Tell him *every* time you feel better.
- Tell him each step you take toward learning more or feeling better.
- Ask for his help. You may be surprised at what he has noticed and can give you feedback on.
- No matter how silly it may seem to you, be prepared to try each of his suggestions. This shows you respect his judgment and welcome his participation.

Why Is He So Quiet When I'm Hurting?

Men are trained from childhood to provide for and protect their mates. A man watching his wife endure severe pain that he can't stop often faces a serious threat to his manhood. He feels helpless to save her from something that is ruining the quality of her life.

A common response to this situation is to withdraw. Your

husband may feel that there is no way to fight the enemy, and so he may throw up his hands wondering what to do. It is so very difficult to comfort someone you feel you have let down. The result may be silence.

To Help Him Reconnect with You:

- Let him know that you don't expect him to fix the problem. Remind him that it's no one's fault that you have endometriosis, and certainly not his.
- Tell him how much his closeness means to you. It will help him to know that just comforting you is meeting his duties as a husband.
- Convince him that he has not let you down.

Intercourse Hurts. Now What?

It is very rare for men to experience anything that interferes with their sex drives. It is even more uncommon for intercourse to cause pain for a man. This makes it hard for a man to understand how pain and the fear of it can interfere with a woman's sex drive. Sometimes the woman suffers through intercourse without saying anything. She loves her husband and wants to satisfy him. However, it's hard to play an enthusiastic, responsive partner when you're in pain. And the man who loves her can often tell that something is wrong, but he doesn't know what. He may assume that he has failed to satisfy her. The couple may move further apart.

Now This:

- Tell your partner everything he does to satisfy your sexual needs. Men and women approach sexuality differently, and he may not understand just how important touching, caressing, and cuddling can be to you. Reassure him often.

▪ Don't let painful intercourse keep you from other forms of sexual expression. Do for your husband all that you can, and let him know the things you like him to do for you. Be creative!

Spend time developing in his mind your determined hope to be able to enjoy physical intimacy to its ultimate. He needs to know that he is still the one you desire above all others.

Friends and Colleagues

Your friendships will also be altered by your endometriosis diagnosis. While some friends may be very concerned and helpful, others may become estranged over a period of time, disturbed by your diagnosis and not knowing how to deal with it. Others may pretend that everything is the same; nothing has changed. These latter types of friends may not understand your complaints of pain or inability to handle former activities and may even dismiss these as exaggerations or attention seeking. These are not suitable candidates for your support network.

However, good friends are treasures. Talk openly to those who are willing to support you about what is going on with you and how they can help. Educate them about the disease and make them aware of what you can and cannot do. If they are your true friends, they will understand and will support you. Seph says:

My friends had mixed reactions. Mostly they were supportive and although at first, like myself, they didn't really understand, they asked questions and were interested to find out more information on endo, which I thought was wonderful. There were a few though who found it hard to deal with, and

I haven't really heard from them since. But like most things in life, difficult times bring out the best and worst in people, and this was no exception.

Elisabet has found that endometriosis can seriously impact various types of relationships. She describes how she deals with the potential impacts:

Endo has affected my relationships and my whole life so much. I always thought that when a person becomes ill, people automatically gather around that person in an effort to help and support. I now know that the very opposite reaction is surprisingly common. I believe that fear is the reason for this. I have been forced to deal with relationships in a new, more mature way.

I have found that two main techniques work best for me. Honesty is the first one. I have always thought of myself as a very honest person. But endo has taught me that there were many times I simply didn't say what I was thinking. I have now learned and refined the art of thinking out loud and not being scared to admit who I really am. I learned this from my friend Carla, who is the other support group leader together with me in the L.A. group. Her honesty was striking from our very first meeting. Having lived with endo for so many years and, on top of that, being a psychologist, she had learned what worked and what didn't work for her. I quickly tried her technique and have not turned back since. Total honesty with people around me works best for me too. If I'm in pain, I say so. If the pain makes me grumpy and not nice, I explain why I'm acting that way. I apologize and keep doing my best to behave maturely (i.e., being grumpy).

Since the alternative treatment I follow involves a lot of special nutritional needs and herbal teas, social life often becomes a casualty or at least more difficult. I had just gotten to know a new friend who kept asking to go out and hang with me. I thought to myself, It's impossible, I can't do it, when would I have the time between my herbal teas? I don't want to admit I have endo because I don't want to be the person who starts a new friendship talking about their uterus. Plus, she's going to think I'm neurotic, only eating special foods etc. etc. So, I didn't return her phone calls and I answered with avoidance whenever she wanted to plan something with me. Then I decided to try total honesty. So, I promptly told my new friend, "This is my life, this is what I suffer from and this is how I deal with it." Take it or leave it. I simply decided to stand for what I am and how I live. I am the person who talks about her uterus, whether I like it or not. Since I was still so insecure about my lifestyle choices, I was sure she'd deem me mad and leave, but instead she started giving me lots of information on alternative treatments for endo and became a good friend. The outcome could not have been better. The relief I felt was enormous. I realized that although I don't like that endo is part of my life. It's a waste of time trying to hide it.

My other strategy is something that I learned on the first endo Web site I visited. Simply put, if I keep talking with a person about endo and it keeps feeling bad, that is, if the conversation makes me sad, low, depressed, or upset, over and over, then there is no real use in discussing the problem with this person. At some point you have to learn to let go of the thought that all people are going to give you support. It's fine, not all people can give an endo sufferer support. You can still be good friends. I have so many other sides to me. So much else going on in my life, so many interests, dreams, and hopes there will be enough to talk about with this person too. It's really not a big deal. If it doesn't make me stronger or happier or feeling like I can deal with endo better, it's only negative, and I don't need more negative in my life right now. So, it actually saves the relationship to stop discussing something that will upset me. This has been a great tool for me. It's liberating and it's a great way of protecting myself from negative energy. I need all the positivity in the world. I can discuss endo with other people. I have so many supportive endo friends, and healthy friends. Talking to them always leaves me with a feeling of renewed energy and relief, not despair. That's what friends are for. It's difficult to explain or define the difference between one good friend and another and their ability to support or not, but you know what I mean when you feel it.

Illness really makes all things in life more crystallized. The friends who understand and support become clearer and those friendships grow deeper, and the people who make things worse are dealt with differently.

Support Groups

Talking with other women with similar situations is very valuable and empowering. In these various support groups, whether in person or online, you will meet other women who share your concerns and problems. You can ask questions of one another and have an understanding of the disease based on their own experiences. This kind of information you cannot get from people who do not have the disease. Amy benefited from these online support groups:

I am finding more info out there about it and some wonderful Web sites offering support and answers to the many questions we all seem to have. I find a lot of comfort in knowing I am not alone. While I have a great man and family in my life, no one but another woman with endo can really understand what it is like.

The ERC and EA offer several in-person support groups across the United States and the world. Contact each organization for a list of their groups to find one near you. Appendix A lists a number of online endometriosis communities you can join.

This is what Danielle had to say about her experience with an online support group:

The Internet soon became my lifeline and my biggest tool in self-education. I began to put the pieces together, and the vastness of this disease unfolded before my eyes. I felt dumbfounded, scared, and depressed both by the medical data I had found and by the stories that were being shared. I soon became part of a family I never knew existed but could now not live without; I was an endo-sister with millions of women worldwide who would lend an ear, give advice, share their battles and their tears for a stranger at the other end of the keyboard.

Elisabet has this to say about her attendance at an in-person support group:

It felt great to get to share and hear what others have gone through, both the tough parts and the more hopeful parts like people actually getting children. It was liberating to bitch about everything we endo sufferers hate, like crazy doctors, bad nurses, crappy hospital experiences, bad "support" from friends and family, weird thoughts in moments of pain, stupid cancer medicines that don't work, the frustration of never being taken seriously. Still, after multiple surgeries, you get people who don't think it's so bad, just some period cramps. The desperation and depression we had all felt and still sometimes feel. The grief of losing unborn children, the frustration of infertility. But also trying to find a solution to-

gether. It does bring you instantly close to everyone in the room. I guess it's the feeling of strength that comes from the unity. So different from the cold loneliness you feel when you sit naked, clad only in a paper gown, waiting for the gynecologist to come in and cause you more pain and then give you more bad news.

Remember, this is your battle, so preparation is the key. First and foremost, educate yourself. Get to know as much as possible about this new skin called endometriosis and you are on your way to effectively treating the disease. Further empower yourself by seeking support from family members, spouses, and significant others, friends and fellow endo-sisters from in-person and online support groups. You will of course happen upon several roadblocks along the way, but remember you need to become an active participant in your health care in order to live well with endometriosis.

I close with an extract from Dr. Mark Perloe's speech at the Endometriosis Walk for Awareness, Washington D.C., 2000:

Don't Let Endometriosis Own You
By Mark Perloe, MD, Medical Director, Georgia Reproductive Specialists

You have two choices, you can let endometriosis control you or you can take control. I say take control and don't let endometriosis own you; you can accept and move beyond the anger you feel.

Don't let endometriosis own you: *You can learn about this condition, and you can learn all you can.*

Don't let endometriosis own you: You can become a partner in that medical care. Insist on a team approach. Your team should include ob-gyn physicians, urologists, GI surgeons, gastroenterologists, pain specialists, general surgeons, and, most importantly, don't forget to be an active member yourself in this team. And all these physicians need to talk to one another.

Don't let endometriosis own you: Develop an endometriosis management plan with your physicians. Learn about your pain medication options, whether it's a medication to control pain on a daily basis or what you are going to do Saturday night at 10:00 when you're in severe pain and your doctor is away on vacation in Washington, maybe speaking, and you don't know what to do. A management plan should have both short-range and long-range options. What are you going to do? How long are you going to try a given therapy before you know if it works? What do you do if this treatment fails? How much does it cost? Will it hurt? Will the insurance company pay for it—if it doesn't, how can I educate the insurance company to look at this and provide the care I need?

Don't let endometriosis own you: What about fertility? Too often many of you have heard that if you just get pregnant endometriosis will go away. We all know that's not true, but it is important to discuss this and make plans and be aware of fertility when considering your options.

Don't let endometriosis own you: Build a support team. This can include counselors who are trained and understand the condition, and it involves your partners or spouse. It involves getting involved in an exercise program, learning about nutrition, participating in stress reduction groups, support groups, *and online discussions. But I want to provide caution because the online support groups can provide a forum to share your horror stories, but sometimes they fail to empower you or take you the next step beyond the pain that's so important to manage the condition.*

AFTERWORD

This book could be called a labor of love or perhaps a mission. Certainly it is a worthy avocation to attempt to help a long-suffering group of women who share this common malady—endometriosis. Kerry-Ann uses her own experience, along with extensive research, "expert" opinion, as well as compelling patient testimony to give the reader a multifaceted view of the impact of endometriosis on the lives of the 30 percent of the female population beset with this disease.

Personally, I was pleased to be asked for contributions to the work on this project and I have been happy to write this afterword. I sincerely hope that the endometriosis public accesses and uses this book and finds information and comfort in the pages composed by an empathetic and sympathetic author. There is always strength in more knowledge. The power granted, along with the fellowship of those who also have gone before, as well as the families that have also gone can make the book a successful venture for us all.

Thanks Kerry-Ann for doing this good deed for those people affected by endometriosis.

—Tom Lyons

Thomas L. Lyons, MD, MS, FACOG, is the Medical Director, Center for Women's Care and Reproductive Medicine, Atlanta, Georgia

Appendices

APPENDIX A:

RESOURCES

This Book's Web Site

The Unveiling Endometriosis Project
http://www.unveilingendometriosis.com

Contact the Author

E-mail the author at webmaster@unveilingendometriosis.com or write
Kerry-Ann Morris
P.O. Box 166
Greater Portmore
St. Catherine
Jamaica

Endometriosis-Related Patient Organizations

United States

Endometriosis Research Center
World Headquarters
630 Ibis Drive
Delray Beach, FL 33444
Toll-free: 800-239-7280
Phone: 561-274-7442

Fax: 561-274-0931
E-mail: AskERC@aol.com

The Endometriosis Research Center (ERC) is an established nonprofit organization founded in 1997. It acts as a resource center for more information about the disease, as well as support. It provides several in-person support groups across the United States, several others across the Caribbean and Canada, as well as the largest online endometriosis support group. Information on endometriosis is available on its Web site, its fact sheets, and in its monthly newsletter and other literature.

Endometriosis Association

International Headquarters
8585 N. 76th Place
Milwaukee, WI 53223
Toll-free: 800-992-3636
Phone: 414-355-2200
Fax: 414-355-6065
URL: http://www.endometriosisassn.org

The Endometriosis Association (EA), the first self-help organization in the world created for women with endometriosis, was founded in 1980 by Mary Lou Ballweg and Carolyn Ketch. The association has published three books and leads the way in many research activities. The association also provides information about endometriosis on its Web site; through its educational brochures available in twenty-eight languages; via a newsletter published four to six times per year, which is free with membership; and through audio and videotapes.

Rest of the World

Endometriosis Group Argentina
Av. Santa Fe 1675 2 A CP 1060
Capital Federal, Buenos Aires
Argentina
Phone: +54-11-4815-4802
Fax: +54-11-4815-4802
E-mail: info@endometriosisgroup.com.ar
URL: http://www.endometriosisgroup.com.ar

Endometriosis Association (Victoria) Inc.
28 Warrandyte Road
Ringwood
Victoria 3134
Australia
Phone: +61-3-9457-2933
Fax: +61-3-9458-4367
E-mail: info@endometriosis.org.au
URL: http://www.endometriosis.org.au

Öesterreichische Endometriose Vereinigung (Austria)
Obere Augartenstrasse 26-28
1020 Wien
Austria
Phone: +43-0-676-4447344
Fax: +43-0-2236-866653
E-mail: office@endometriose-wien.at
URL: http://www.endometriose-wien.at

Associação Brasileira de Endometriose (ABEND—Brazil)
Rua Claro de Camargo Sobrinho, 89
Vila Pouso Alegre—Barueri
SP Cep 06402-050
Brazil
Phone: +55-11-4198-7456
Fax: +55-11-4163-5086
E-mail: abend@abend.org.br
URL: http://www.abend.org.br

Endometriose Foreningen Denmark (Endometriosis Association)
Kvorupvej 1, Åsted
6800 Varde
Denmark
Phone: +45-2172-4300
Fax: +45-7525-4455
E-mail: info@endo.dk
URL: http://www.endo.dk

Endometrioosiyhdistys Finland (Endometriosis Association)
PL 142
00531 Helsinki
Finland
Phone: +358-0-50-380-6715
Fax: +358-0-50-380-6715
E-mail: endo@endometrioosiyhdistys.fi
URL: http://www.endometrioosiyhdistys.fi

Association EndoFrance (France)
17, allée des Eguerêts
F-95280 Jouy le Moutier
France
E-mail: contact@endofrance.org
URL: http://www.endofrance.org

The Endometriose-Vereinigung Deutschland e. V (Germany)
Counselling centre Leipzig
Bernhard-Göring-Str. 152
04277 Leipzig
Germany
Phone: +49-0-341-3-06-53-04
URL: http://www.endometriose-vereinigung.de

Endometriosis Society India (India)
6A & 6F Needlamber
28B Shakespeare Sarani
Kolkata 700 017
India
Phone: 033-2865-0364, 033-2240-4463
Fax: 91-33-2281-1639
E-mail: mail@endosocindia.org
URL: http://www.endosocindia.org

Endometriosis Association of Ireland
Carmichael Centre
North Brunswick Street
Dublin 7
Ireland
Phone: +353-1-8735702
Fax: +353-1-8735737
E-mail: info@endo.ie
URL: http://www.endo.ie

L'Associazione Italiana Endometriosi ONLUS (AIE—Italy)
Casella Postale 114
I-20014 Nerviano (MI)
Italy
Phone: +39-0331-589800
Fax: +39-0331-589800
E-mail: info@endoassoc.it
URL: http://www.endoassoc.it

The Japan Endometriosis Association (JEMA—Japan)
3-36-26-201 Kugayama
Suginami-ku, Tokyo
168-0082 Japan
Phone: +81-3-5938-1850
Fax: +81-3-5938-1850
E-mail: jema@japan.intera.or.jp
URL: http://www.interq.or.jp/japan/jema/

Asociación de Endometriosis Capítulo Mexicano, A.C (Mexico)
Phone: +52-55-51-49-04-68
E-mail: mexendometriosis@yahoo.com.mx
URL: http://www.mexendometriosis.com

Endometriose Stichting (The Netherlands)
Endometriose Stichting
Antwoordnummer 1789
2000 VC Haarlem
The Netherlands
Phone: +31 0900-0400481
Fax: + 31 046-4586028
Email: info@endometriose.nl
URL: http://www.endometriose.nl

The New Zealand Endometriosis Foundation Incorporated (NZEF)
New Zealand Endometriosis Foundation Inc.
PO Box 1673
Palmerston North 5301
New Zealand
Phone: +64-0-3-379-7959
Fax: +64-0-3-379-7969
Support Line: +64-0800-733-277
E-mail: nzendo@xtra.co.nz
URL: http://www.nzendo.co.nz

Endometrioseforeningen (Norway)
Postboks 4391 Lura
N-4301 Sandnes
Norway
E-mail: endonorge@yahoo.com
URL: http://www.endonorge.org

Endometriosis Association (Singapore)
c/o Mount Alvernia Hospital
820 Thomson Road
Singapore 574623
Phone: +65-63476640
Fax: +65-62505138
E-mail: support@endometriosis.org.sg
URL: http://www.endometriosis.org.sg

The Endometriosis Society of South Africa
PO Box 3389
Parklands
2121 Johannesburg
South Africa
Phone: +27-0-11-646-0449
Fax: +27-0-11-646-0449

Asociación Endometriosis España (AEE—Spain)
Calle Mayor, 29
E–17455 Caldes de Malavella
Spain
E-mail: endospain@hotmail.com
URL: http://www.endoinfo.info

Svenska Endometriosföreningen (Sweden)
Box 14087
S-167 14 Bromma
Sweden
E-mail: endo@sverige.nu

National Endometriosis Society (United Kingdom)
50 Westminster Palace Gardens
Artillery Row
London SW1P 1RL
United Kingdom
Phone: +44-0-20-7222 2781
Help line: 0808-808-2227
Fax: +44-0-20-7222-2786
E-mail: nes@endo.org.uk
URL: http://www.endo.org.uk

Endometriosis SHE Trust (United Kingdom)
14 Moorland Way
Lincoln
LN6 7JW
United Kingdom
Phone: 0870-7743665/4
Fax: 0870-774366/4
E-mail: shetrust@shetrust.org.uk
URL: http://www.shetrust.org.uk

Endometriosis-Related Medical Organizations

American Society for Reproductive Medicine (ASRM)
1209 Montgomery Highway
Birmingham, Alabama 35210-2809
Phone: 205-978-5000
Fax: 205-978-5005
E-mail: asrm@asrm.org
URL: http://www.asrm.org

The American Society for Reproductive Medicine (ASRM), formerly the American Fertility Society, is a nonprofit, multidisciplinary organization that focuses on the advancement and practice of reproductive medicine in the United States. It provides educational programs/material for the public as well as continuing education for medical professionals. On its Web site, patients can find information on reproductive health issues, including fertility, menopause, assisted reproductive technologies (ART) and endometriosis. Information for the lay public is presented as Patient Fact Sheets and Patient Booklets.

American College of Obstetricians and Gynecologists (ACOG)
409 12th Street, SW, PO Box 96920
Washington, D.C. 20090-6920
Phone: 202-638-5577
URL: http://www.acog.org

The American College of Obstetricians and Gynecologists (ACOG) is a private, voluntary, nonprofit membership organization made up of medical professionals who provide health care for women. The group serves as a strong advocate for quality health care. On its Web site patients can find educational materials about various aspects of medical issues specifically concerning women. Gynecologists are certified by ABOG, and patients can find out more information about a particular physician by using the ACOG's "Find an Ob-Gyn" link.

Endometriosis Web Sites

Endometriosis.org
http://www.endometriosis.org

A comprehensive Web site with informative articles about various aspects of endometriosis, the latest medical and scientific news about endometriosis, and related topics with links to support groups, online forums, and various other related Web sites.

Endometriosis Awareness and Information
http://www.hcgresources.com/endoindex.html

Begun and maintained by Heather C. Guidone, director of operations of the Endometriosis Research Center, this site offers a plethora of informative and advice-filled articles about any and every aspect of endometriosis. The site also features news and the latest information about endometriosis-related breakthroughs for educational purposes, and links to other well-respected Web sites about endometriosis.

Georgia Reproductive Specialists
http://www.ivf.com/endohtml.html

This is the Web presence of Dr. Mark Perloe's practice, Georgia Reproductive Specialists (GRS), located in Atlanta, Georgia. Dr. Perloe and his colleagues at GRS, while primarily involved in the treatment of infertile patients, do provide comprehensive treatment services to all endometriosis patients. The Web site provides information about the disease and its various treatment options.

MedlinePlus: Endometriosis
http://www.nlm.nih.gov/medlineplus/endometriosis.html

MedlinePlus provides links to endometriosis-related information such as symptoms, diagnosis, treatments, latest news, and clinical trials.

The National Women's Health Information Center (NWHIC)
http://www.4woman.gov/faq/endomet.htm

This section of the National Women's Health Information Center's Web site (NWHIC) provides basic information about endometriosis in a fact sheet titled "Endometriosis." The NWHIC is a project of the U.S. Department of Health and Human Services, Office on Women's Health.

Center for Women's Care and Reproductive Surgery
http://www.thomasllyons.com

The Web presence of the Center for Women's Care and Reproductive Surgery, headed by Dr. Thomas L. Lyons. This site features articles written by Dr. Lyons about various aspects of endometriosis treatments, hysterectomy, endometrial ablation, and incontinence.

Center for Endometriosis Care (CEC)
http://www.centerforendo.com

The web site for the Center for Endometriosis Care (CEC), an endometriosis treatment center located in Atlanta, which provides online visitors with articles written about endometriosis by its doctors, including Dr. Robert Albee, Dr. Ken Sinervo, and Dr. Thomas L. Lyons.

MayoClinic.com
http://www.mayoclinic.com/invoke.cfm?id=DS00289

This section of the MayoClinic Web site features a comprehensive article about endometriosis with the following sections: overview, signs and symptoms, causes, risk factors, screening and diagnosis, complications, treatment, prevention, and coping skills.

Vital Care Institute of Health
http://www.pelvicpain.com

This is the Web presence of the Vital Care Institute of Health, headed by Dr. Andrew Cook. It has the popular "Ask Dr. Cook," which features Dr. Cook's answers to questions posed by endometriosis patients. Questions cover the gamut of the endometriosis experience from symptoms to diagnosis, pain management, hysterectomy, adhesions, and much more.

Endometriosis Resolved
http://www.endo-resolved.com

Created and maintained by Carolyn Levett, author of the self-published *Recipes for the Endometriosis Diet* (2005), this Web site features very detailed articles concerning the nutritional aspects of living well with endometriosis and has a strong emphasis on alternative treatment/lifestyle options. Visitors to the Web site can read about alternative treatments for endometriosis, diet and endometriosis, overview of pain and endometriosis, endometriosis and our immune systems, and much more.

The National Institute of Child Health and Human Development (NICHD) Endometriosis Information
http://www.nichd.nih.gov/publications/pubs/endometriosis/sub2.htm

This subsite of the National Institutes of Health (NIH) presents a detailed article about endometriosis, its symptoms, diagnosis, and treatment options. The article is presented in a question-and-answer format. Some questions include: What is endometriosis? In what places, outside of the uterus, do areas of endometriosis grow? What are the symptoms of endometriosis? Who gets endometriosis? Does having endometriosis mean I'll be infertile or unable to have children? This is a good overview of the many aspects of endometriosis.

Endometriosis Association of Victoria (EAV)
http://www.endometriosis.org.au

This is the Web presence of Australia's national endometriosis patient support organization, the Endometriosis Association of Victoria (EAV). The Web site provides information to endometriosis patients about symptoms, diagnosis, and treatments, and includes information leaflets that can be downloaded or ordered from the EAV.

St. Charles Endometriosis Treatment Program
http://www.endometriosistreatment.org

Directed by Dr. David Redwine, renowned endometriosis specialist, the Web presence of the St. Charles Endometriosis Treatment Program in Bend, Oregon, features articles written by Dr. Redwine and others in its publication, the *St. Charles Medical Center Endometriosis Newsletter*. There is also an "Answers to Common Questions" section, which gives answers to some of the basic questions that concern endometriosis patients, such as: Is my pain due to endometriosis? Does endometriosis "come back" after surgical treatment?

Endometriosis Research Center (ERC)
http://www.endocenter.org

The Endometriosis Research Center (ERC) provides support and education to women diagnosed with endometriosis, to loved ones indirectly affected by the disease, and to health care providers. Visitors can download the ERC's order form to purchase additional publications. Funds go toward the center's awareness and education programs.

Endometriosis Association (EA)
http://www.endometriosisassn.org/index2.html

The Web site of the Endometriosis Association (EA) is a comprehensive, jam-packed portal of information about the association and the work it does within the endometriosis community. Web visitors are encouraged to contact the association to receive a free information package and details about becoming a member.

Endometriosis Zone
http://www.endozone.org

The Endometriosis Zone is a true information portal and database of all things endometriosis. Visitors to the site are kept up to date about medical and scientific breakthroughs via news items, conference coverage, interviews, and reviews. The Coping Zone features articles on day-to-day aspects of endometriosis for those living with the disease's insidious effects. Educational tools include an image library, case histories, and PowerPoint presentations. Expert views of medical practitioners touch on such aspects of the disease as the pathogenesis and theories, surgical treatment, medical therapies, and much more.

A.D.A.M Healthcare Center at About.com
http://adam.about.com/reports/000074_3.htm?terms=endometriosis

This section of About.com features an in-depth report by A.D.A.M Inc., on the causes, diagnosis, treatment, and prevention of endometriosis.

MENDO—Men and Endometriosis
http://www.geocities.com/HotSprings/Spa/8449

A site created by John Blondin (whose wife, Carey, has endometriosis) specifically targeting men who love and live with women who have endometriosis. The site provides information about the male side of the disease through articles written by John as well as the words of other men.

Women's Surgery Group Endometriosis Page
http://www.womenssurgerygroup.com/conditions/Endometriosis/
   overview.asp

This page of the Women's Surgery Group Web site features a comprehensive article about endometriosis. Sections of the article include overview, diagnosis, treatment, photos, myths, FAQs, and so forth. The Women's Surgery Group is a group of laparoscopic gynecologic surgeons who are widely known as pioneers in the field of gynecologic laparoscopy.

The Endometriosis Center at the Sher Institute for Reproductive Medicine
http://www.treatendo.com/default.htm

This Web site of the Endometriosis Center at the Sher Institute for Reproductive Medicine (SIRM) features articles on endometriosis-associated infertility and the work of the center in the treatment of endometriosis patients.

National Women's Health Resource Center (NWHRC)
http://www.healthywomen.org/content.cfm?L1=3&L2=24

This section of the National Women's Health Resource Center (NWHRC) provides a comprehensive overview about specific aspects of endometriosis, including diagnosis, treatment, prevention, lifestyle tips, and others.

Online Forums and Discussion Groups

ERC—Endometriosis Research Center
http://health.groups.yahoo.com/group/erc

This is the largest endometriosis online discussion group. Started by the Endometriosis Research Center in 1998, the forum provides women and loved ones a chance to share with others their experiences with endometriosis, as well as an opportunity to learn.

ERC Girl Talk
http://health.groups.yahoo.com/group/ERCGirlTalk

This online discussion forum is a project of the ERC's Girl Talk Program. This program specifically addresses the needs of women twenty-five years and younger who have or think they might have endometriosis. ERC Girl Talk online discussion listserv aims to encourage collaboration and sharing of support, information, ideas, and experiences among its targeted members.

Goddesses of Endometriosis
http://health.groups.yahoo.com/group/Goddesses_Of_Endometriosis

This is another popular online discussion forum for endometriosis patients to vent their frustrations with this disease and to learn from others.

Endometriosis and the Military
http://groups.msn.com/EndometriosisandtheMilitary/home.htm

This discussion list particularly serves the needs of women with endometriosis who are serving in the army. It is an official online group of the Endometriosis Research Center.

The Endometriosis Forum at OBGYN.net
http://forums.obgyn.net/endo

This is another large online endometriosis discussion forum created specifically for women and those affected by the disease. Here, visitors share with one another experiences and ideas about life with endometriosis.

The Endometriosis Quilt
http://www.endozone.org/quilt/endo.cfm

While not an online discussion forum, the endometriosis quilt is a compilation of information from hundreds of women across the world with endometriosis. Information presented includes time of onset of symptoms, date when diagnosed, treatments tried, etc. The main purpose of the quilt is to symbolize the need for proper education to assist in the timely diagnosis of the disease.

MendoMen
http://health.groups.yahoo.com/group/mendomen

This is the online discussion forum for MENDO, created by John Blondin. This discussion forum is only for men who live with and love women with endometriosis.

Endometriosis Books

Endometriosis: The Complete Reference for Taking Charge of Your Health
Mary Lou Ballweg and the Endometriosis Association (editors)

An informative, up-to-date guide on treatments for endometriosis, with new information about endometriosis's link to autoimmune diseases and conditions.

Endometriosis: A Key to Healing Through Nutrition
Dian Shepperson Mills and Michael Vernon

An informative look at the nutritional aspect of overcoming endometriosis, including recipes and details about alternative treatment strategies.

Coping with Endometriosis: Sound, Compassionate Advice for Alleviating the Physical and Emotional Symptoms of This Frequently Misunderstood Illness
Glenda Motta and Robert Phillips

Specifically deals with the stress of endometriosis and ways in which patients can cope with the disease on a daily basis.

What to Do When the Doctor Says It's Endometriosis: Everything You Need to Know to Stop the Pain and Heal Your Fertility
Thomas L. Lyons, MD, and Cheryl Kimball

As the medical director of the Center for Women's Care and Reproductive Surgery in Atlanta, Georgia, Dr. Lyons teams with health writer Cheryl Kimball to demystify endometriosis, from treatments to alternative therapies, but with an emphasis on pain-management strategies.

The Endometriosis Sourcebook
Mary Lou Ballweg and the Endometriosis Association (editors)

Described as the "definitive guide to current treatment options, the latest research, common myths about the disease, and coping strategies," the book offers readers an informative collection of articles by various authors about every aspect of the disease up to the time of its publication.

Explaining Endometriosis
Lorraine Henderson and Ros Wood

As the name suggests, this handbook explains the various aspects of endometriosis: the possible causes, diagnosis, surgeries, and conventional and alternative treatment options for the disease. In addition the book offers advice to help women make decisions about treatments.

Endometriosis: A Natural Approach
Jo Mears

This 170-page book answers some of the basic questions concerning endometriosis: causes, diagnosis, and conventional and alternative treatment options.

Endometriosis: One Woman's Journey
Jennifer Marie Lewis

Jennifer Marie Lewis provides a personal account of her everyday life with endometriosis, from symptoms and diagnosis to treatments. She uses her life as a road map to which other endometriosis patients may refer.

Fibroid Tumors & Endometriosis Self Help Book
Susan M. Lark, MD

Based on her more than twenty years experience in women's health care and preventive medicine, Dr. Susan M. Lark provides readers with information about the causes of endometriosis and fibroid tumors, a weekly self-evaluating workbook for readers to assess their symptoms, and advice on what they can do to help themselves, such as vitamins, herbs, minerals, acupressure, and yoga.

Endometriosis and Other Pelvic Pain
Susan Evans, MD

This book sets out information about endometriosis and other pelvic pain disorders and reviews current treatment choices to deal with these conditions.

Endometriosis Video

Endometriosis: The Inside Story
Belle Browne and Monica Flores

Belle Browne from Australia and Monica Flores from the United States show what life is really like living with endometriosis and what to do to get help in managing the disease.

Pelvic Pain Resources

International Pelvic Pain Society
Phone: 205-877-2950 or 800-624-9676
URL: http://www.pelvicpain.org

The International Pelvic Pain Society (IPPS) is a group of physicians who treat women who suffer from conditions or diseases that cause chronic pelvic pain, such as endometriosis. Their Web site features informative articles on various aspects of chronic pelvic pain, such as diagnosing and treating those conditions that cause it. Articles are targeted at both patients and medical professionals.

National Pain Foundation (NPF)

The National Pain Foundation
300 East Hampden Avenue, Suite 100
Englewood, CO 80113
E-mail: aardrup@nationalpainfoundation.org
URL: http://www.painconnection.net

The National Pain Foundation is nonprofit organization formed in 1998 to inform, educate, and support persons dealing with chronic pelvic pain and to promote functional recovery of persons disabled by pain. Their Web site includes informative articles about pain and interactive tools, such as an online pain journal, women can use to assess their pain.

American Pain Foundation

http://www.painfoundation.org

The American Pain Foundation (APF) is a nonprofit organization that educates, advocates for, and supports people who live with pain. It aims to improve these individuals' quality of life through public awareness programs, the provision of practical advice, and advocation for increased access to effective pain management. The Web site features articles about pain and pain management, as well as discussion boards.

MayoClinic.com

http://www.mayoclinic.com/invoke.cfm?id=DS00571

This section of the MayoClinic Web site features a very detailed and informative article about chronic pelvic pain. The article is divided into different subtopics: signs and symptoms, causes, when to seek medical advice, screening and diagnosis, treatments, and others.

WebMD Health
http://my.webmd.com/hw/chronic_pelvic_pain/tv2265.asp

This extensive consumer health Web site features a very comprehensive and detailed health guide titled *Female Chronic Pelvic Pain*. Sections of the guide include causes, symptoms, what happens, what increases your risk, when to call a doctor, and treatment overview, to name a few.

OBGYN.net's Women's Health Pelvic Pain Section
http://www.obgyn.net/cpp/cpp.asp

In keeping with OBGYN.net's consumerist health approach, this Web site features a section dealing with chronic pelvic pain, a common condition in women. This section is just one of many topics related to female reproductive disorders and diseases. The pelvic pain section is divided into subsections all dealing with some aspect of pelvic pain: articles, interviews, latest news items, PowerPoint presentations, among others.

Infertility Resources

RESOLVE: The National Infertility Association
National Headquarters
7910 Woodmont Avenue, Suite 1350
Bethesda, MD 20814
Phone: 301-652-8585
Fax: 301-652-9375
E-mail: info@resolve.org
URL: http://www.resolve.org

RESOLVE is a nonprofit organization that promotes reproductive health and advocates equal access to family-building options for men and women who are experiencing infertility. It also provides education, support, and physician referral to patients. The Web site features informative articles about ovulation, infertility treatment options, coping strategies, and other related issues.

OBGYN.net Infertility Section
http://www.obgyn.net/infertility/infertility.asp

This section of OBGYN.net's women's health section features various types of information related to infertility, taken from a variety of sources. The categories include articles, interviews, the latest news items, PowerPoint presentations, and others.

American Fertility Association
656 Fifth Avenue, Suite 278
New York, NY 10103
Phone: 888-917-3777
Fax: 718-601-7722
E-mail: info@theafa.org
URL: http://www.theafa.org

The American Fertility Association (AFA) was founded in 1999. Through educational and awareness programs about infertility, the organization works to change the lives of couples who face infertility. It also strives for legislative and social changes surrounding the issues of infertility and adoption.

InterNational Council on Infertility Information Dissemination (INCIID)
PO Box 6836 Arlington, VA 22206
Phone: 703-379-9178
Fax: 703-379-1593
E-mail: inciidinfo@inciid.org
URL: http://www.inciid.org

InterNational Council on Infertility Information Dissemination (INCIID) is a nonprofit organization that helps individuals and couples explore their family-building options. The Web site provides current information and immediate support regarding the diagnosis, treatment, and prevention of infertility and pregnancy loss, as well as other guidance to those considering adoption or child-free lifestyles.

Infertility at About.com
http://infertility.about.com

About.com offers several articles on infertility such as infertility drugs, treatments, surrogacy, adoption, etc.

Infertility Resources Web Site
http://www.ihr.com/infertility

This comprehensive Web site provides information about assisted reproductive techniques (ART) such as in vitro fertilization (IVF); information about infertility clinics, diagnosing infertility, and other infertility-related information.

Fertility Neighborhood: A Service of Freedom Drug
http://www.fertilityneighborhood.com

This is an online educational resource about infertility, infertility treatment options, support, and financial aspects of infertility. There is also a message board and a chat room where infertile patients can talk to one another, share experiences, and support one another.

Adhesion Resources

International Adhesions Society (IAS)
David Wiseman, PhD, MR, PharmS
Synechion, Inc.
6757 Arapaho Road, Suite 711 #238
Dallas, TX 75248
Phone: 972-931-5596
Fax: 972-931-5476
E-mail: david.wiseman@adhesions.org
URL: http://www.adhesions.org

This organization with more than fifty support groups around the world provides support and advocacy for patients who suffer from adhesions and related disorders (ARD). It also provides educational materials, research, and product information about ARD, and publishes *Connections Newsletter*, which provides additional information and resources to all ARD sufferers.

The Australian Adhesions Support Group Inc.
Joanne Eslick (Founder)
PO Box 1919
Bathurst, NSW 2795
Australia
Phone: +61-02-6334-2635
E-mail: joanne@bombobeach.com
URL: http://www.bombobeach.com

This is an international adhesions awareness and support group for sufferers, family members, and caregivers, with a chapter in the United States.

The American Adhesions Support Group, Inc.
Anthea Nesbitt (Cofounder)
PO Box 152
1215 Polaris Parkway
Columbus, OH 43240
E-mail: nesbittan@yahoo.com
URL: http://www.bombobeach.com

Hysterectomy Resources

HysterSisters.com
http://www.hystersisters.com

A Web site created and maintained by women who had hysterectomies to support other women in recovery from the surgery. The Web site is chock-full of information about hysterectomy, including articles about pre- and post-op issues, effects of hysterectomy on sexual function, and much more. Visitors to the site can also interact with other hysterectomy patients on the hystersisters.com message boards. The site offers a very entertaining yet educational approach to recovery from hysterectomy surgery with the main emphasis on supporting women who have to go through the surgery at any time.

HERS Foundation
422 Bryn Mawr Avenue
Bala Cynwyd, PA 19004
Phone: 610-667-7757
Fax: 610-667-8096
E-mail: hersfdn@earthlink.net
URL: http://www.hersfoundation.com

The HERS Foundation is an independent, international nonprofit organization that provides information about hysterectomy and the alternatives available to women. HERS also provides the following services: free information by mail, telephone counseling, physician referrals, lawyer referrals, CDs and audio and videotapes about hysterectomy, a reading list of suggested books and medical journal articles, as well as a free lending library. You can order publications from the foundation's Web site.

MayoClinic.com
http://www.mayoclinic.com/invoke.cfm?id=HQ00905

This section of the MayoClinic Web site features a comprehensive article about the benefits of and alternatives to hysterectomy. Extensive information is provided on who may have a hysterectomy; how to prepare for a hysterectomy; types of hysterectomies, post-op issues, and alternatives to hysterectomy.

Hysterectomy at About.com
http://womenshealth.about.com/cs/hysterectomy/

This section of About.com features in-depth Guide Picks—links to many articles—on hysterectomy and alternatives to hysterectomy.

WebMD Health
http://my.webmd.com/hw/womens_conditions/aa68979.asp?src=
  Inktomi&condition=healthwise

This extensive consumer health Web site features a very comprehensive and detailed health guide titled *Hysterectomy*. Sections of the guide include why it is done, hysterectomy types, comparison of hysterectomy procedures, risks, preparing for a hysterectomy, and other subtopics.

MedlinePlus: Hysterectomy
http://www.nlm.nih.gov/medlineplus/hysterectomy.html

MedlinePlus provides links to hysterectomy-related information, such as the latest news, overview about the procedure, alternatives to hysterectomy, clinical trials, current research, and organizations.

The National Women's Health Information Center (NWHIC)
http://www.4woman.gov/faq/hysterectomy.htm

This section of the Web site for the National Women's Health Information Center (NWHIC) provides basic information about hysterectomy in a fact sheet titled *Hysterectomy*. The NWHIC is a project of the U.S. Department of Health and Human Services, Office on Women's Health.

OBGYN.net Hysterectomy & Alternatives Section
http://www.obgyn.net/ah/ah.asp

This section of OBGYN.net features various types of information dealing with hysterectomy and alternatives to hysterectomy. The Hysterectomy & Alternatives Section is divided into subsections all dealing with some aspect of hysterectomy: articles, interviews, latest news items, PowerPoint presentations, among others.

APPENDIX B:

GLOSSARY

Abdominal hysterectomy—removal of the uterus through an abdominal incision.

Ablation—destruction of endometrial implants by any surgical means.

Add-back therapy—adding small doses of estrogen while undergoing gonadotropin-releasing hormone (GnRH) therapy to reduce menopausal symptoms and bone mineral density (BMD) loss as a result of blocked estrogen production.

Adhesion—the medical term for scar tissue that forms an abnormal connection between normally separate organs.

Amenorrhea—absence of menstrual cycles.

Analgesic—the general name for painkillers.

Angiogenesis—natural formation of new blood vessels.

Antibodies—substances produced by B cell lymphocytes that surround bacteria, viruses, and foreign matter and mark them for destruction.

Anticoagulant—an agent that prevents the clotting of blood.

Antioxidant—a substance that neutralizes free radicals.

Antiphospholipid antibodies (APAs)—antibodies formed against phospholipids that make up part of the membrane in all cells of the body.

Apoptosis—the natural process of removing unwanted cells in the body; also referred to as cell death.

Aromatase—an enzyme that can convert testosterone to estradiol.

Aromatase inhibitor—chemical that blocks aromatase activity in endometrial implants.

Assisted reproductive techniques (ART)—procedures that are used to fertilize an egg and increase the chances of conception.

Asymptomatic—not showing any symptoms of a disease.

Autoantibodies—antibodies produced by B cell lymphocytes that detect the body's own cells as foreign matter/bacteria and mark them for destruction.

Autoimmunity—the process of an immune system attack against the body's own cells, tissues, etc.; also referred to as self-immunity.

Basal body temperature (BBT)—the lowest temperature that a healthy person experiences on any given day; can be used to determine the most fertile days because hormonal changes during the menstrual cycle lower a woman's body temperature one or two days before ovulation and increase it one or two days after. Ovulation increases BBT by 0.4°F (0.2°C) and remains high for a week.

B cell lymphocytes—produces circulating antibodies to trap foreign matter.

Bilateral salpingo-oophorectomy—removal of fallopian tubes and ovaries and, often, the uterus and the cervix.

Blastocyst—an early stage of an embryo's development; five-day-old embryos.

Blastocyst transfer—the transfer of five-day-old embryos into the uterus.

CA 19-9—serum cancer antigen 19-9 is a marker for ovarian cancer that is found in elevated levels in women with endometriosis.

CA-125—serum cancer antigen 125 is found in many normal tissues such as the endometrium. High levels have been found in women with endometriosis. It is also a marker for ovarian cancer.

Catamenial hemoptysis—coughing up blood or bloody sputum.

Catamenial pneumothorax—accumulation of air in the pleural cavity that can lead to lung collapse.

Chronic pelvic pain—debilitating noncyclical pain that lasts for six months and requires medical attention.

Cilia—tiny hairs in the fallopian tubes that help the egg travel toward sperm.

Complement system—a combination of about twenty-five proteins that work together to complement the work of antibodies in destroying bacteria and foreign matter and help rid the body of antibody located antigens, produce inflammation at the site of infection, and regulate immune functions.

Controlled ovarian hyperstimulation (COH)—ovulation induction using potent fertility drugs; monitored by a doctor.

Controlled ovarian hyperstimulation and intrauterine insemination (COH-IUI)—a combined fertility treatment method to increase the chance of conception.

Corpus luteum—Latin for "yellow body," formed from the burst follicle that releases a mature egg during the luteal phase of the menstrual cycle.

COX-2 inhibitors—a new generation of NSAIDs with the same prostaglandin-blocking action but reduced gastrointestinal side effects.

Computerized tomography scan (CT Scan)—a form of X-ray that involves producing three-dimensional (3D) computerized images of a section of a body via a CT scanner, which rotates around the body part to be scanned.

Cul-de-sac—also called the pouch of Douglas; the area between the vagina and the cervix.

Cytokines—chemical messengers that communicate with other components of the immune system and communicate between the immune system and other systems of the body.

Danazol—synthetic testosterone that inhibits release of gonadotropin-releasing hormone (GnRH) from the hypothalamus and follicle-stimulating hormone (FSH) and luteinizing hormone (LH) from the pituitary gland.

Diaphragm—dome-shaped muscle that separates the chest cavity from the abdominal cavity.

Differentiation—conversion of cells and tissue into specialized cells and tissue.

Dioxin—an environmental pollutant that disrupts the normal functioning of the endocrine system, resulting in hormone imbalances in humans.

Dyschezia—painful bowel movement.

Dysmenorrhea—extremely painful menstruation.

Dyspareunia—painful sexual intercourse.

Dyspnea—difficult or labored breathing.

Dysuria—difficult or painful urinating.

Ectopic pregnancy—abnormal development of a fetus in a site other than the uterus; most common type of ectopic pregnancy occurs in a fallopian tube (tubal pregnancy) if the tube is blocked or inflamed, obstructing the path of the egg to the uterus.

Electrocoagulation—destruction of implants by heating or drying the tissues using any electrical surgical tool.

Extracellular matrix modulators (EMMs)—chemicals that block MMP activity in implants to prevent implantation and development in ectopic locations.

Endocrine gland—this type of gland produces one or more types of hormones and secretes them directly into the bloodstream; an example is the pituitary gland, which secretes the follicle-stimulating hormone (FSH) and luteinizing hormone (LH) to the ovaries.

Endometrioma—chocolate cyst found on the ovaries that is filled with menstrual debris from past menstrual shedding.

Endometrium—tissue that lines the walls of the uterus.

Endorphins—chemical compounds that occur naturally in the brain with pain-relieving properties similar to opiates.

Endostatin—a new type of medical therapy being investigated to inhibit the development of new blood vessels around endometriotic implants.

Environmental endocrine disruptors—external agents such as chemical pollutants that disrupt the synthesis, secretion, and action of natural hormones in the body; TCDD (dioxin) is a harmful endocrine disruptor.

Essential fatty acid (EFA)—part of a group of unsaturated fatty acids, found in certain herbs and foods, that is needed by the body.

Estrogen replacement therapy (ERT)—administration of estrogen to those who had a hysterectomy; used to suppress menopausal symptoms.

Estradiol—a powerful form of estrogen produced by the maturing follicles during the follicular phase of the menstrual cycle; this hormone also controls female sexual development and female characteristics such as breast development.

Excision—to cut out entire disease implants by hand while preserving healthy portions of the affected organ.

Expectant management—using natural family-planning techniques to predict a woman's most fertile days to attempt conception.

Free radicals—naturally occurring unstable oxygen molecules that acquire healthy molecules from healthy cells to balance themselves and, in the process, damage the cells and tissues of the body.

Follicular phase—occurs during the first half of the menstrual cycle: a number of follicles are stimulated by follicle-stimulating hormone (FSH) to start maturing; maturing follicles produce estradiol that prepares the endometrial lining.

Follicle-stimulating hormone (FSH)—hormone secreted by the pituitary gland to trigger maturation of follicles in the ovaries.

Fibromyalgia—a condition associated with chronic fatigue and widespread joint and muscle pain and stiffness.

Fulguration—superficial burning of implants using any electrical surgical tool.

Gamete—a mature sex cell: the ovum of the female and the sperm of the male.

Gamete intrafallopian transfer (GIFT)—a form of in vitro fertilization (IVF) in which eggs are harvested, mixed with sperm, and immediately injected back into the uterus, in the exact area where they would be in natural fertilization.

Gamma-linolenic acid (GLA)—an essential fatty acid found in the oil of the evening primrose plant; used by the body to produce anti-inflammatory prostaglandins; also suppresses the production of inflammatory prostaglandins.

Gestrinone—an anti-estrogen and anti-progesterone steroid that increases male hormones in the body.

Gland—an organ or group of cells in humans that is specifically responsible for synthesizing chemical substances and secreting them for the body to use or eliminate.

Gonadotrophin-releasing hormone (GnRH)—hormone released by the hypothalamus that stimulates the pituitary gland to release follicle-stimulating hormone (FSH) and luteinizing hormone (LH).

Gonadotropin-releasing hormone (GnRH) agonists—a group of chemicals that mimics the body's own hormone after which it is named; acts by first overloading the pituitary gland with chemical messages to release more follicle-stimulating hormone (FSH) and luteinizing hormone (LH) then gradually down-regulates the ovaries to stop estrogen production; also prescribed during gonadotropin therapy to prevent premature ovulation.

Gonadotropin-releasing hormone (GnRH) antagonists—drugs that block the pituitary gland from releasing follicle-stimulating hormone (FSH) and luteinizing hormone (LH) needed for the ovulatory cycle.

Gonadotropins—very potent fertility drugs that directly act on the ovaries and stimulate follicular maturation and development of multiple eggs

Growth factors—chemicals that stimulate new cell growth and cell maintenance.

Hematochezia—blood in stool.

Hematuria—blood in urine.

Hemothorax—collection of blood in the pleural cavity.

Heparin—an anticoagulant medication.

High density lipoprotein (HDL)—also known as good cholesterol.

Hormone—a chemical substance produced an endocrine gland; for example, estrogen, which is produced by the ovaries and is secreted into the bloodstream and carried to specific organs and tissues on which it has a specific effect.

Human chorionic gonadotropin (hCG)—mimics the natural luteinizing hormone (LH) surge during the luteal phase of the menstrual cycle to trigger release of an egg from the mature follicle during ovulation.

Hypertension—high blood pressure.

Hypotension—low blood pressure.

Hypothalamus—region of the brain, attached to the pituitary gland, that sends chemical messages to the gland to release hormones for different bodily functions to take place; for instance, the hypothalamus sends chemical messages—gonadotropin-releasing hormone (GnRH)—to the pituitary gland to release luteinizing hormone (LH) and follicle-stimulating hormone (FSH) into the blood to kick-start ovulation.

Hysterectomy—surgical removal of the uterus.

Immune system—the body's first line of defense against bacterial and viral infections and other foreign matter.

Immune tolerance—ability of the body's immune system to recognize the body's cells as a part of self and not as bacteria or viruses to be destroyed.

Immunoglobulin (Ig)—a protein derived from human blood that works by suppressing natural killer (NK) cell activity and antiphospholipid antibody (APA) production.

Immunomodulator—a type of medication that targets the hyperstimulated immune system with the aim to normalize the immune response.

Incontinence—involuntary urine leakage.

Infertility—inability in a woman to conceive.

Inflammation—the body's reaction to injury or infection, characterized by pain, redness, and swelling at the site.

Inhibin—substance secreted by the most mature follicle that reduces the secretion of follicle-stimulating hormone (FSH) to the other follicles in the ovary.

Insomnia—inability to fall asleep or stay asleep for adequate lengths of time.

Integrin—a group of proteins that facilitates the attachment of the embryo to the uterine wall; also referred to as cell-to-cell adhesion molecules.

Interferons—substances produced by the body's cells when infected with a virus; have the ability to interfere with viral growth.

Interleukins (IL)—proteins produced by white blood cells that regulate the interaction between lymphocytes and other white blood cells.

Interstitial cystitis (IC)—chronic inflammation of the wall of the bladder in the absence of bacteria; results in bladder pain and frequent urgent desires to pass urine.

In vitro fertilization (IVF)—fertilization of an egg outside of the body.

Intracytoplasmic injection (ICSI)—this involves harvesting eggs and using microscopic instruments to inject a single sperm into the center of an egg to induce fertilization; fertilized egg is then transferred to the woman's uterus and a blood test done two weeks later to confirm pregnancy.

Intrauterine insemination (IUI)—a form of assisted reproduction technique (ART) in which healthy sperm are placed inside the uterine cavity around the time of ovulation.

Intravenous immunoglobulin g (IVIg) therapy—involves using sterile intravenous immunoglobulin (IVIg) to normalize natural killer (NK) cell activity and deactivate antiphospholipid antibody (APA) production to enhance embryo implantation.

Laparoscope—a thin, lighted instrument, fitted with a telescope lens, that is inserted into the abdominal cavity during a laparoscopy and transmits images to a video monitor.

Laparoscopy—a minimally invasive outpatient surgical procedure in which the surgeon makes a tiny incision in or near the belly button and inserts a laparoscope to view the abdominal cavity and make diagnoses; additional small incisions are also made through which other instruments are inserted to treat the condition, such as excising any endometrial implants found.

Laparotomy—conventional open surgery under general anesthesia in which a wide incision is made in the abdomen.

Laser vaporization—destruction of implants using a high-power laser that directs a concentrated packet of light energy that instantly boils the cellular water in implants.

Laparoscopic assisted vaginal hysterectomy (LAVH)—hysterectomy through the vagina using a laparoscope.

Laparoscopic supracervical hysterectomy (LSH)—hysterectomy through an abdominal incision in which the uterus and a portion of the cervix is removed, leaving the ligaments that support the vagina and cervix intact.

Laparoscopic uterosacral nerve ablation (LUNA)—a surgical procedure in which a small nerve near the back of the uterus is severed to block pain transmission from the uterus.

Levonorgestrel—synthesized form (progestin) of the female sex hormone progesterone administered as a slow-releasing intrauterine device (IUD), used in the treatment of endometriosis.

Lipotropic combinations—nutritional supplements made up of several different ingredients that complement one another and are designed to enhance the liver's functions; in the case of women with endometriosis, lipotropic combinations help the liver process excess estrogen from the body.

Low density lipoprotein (LDL)—also known as bad cholesterol.

Luteal phase—occurs during the second half of the menstrual cycle; fully mature follicle secretes enough estradiol into the bloodstream to trigger the release of a large amount of luteinizing hormone (LH), which weakens the follicular wall and releases the mature egg.

Luteinizing hormone (LH)—hormone that triggers the release of the mature egg from the most mature ovarian follicle.

Lymph—a clear fluid that bathes the tissues of the body and carries the immune cells and foreign molecules into the bloodstream.

Lymphocytes—a variety of white blood cells that are a part of the body's immune system; filter the body of bacteria.

Lymphoid organs—the organs that make up the immune system involved in the production of lymphocytes and antibodies.

Lysosomal—an enzyme that induces tissue damage and pain.

Macrophage—a type of phagocyte found in tissues throughout the body, scavenger cells that rid tissues of worn-out cells, debris, bacteria, and other foreign matter.

Magnetic resonance imaging (MRI)—analysis of the absorption and transmission of high frequency radio waves by hydrogen in water molecules and other components of body tissue once placed in a strong magnetic field.

Major histocompatibility complex (MHC)—a type of antigen found on the surface of cells that is recognized by T cell lymphocytes.

Matrix metalloproteinase (MMP)—an enzyme that plays an important role in tissue remodeling associated with angiogenesis.

Medroxyprogesterone acetate (MPA)—synthesized form (progestin) of the female sex hormone progesterone administered as a tablet or an injection.

Menorrhagia—extensive blood loss during menstruation.

Mesothelium—a simple layer of cells that lines smooth, transparent membranes such as the peritoneum of the abdomen.

Mesoprogestins—a third category of progestins that mimics and blocks progesterone activity in the body.

Metaplasia—transformation of one type of cell into another.

Microlaparoscopy—a minimally invasive diagnostic surgical laparoscopy that involves the use of microlaparoscopes to make diagnosis.

Miscarriage—loss of an embryo or fetus from the uterus at a stage of the pregnancy in which it cannot survive on its own.

Monocyte—a type of phagocyte that circulates in the blood and swallows and digests microbes and other foreign matter; scavengers cell.

Motility—spontaneous movement of sperm in the uterus.

Myalgia—pain in the muscle.

Natural killer (NK) cells—detects, identifies, and destroys cells or organisms that are foreign to the body or that stray out of their usual domain.

Nonsteroidal anti-inflammatory drugs (NSAIDs)—a group of painkillers that block prostaglandin production in the body to alleviate pain, swelling, and inflammation.

Ovarian hyperstimulation syndrome (OHSS)—a complication of controlled ovarian hyperstimulation (COH) when the ovaries overrespond to therapy and produce so many eggs that the ovaries become swollen, enlarged, and very painful.

Ovulation—process of releasing a mature egg from a mature follicle.

Ovulation induction—using medication to stimulate the development of ovarian follicles to produce more than one egg.

Ovum—a ripened egg.

Pain map—a simple grid on which patients can pinpoint the precise locations of their pain.

Pathogenesis— the development of a disease.

Patient-assisted laparoscopy (PAL)—a laparoscopic technique in which the patient is awake during the procedure so she can pinpoint to the surgeon which areas, when touched by a probe, duplicate her pain.

Peritoneal fluid—fluid found in the abdominal and pelvic cavities that lubricates the organs in these areas.

Peritoneum—smooth surface lining that covers the entire abdominal wall and is folded inward over the organs in the pelvic area.

Phagocytes—large white blood cells that can swallow and digest microbes and other foreign matter; scavengers cells.

Phospholipids—a group of fatty compounds found in all tissues and organs of the body.

Photosensitivity—abnormal reaction to sunlight that can result in severe sunburns or skin rashes.

Phytoestrogen—plant estrogen that, when introduced into a woman's body, binds to estrogen receptors in organs such as the uterus and breasts and mimics estrogen's effects.

Pituitary gland—a gland located at the base of the brain that stores and secretes several different hormones for different functions in the body, such as the follicle-stimulating hormone (FSH) and luteinizing hormone (LH) for the menstrual cycle.

Pleural effusion—water on the lungs.

Pneumomediastinum—accumulation of air in the chest cavity.

Premenstrual syndrome (PMS)—a group of symptoms that occur in women the week or two before menstruation; include breast tenderness, headache, bloating, fatigue, irritability and other mood changes, among others.

Presacral neurectomy (PSN)—a surgical procedure in which the nerves in the back of the uterus are severed to block pain transmission from the uterus.

Progestin—synthesized progesterone that mimics progesterone's actions on the endometrial lining of the uterus.

Progesterone supplementation—administered during controlled ovarian hyperstimulation (COH) gonadotropin therapy to mimic a regular menstrual cycle.

Prolactin—a female hormone produced by the pituitary gland that stimulates the corpus luteum in the ovary to produce progesterone and also stimulates breast milk production after childbirth.

Proliferation—growth of new cells.

Prostaglandin—hormonelike chemicals that can cause inflammation and induce pain (inflammatory prostaglandins); also have a beneficial role in the body and are present in a wide variety of tissues; for instance, prostaglandins in the stomach are involved in the production of mucus, which protects the muscles and tissues against acid gastric juice.

Pseudomenopause—using chemicals derived from the body's own hormones to trick the body into thinking that the ovaries are no longer functioning.

Pseudopregnant—using chemicals derived from the body's own hormones to trick the body into thinking that a growing fetus is in the uterus.

Radical hysterectomy—total removal of uterus, ovaries, cervix, fallopian tubes, upper part of the vagina, the surrounding tissue, and sometimes the pelvic lymph nodes.

Rectovaginal septum—dividing wall/membrane between the rectum and the vagina.

Retrograde flow—menstrual blood that flows backward through the fallopian tubes instead of out through the vagina.

Sclerotherapy—the treatment/removal of ovarian endometriomas by first aspirating the cyst, then injecting an irritant solution, such as tetracycline solution, into the cyst cavity, destroying all viable cells and preventing cyst recurrence.

Self—organs, tissue, blood, etc., in the human body.

Selective estrogen receptor modulators (SERMs)—designer estrogens that mimic the effects of estrogen where it is needed and block the effects of estrogen in other areas.

Selective immunotherapy—an immunologically based treatment that normalizes natural killer (NK) cell activity and suppresses binding actions of antiphospholipid antibodies (APA) on integrins to increase the chances of conceiving.

Staging—the criteria given to disease based on its location, size, depth, and amount.

Stress incontinence—urine leakage brought on by a sneeze, laugh, or cough.

Stroma—the supportive connective framework of a cell, tissue, or organ.

Supracervical hysterectomy—removal of upper part of the uterus.

Suprapubic—pain experienced above the pelvic bone.

Tachycardia—an increase in the heart rate above normal.

TCDD—the acronym for 2,3,7,8-tetrachlorodibenzo-para-dioxin, a dioxin found responsible for increasing the risk of developing endometriosis.

T cell lymphocytes—small white blood cells that destroy infected cells and coordinate the body's overall immune response.

Testosterone—the major male sex hormone responsible for the development of male sex organs and secondary male sex characteristics such as voice change and facial hair growth.

Thoracic endometriosis syndrome (TES)—the collection of symptoms of endometriosis involving the lung.

Tinnitus—ringing in the ears experienced in the absence of any external sources of sound.

Topical—application of a gel or cream directly on the skin.

Total hysterectomy—removal of uterus and cervix.

Transvaginal laparoscopy (TL)—minimally invasive diagnostic procedure like a standard laparoscopy but through a needle puncture in the vagina.

Trophoblast—the tissue that forms the wall of the blastocyst.

Tumor necrosis factors alpha and beta (TNF-α and TNF-β)—proteins involved in the destruction of tumor cells.

Ultrasonography (ultrasound)—the projection of high-frequency sound waves, inaudible to the human ear, through a section of a body, which then produces images on a video monitor.

Uterosacral ligaments—ligaments that support the uterus.

Urge incontinence—urine leakage that occurs when you feel the urge to urinate but may not have enough warning to get to the bathroom on time.

Vaginal hysterectomy—hysterectomy through an incision in the vagina.

Vascular endothelial growth factor (VEGF)—chemicals involved in the invasive process of tumors, includes the formation of new blood cells critical to the growth and maintenance of endometrial implants.

Xenohormone—a class of hormones found in substances such as environmental pollutants like dioxin which, when introduced into the body, mimics the body's own natural hormones, upsetting the body's hormone balance.

Zygote—a fertilized egg.

Zygote intrafallopian transfer (ZIFT)—a form of in vitro fertilization (IVF) in which eggs are harvested, mixed with sperm, and fertilized in the laboratory; fertilized eggs are then introduced into the fallopian tubes.

APPENDIX C:

REFERENCES

Chapter 1

Endometriosis Research Center (ERC), Press Release: Groundbreaking Endometriosis Resolution Passed: House of Representatives Overwhelmingly Supports H. Con. Res. 291 in Session of 107th Congress, http://www .endocenter.org.

Redwine, David, "Endometriosis: Ignorance, Politics and 'Sophie's Choice,'" Gynecology Forum, vol. 8, no 1, 2003, http://www.medforum.nl/gynfo/ endometriosis_ignorance,_politics_and_.htm.

Chapter 2

A.D.A.M.S. Inc, Endometriosis, A.D.A.M.S. Inc. Well-Connected Series, December 2004, http://www.enh.org/healthandwellness/encyclopedia/well connected/000074.asp.

Editorial Perspectives from the 1999 World Congress on Endometriosis, http://www.ivf.com/article1.html.

Endometriosis Research Center (ERC), 2001: "The Future of Research and Treatment," http://www.endocenter.org.

———, "Endometriosis and You: Education and Encouragement for Young Women and Their Families," http://www.endocenter.org.

———, "Understanding Endometriosis: Past, Present and Future: How Far Have We Come? How Much Further Must We Go?," http://www.endo center.org.

Howard, Fred M., MS, MD, "Chronic Pelvic Pain," *Obstetrics and Gynecology*, vol. 101, no.3, March 2003.

Johnson, Ellen T., "What Is Endometriosis?," http://www.endozone .org/display.asp?page=what_is_endometriosis.

Lee, John, *What Your Doctor May Not Tell You About Menopause*, New York: Warner Books, 2005.

Seli, Emre, Murat Berkkanoglu, and Ayolin Arici, "Pathogenesis of Endometriosis," *Obstetrics and Gynecology Clinics of North America*, vol. 30, no.1, March 2003.

Winkel, Craig A., "Evaluation and Management of Women with Endometriosis," *Obstetrics and Gynecology*, vol. 102, no.2, August 2003.

Chapters 3 and 4

"Aromatase in Endometriosis," http://www.endozone.org/display.asp?page =congress_ESHRE2003_dhooge-bulun.

Birnbaum, Linda S., and Audrey M. Cummings, "Dioxins and Endometriosis: A Plausible Hypothesis," *Environmental Health Perspectives*, vol. 110, no. 1, January 2002, http://ehp.niehs.nih.gov/members/2002/ 110p15-21birnbaum/birnbaum-full.html.

"Changes in Immune and Endocrine System in Women with Endometriosis," http://www.endozone.org/display.asp?page=congress_ASRM2002- Ballweg-01.

"Coffee Increases Estrogen in Women," http://www.mercola.com/fcgi/ pf2001/dec/8/coffee_estrogen.htm.

Cramer, Daniel W., et al., "The Relation of Endometriosis to Menstrual Characteristics, Smoking and Exercise," *Journal of the American Medical Association*, vol. 255, no. 14, April 11, 1986.

Crisp, Thomas M, et al., "Environmental Endocrine Disruption: An Effects Assessment and Analysis," *Environmental Health Perspectives*, vol. 106, Supplement 1, February 1998, http://ehp.niehs.nih.gov/realfiles/members/ 1998/Suppl-1/11-56crisp/full2.html.

"Endometrial Cells Can Originate from Donor-Derived Bone Marrow Cells," http://www.endozone.org/display.asp?page=news_0407_endome trial_cells.

Guidone, Heather C., "Building the Typical Endometriosis Patient Profile," http://www.hcgresources.com/profile.htm.

Harrar, Sarí N., "Redheads Feel More Pain: Genetic Glitch Has Hidden *Ouch* Factor," http://www.prevention.com/article/0,5778,s1-1-77-169-2444-1,00.html?.

Harada, Tasuku, et al., "Role of Cytokines in Progression of Endometriosis," *Gynecologic and Obstetric Investigation*, vol. 47, Supplement 1, 1999.

Healy, D. L., P. A. W. Rogers, L. Hii, and M. Wingfield, "Angiogenesis: A New Theory for Endometriosis," *Human Reproduction Update*, vol. 4, no. 5, 1998.

Hemmings, Robert, et al., "Evaluation of Risk Factors Associated with Endometriosis," *Fertility and Sterility*, vol. 81, no. 6, June 2004.

"High-Intensity Physical Activity Reduces Endometrioma Risk," http://www.endozone.org/display.asp?page=news_0310_high-intensity-physical-activity.

"Is Endometriosis Angiogenesis Dependent?" http://www.endozone.org/display.asp?page=congress_WCGE2004-greb-taylor.

"Italian Research Links Diet with Endometriosis Risk," http://www.eurekalert.org/pub_releases/2004-07/esfh-ir/071204.php.

Kirshon, Brian, and Alfred N. Poindexter III, "Contraception: A Risk Factor for Endometriosis," *Obstetrics and Gynecology*, vol. 71, no. 6, part 1, June 1988.

Kyama, Cleophas M., et al., "Potential Involvement of the Immune System in the Development of Endometriosis," *Reproductive Biology and Endocrinology*, January 2003, http://www.rbej.com/content/1/1/123.

Lebovic, Dan I., "Immunobiology of Endometriosis," *Fertility and Sterility*, vol. 75, no. 1, January 2001.

McLaren, J., "Vascular Endothelial Growth Factor and Endometriotic Angiogenesis," *Human Reproduction Update*, vol. 6, no. 1, January 2000.

Missmer, Stacey A., and Daniel W. Cramer, "The Epidemiology of Endometriosis," *Obstetrics and Gynecology Clinics of North America*, vol. 30, no.1, March 2003.

Redwine, David, "The Immune System and Sin #4," *St. Charles Medical Center Endometriosis Newsletter*, Spring 1997, http://www.endometriosistreatment.org/html/reprint10.html.

Seli, Emre, Murat Berkkanoglu, and Ayolin Arici, "Pathogenesis of Endometriosis," *Obstetrics and Gynecology Clinics of North America*, vol. 30, no.1, March 2003.

Sinaii, N. et al., "High Rates of Autoimmune and Endocrine Disorders, Fibromyalgia, Chronic Fatigue Syndrome and Atopic Diseases Among Women with Endometriosis: A Survey Analysis," *Journal of Human Reproduction*, vol. 17, no. 10, October 2002.

Stefansson, H., et al., "Genetic Factors Contribute to the Risk of Developing Endometriosis," *Journal of Human Reproduction*, vol. 17, no. 3, 2002.

U.S. Department of Health and Human Services/National Institutes of Health, "Understanding the Immune System: How It Works," National Institute of Allergy and Infectious Disease and the National Cancer Institute, September 2003, http://www.niaid.nih.gov/publications/immune/the_immune_system.pdf.

"U.S. Researchers Find Endometriosis Associated with Wide Range of Diseases Including Autoimmune, Endocrine, Allergic and Chronic Pain and Fatigue Disorders," http://www.endozone.org/display.asp?page=pr_sinaii.

Woodworth, Steven H., et al., "A Prospective Study on the Association Between Red Hair Color and Endometriosis in Infertile Patients," *Fertility and Sterility*, vol. 64, no. 3, September 1995.

Chapter 5

"ACOG Issues New Practice Bulletin on Chronic Pelvic Pain in Women," http://www.endozone.org/display.asp?pages=ews_0403_acog.

Ballweg, Mary Lou, and the Endometriosis Association (eds.), *The Endometriosis Sourcebook*, Chicago: Contemporary Books, 1998.

Carter, E. Jane, and David B. Ettensohn, "Catamenial Pneumothorax," *Chest*, vol. 98, no. 3, September 1990.

"Catamenial Pneumothorax—What Is It?," http://www.catamenialpneumothorax.com/id2.htm.

"Endometriotic Lesions Grow Nerves," http://www.endozone.org/display.asp?page=news_0407_nerves.

Guidone, Heather, "Building the Typical Endometriosis Patient Profile," http://www.hcgresources.com/profile.htm.

———, "The Encounter or How to Get Your Doctor to Listen," http://www.hcgresources.com/talktodoctor.html.

———, "Uncommon Manifestations: Sciatic and Thoracic Endometriosis," http://www.hcgresources.com/sciaticthoracic.html.

Johnson, Margaret M., "Catamenial Pneumothorax and Other Thoracic Manifestations of Endometriosis," *Clinics in Chest Medicine,* vol. 25, no. 2, June 2004.

Joseph, Jos, and Steven A. Sohn, "Thoracic Endometriosis Syndrome: New Observations from an Analysis of 110 Cases," *American Journal of Medicine*, vol. 100, no. 2, February 1996.

"Kissing Ovaries Predict Severe Endometriosis," http://www.endozone.org/display.asp?page=news_0502_kissing-ovaries.

"Link Between Migraine, Endometriosis Found," http://www.endozone.org/display.asp?page=news_0502_migraine.

Matalliotakis, Ioannis M., et al., "Pulmonary Endometriosis in a Patient with Unicornuate Uterus and Noncommunicating Rudimentary Horn," *Fertility and Sterility*, vol. 78, no. 1, July 2002.

Nezhat, Camran, et al., "Laparoscopic Surgical Management of Diaphragmatic Endometriosis," *Fertility and Sterility*, vol. 69, no. 6, June 1998.

Nirula, Raminder, and Gregory C. Greaney, "Incisional Endometriosis: An Underappreciated Diagnosis in General Surgery," *Journal of the American College of Surgeons*, April 2000, http://www.facs.org/jacs/lead_articles/apr00lead.html.

Parade/Research!America, Taking Our Pulse: The Parade/Research!America Health Poll, 2004, http://www.researchamerica.org/polldata/2004/paradewomenshealth04.pdf.

"Quality of Sex Life in Women with Endometriosis and Deep Dyspareunia," http://www.endometriosis.org/research0405.html.

Redwine, David B., "Diaphragmatic Endometriosis—Similar but Different," *St. Charles Medical Center Endometriosis Newsletter*, Winter 1994, http://www.endometriosistreatment.org/html/reprint9.html.

———, "Intestinal Endometriosis," http://www.endometriosiszone.org.display.asp?page=expert/intestinal_endometriosis.

Roberts, Lisa M., Jay Redan, and Harry Reich, "Extraperitoneal Endometriosis, Catamenial Pneumothorax, and Review of the Literature," http://www.endometriosiszone.org/display.asp?page=/expert/extraperitoneal_endometriosis.htm.

Seli, Emre, Murat Berkanoglu, and Aydin Arici, "Pathogenesis of Endometriosis," *Obstetrics and Gynecology Clinics of North America*, vol. 30, no. 1, March 2003.

Sinervo, Ken, "Endometriosis and Bowel Symptoms," http://www.centerforendo.com/news/bowel%20endo/bowel%20endo.htm.

Smith, Susan A., "Double Trouble: The Axis of Pain and Depression," *Psychology Today*, July–August 2004.

"U.S. Researchers Find Endometriosis Associated with Wide Range of Diseases Including Autoimmune, Endocrine, Allergic and Chronic Pain and Fatigue Disorders," http://www.endozone.org/display.asp?page=pr_sinaii.

"Women Report Chronic Pelvic Pain Not Taken Seriously, Survey Shows," http://www.obgyn.net/newsheadlines/women_health-endometriosis-20021114-22.asp.

Wood, Ros, "Bowel Symptoms," http://www.endometriosis.org/bowel-symptoms.html

Chapter 6

American College of Surgeons, "About Hysterectomy: Surgical Removal of the Uterus or Womb," http://www.facs.org/public_info/operation/hysterectomy.pdf.

Ballweg, Mary Lou, and the Endometriosis Association (eds.), *The Endometriosis Sourcebook*, Chicago: Contemporary Books, 1995.

Benn, Linda, "Alternatives to Hysterectomy: New Technologies, More Options," *FDA Consumer Magazine*, vol. 35, no. 6, November–December, 2001.

"Breakthrough Endometriosis Pain Treatment: Menastil," http://www.immediate-relief.com.

Cook, Andrew, "Ask Dr. Cook: How are Adhesions Treated?," http://www.drcook.com/adca17.html.

———, "Ask Dr. Cook: What Are Adhesions?," http://www.drcook.com/adca15.html.

———, "Ask Dr. Cook: What Causes Adhesions?," http://www.drcook.com/adca16.html.

Endometriosis Research Center (ERC), "Understanding Hysterectomy," http://www.endocenter.org/.

"Endometriosis Symptoms Improve Dramatically After Surgery for Most Women—UB Prospective Study Finds," http://www.scienceblog.com/community/older/1997/B/199701310.html.

"Evaluating Adjustment Presacral Neurectomy for the Treatment of Dysmenorrhea Associated with Endometriosis," http://www.endozone.org/display.asp?page=news_0405_evaluating-adjuvant.

Gambone, Joseph C., et al., "Consensus Statement for the Management of Chronic Pelvic Pain and Endometriosis: Proceedings of an Expert-Panel Consensus Process," *Fertility and Sterility*, vol. 78, no. 5, November 2002.

Georgia Reproductive Specialists, "Endometrial Ablation," http://www.ivf.com/eablate.html.

Guidone, Heather C., "The Hysterectomy Decision," http://www.hcgresources.com/hysts.htm.

———, "Tell Me Where It Hurts—Patient-Assisted Laparoscopy (Pain Mapping): Pointing Out the Pain," http://www.hcgresources.com/Pain Mapping.html.

———, "Understanding LUNA and PSN," http://www.hcgresources.com/LUNAPSN.htm.

"Laparoscopic Excision of Endometriosis a Long-Term Success," http://www.endozone.org/display.asp?page=news_0309_laparoscopic-excision-of-endometriosis.

Martin, Dan C., and Daniel T. O'Connor, "Surgical Management of Endometriosis-Associated Pain," *Obstetrics and Gynecology Clinics of North America*, vol. 30, no.1, March 2003.

"Microlaparoscopy for Women with Chronic Pelvic Pain and Pain Mapping," http://www.obgyn.net/displaytranscript.asp?page=/avtranscripts/aagl998-demco.

National Women's Health Information Center (NWHIC), "Frequently Asked Questions About Hysterectomy," http://www.4woman.gov/faq/infertility.htm.

Perloe, Mark, "What Is Microlaparoscopy?," http://www.ivf.com/microlap.html.

"Recurrent Endometriosis Pain Following Hysterectomy," http://www.endometriosiszone.org/display.asp?page=/congress_ISGE2004_hysterectomy.htm.

St. Johns Mercy Hospital, "Tests and Procedures—Endometrial Ablation," http://www.stjohnsmercy.org/healthinfo/test/gyn/TP113.asp.

U.S. Food and Drug Administration, "FDA Approves New Anti-Adhesion Treatment for Gynecologic Surgery," *FDA Talk Paper*, November 19, 2001, http://www.fda.gov/bbs/topics/ANSWERS/2001/ANS01117.html.

"Uterosacral Ligament Resection Has No Extra Dysmenorrhea Benefit," http://www.endozone.org/display.asp?page=news_0309_uterosacral-ligament-resection.

Winkel, Craig A., "Evaluation and Management of Women with Endometriosis," *Obstetrics and Gynecology*, vol. 102, no. 2, August 2003.
Wiseman, David M., "A Patient's Guide to Adhesions and Related Pain,"
http://www.obgny.net/cpp/cpp.asp?page=/CPP/articles/cpp_wiseman
_0399#what%20are%20ADHESIONS.

Chapter 7

American Academy of Allergy, Asthma and Immunology (AAAAI), "Tips
to Remember: What Is Allergy Testing?," http://www.aaaai.org/
patients/publicedmat/tips/whatisallergytesting.stm.
———, "Tips to Remember: What Are Allergy Shots?," http://www.aaaai
.org/patients/publicedmat/tips/whatareallergyshots.stm.
"Angiogenesis Therapy for Endometriosis," http://www.endometriosis
zone.org/display.asp?page=/news/news_0403_angiogenesis.htm.
"Asoprisnil Looks Promising for Endometriosis and Uterine Fibroids,"
http://www.endometriosiszone.org/display.asp?page=/news_0402_asopris
nil.htm.
Ballweg, Mary Lou, and the Endometriosis Association (eds.), *The Endometriosis Sourcebook*, Chicago: Contemporary Books, 1995.
Barberie, Robert L., "Gonadotropin-Releasing Hormone Agonists: Treatment of Endometriosis," *Clinical Obstetrics and Gynecology*, vol. 36, no.
3, September 1993.
Bulun, Serder E., et al., "Aromatase and Endometriosis," *Seminars in Reproductive Medicine*, vol. 22, no. 1, January 2004.
Chabbert-Buffet, Nathalie, et al., "GnRH Antagonists," *Clinical Obstet-
rics and Gynecology*, vol. 46, no. 2, June 2003.
"Endometriosis: Could Angiostatic Therapy Be the New Treatment of the
Future?," http://www.endometriosiszone.org/display.asp?page=/news
_0407_angiostatic-therapy.htm.
FDA News, "FDA Announces Series of Changes to the Class of Marketed
Non-Steroidal Anti-Inflammatory Drugs (NSAIDs)," http://www.fda.gov/
bbs/topics/news/2005/NEW01171.html.
Frackiewicz, Edyla J., "Endometriosis: An Overview of the Disease and Its
Treatment," *Journal of the American Pharmaceutical Association*, vol.,
40, no. 5, May 2000.
French, Linda, "Dysmenorrhea," *American Family Physician*, vol. 71, no.
2, January 15, 2005.

Gambone, Joseph C., et al., "Consensus Statement for the Management of Chronic Pelvic Pain and Endometriosis: Proceedings of an Expert-Panel Consensus Process," *Fertility and Sterility*, vol. 78, no. 5, November 2002.

Giudice, Linda C., and Lee C. Kao, "Endometriosis," *The Lancet*, vol. 364, no. 9447, November 13–19, 2004.

"Great News for Menstrual Cramp Sufferers: Menastil," *Business Wire*, October 10, 2001.

Guidone, Heather C., "RU-486 Explained," http://www.hcgresources.com/RU486.htm.

"Immune Treatment for Endometriosis," http://www.obgyn.net/endo/articles/immune-endo.htm.

Kirn, Timothy F., "Heat Therapy Equal to Ibuprofen for Dysmenorrhea," *Family Practice News*, February 1, 2000.

Lessey, Bruce A., "Medical Management of Endometriosis and Infertility," *Fertility and Sterility*, vol. 73, no. 6, June 2000.

"Letrozole May Help Women with Endometriosis," http://www.endometriosiszone.org/display.asp?page=/news_0402_letrozole.htm.

Mahutte, Neal G., and Aydin Arici, "Medical Management of Endometriosis-Associated Pain," *Obstetrics and Gynecology Clinics of North America*, vol. 30, no. 1, March 2003.

Martin, Dan C., and Daniel T. O'Connor, "Surgical Management of Endometriosis-Associated Pain," *Obstetrics and Gynecology Clinics of North America*, vol. 30, no.1, March 2003.

Mayo Clinic Staff, "Over-the-Counter Pain Reliever Guide: Compare Before Choosing," http://www.mayoclinic.com/invoke.cfm?id=PN00061.

———, "Pain Centers and Clinics: Turn to the Specialists," http://www.mayoclinic.com/invoke.cfm?id=PN00047.

———, "Topical Painkillers: Rubbing in Relief," http://www.mayoclinic.com/invoke.cfm?id=PN00041.

MedlinePlus, "Drug Information: Acetaminophen," http://www.nlm.nih.gov/medlineplus/druginfo/uspdi/202001.html.

———, "Drug Information: Narcotic Analgesics," http://www.nlm.nih.gov/medlineplus/druginfo/uspdi/202390.html.

———, "Drug Information: Non-Steroidal Anti-Inflammatory Drugs," http://www.nlm.nih.gov/medlineplus/druginfo/uspdi/202743.html.

"Mesoprogestins (Asoprisnil) in the Treatment of Endometriosis," http://www.endometriosiszone.org/display.asp?page=/congress_WCGE 2004-croxatto.htm.

Metzger, Deborah A., J. Francher, and A. J. Kresch, "Immunotherapy as a Treatment for Endometriosis: A Novel and Cost Effective Approach," http://www.harmonywomenshealth.com/web/FramedArticle.aspx?Bar=MoreInfo&ArticleId=HwhEndometriosisImmunotherapy.

National Pain Foundation (NPF), "Tips for Finding a Pain Physician," http://www.painconnection.net/MyPain/TipsForFindingAPainPhysician.asp.

"Oral Contraceptive Regimen Reduces Endometriosis Dysmenorrhea," http://www.endometriosiszone.org/display.asp?page=/news_0310_oral-contraceptive-regimen-reduces-endo-dysmenorrhea.htm.

Vercellini, Paolo, et al., "Endometriosis Perspective and Postoperative Medical Treatment," *Obstetrics and Gynecology Clinics of North America*, vol. 30, no. 1, March 2003.

Winkel, Craig A., "Evaluation and Management of Women with Endometriosis," *Obstetrics and Gynecology*, vol. 102, no. 2, August 2003.

Wood, Ros, and Ellen T. Johnson, "Managing Endometriosis Pain with NSAIDs," http://www.endometriosis.org/nsaids.html.

Zupi, Errico, et al., "Add-Back Therapy in the Treatment of Endometriosis-Associated Pain," *Fertility and Sterility*, vol. 82, no. 5, November 2004.

Chapter 8

American Society for Reproductive Medicine (ASRM), "Assisted Reproductive Technologies: A Guide for Patients," 2003, http://www.asrm.org/Patients/patientbooklets/ART.pdf.

———, "Ovulation Drugs: A Guide for Patients," 2000, http://www.asrm.org/Patients/patientbooklets/ovulation_drugs.pdf.

Ballweg, Mary Lou, and the Endometriosis Association, (eds.), *The Endometriosis Sourcebook*, Chicago: Contemporary Books, 1998.

Cahill, D. J., "What Is the Optimal Medical Management of Infertility and Minor Endometriosis," *Journal of Human Reproduction*, vol. 17, no. 5, May 2002.

The Endometriosis Treatment Center (a Division of Sher Institute for Reproductive Medicine), "Advanced Treatment for Endometriosis Associated Infertility," http://www.treatendo.com/advinferttreat.htm.

———, "Immune Disorders and Endometriosis Associated Infertility," http://www.treatendo.com/immunedis.htm.

———, "Sclerotherapy: Non-Surgical Treatment of Endometriomas," http://www.treatendo.com/sclerotherapy.htm.

————, "Toxic Pelvic Fluid Environment and Endometriosis Associated Infertility," http://www.treatendo.com/toxicfluid.htm.

————, "Use of Trental for the Treatment of Endometriosis Chronic Pelvic Pain," http://www.treatendo.com/trental.htm.

————, "Uterine Receptivity and Endometriosis Associated Infertility," http://www.treatendo.com/uterinerecpt.htm.

Fisch, Jeffrey, and Geoffrey Sher, "Sclerotherapy with 5% Tetracycline Is a Simple Alternative to Potentially Complex Surgical Treatment of Ovarian Endometriomas Before In Vitro Fertilization," *Fertility and Sterility*, vol. 82, no. 2, August 2004.

"Gene Defect Implicated in Endometriosis-Related Infertility," http://www.endozone.org/display.asp?page=news_0306_gene-defect-implicated.

Gruppo Italiano per lo Studio dell'Endometriosi, "Ablation of Lesions or No Treatment in Minimal–Mild Endometriosis in Infertile Women: A Randomized Trial," *Journal of Human Reproduction*, vol. 14, no. 5, May 1999.

Guidone, Heather C., "Infertility and Endometriosis," http://www.hcgresources.com/infert.htm.

"The Immune System and Infertility in Women with Endometriosis," http://www.endozone.org/display.asp?page=congress_ISGE2003-Dmowski.

"In Vitro Fertilization," http://www.fertilitext.org/p2_doctor/ivf.html.

Kontrik, Susan, "Understanding the Role of Progesterone Therapy in the Management of Infertility," http://www.cvsprocare.com/content/fertility/clinical/progesteron.html.

Kovacs, Peter, "Conference Report: Highlights from the American Society for Reproductive Medicine 60th Annual Meeting, October 16–20, 2004, Philadelphia, Pennsylvania," http://www.medscape.com/viewarticle/492951?src=search.

————, "Endometriosis and Infertility," http://www.medscape.com/viewarticle/469217.

Larkin, Marilynn, "Endometriosis-Infertility Link Explained?" *The Lancet*, vol. 356, July 8, 2000.

Lessey, Bruce A., "Medical Management of Endometriosis and Infertility," *Fertility and Sterility*, vol. 73, no. 6, June 2000.

Marcoux, Sylvie, et al., "Laparoscopic Surgery in Infertile Women with Minimal or Mild Endometriosis," *The New England Journal of Medicine*, vol. 337, no. 4, July 24, 1997.

Martínez-Román, Sergio, et al., "Immunological Factors in Endometriosis-Associated Reproductive Failure: Studies in Fertile and Infertile Women with and Without Endometriosis," *Journal of Human Reproduction*, vol. 12, no. 8, August 1997.

Onmland, A. K., et al., "Natural Cycle IVF in Unexplained, Endometriosis-Associated and Tubal Factor Infertility," *Journal of Human Reproduction*, vol. 16, no. 12, December 2001.

Peris, Anna, "Ovulation Induction," http://www.fertilitext.org/pg2_doctor/induction.html.

PharmaCare, "Treatment of Infertility: Available Drugs," http://www.stadtlander.com/content/fertility/fertilmeds.html.

Reeve, L., H. Lashen, and A. A. Pacey, "Endometriosis Affects Sperm-Endosalpingeal Interactions," *Journal of Human Reproduction*, vol. 20, no. 2, February 2005.

Science Blog, "Missing Proteins in the Uterus Tied to Infertility in Women with Endometriosis," http://www.scienceblog.com/community/older/2000/E/200004760.html.

Sher Institute for Reproductive Medicine (SIRM), "Endometriosis and Immunologic Implantation Failure: A Rational Basis for IVF with Immunomodulation Therapy," http://haveababy.com/infert/immunomod.asp?site=.

———, "Endometriosis and Infertility," http://haveababy.com/infert/endometriosis.asp

———, "Immunologic Implantation Failure: Why It Often Leads to IVF Failure and the Role of Selective Immunotherapy," http://haveababy.com/infert/immunesci.asp?site=.

———, "Immunologic Testing and Selective Immunotherapy in Women Undergoing In Vitro Fertilization for Female Causes of Infertility," http://haveababy.com/infert/immunett.asp?site=.

———, "Management of Infertility Associated with Endometriosis," http://haveababy.com/infert/endoman.asp?site=.

———, "New Research Discovers Link Between Specific Antibodies in Women and Unsuccessful In Vitro Pregnancies," http://haveababy.com/infert/immunebreak.asp?site=.

———, "The Role of Antiphospholipid Antibodies (APA), Natural Killer (NK) Cells and Endometrial Cytokines in Immunologic Implantation Failure," http://haveababy.com/infert/implantfail.asp?site=.

———, "Sclerotherapy for the Treatment of Ovarian Endometriotic Cysts (Endometriomas) Prior to IVF," http://haveababy.com/infert/sclero.asp ?site=.

Surrey, Eric S., and William B. Schoolcraft, "Management of Endometriosis-Associated Infertility," *Obstetrics and Gynecology Clinics of North America*, vol. 30, no. 1, March 2003.

Van Loenen, André C.D., et al., "GnRH Agonists, Antagonists and Assisted Conception," *Seminars in Reproductive Medicine*, vol. 20, no. 4, April 2002.

WebMD, "Fertility Awareness," http://my.webmd.com/hw/infertility _reproduction/hw214032.asp.

Women's Surgery Group, "Hormonal Therapy," http://www.womenssurgery group.com/conditions/Infertility/treatment.asp

Chapter 9

Chiang, Jeanne, "Supplement Recommendations for Endometriosis," http:// www.wholehealthmd.com/print/view/1,1560,RA_460_supp,00.html

De Smet, Peter A. G. M, "Herbal Remedies," *New England Journal of Medicine*, vol. 347, no. 25, December 2002.

Douglas, David, "Black Cohosh Extract Relieves Hot Flashes," *Reuters Health*, http://www.nlm.nih.gov/medlineplus/news/fullstory_24768.html.

"Endometriosis: Healing with Herbs, Vitamins and Minerals," http://www.herbs2000.com/women/herbs_w_13.htm.

Feinstein, Alice (ed.), *Prevention's Healing with Vitamins: The Most Effective Vitamin and Mineral Treatments for Everyday Health Problems and Serious Diseases*, Emmaus, Pennsylvania: Rodale Books, 1996.

Food and Nutrition Board of the Institute of Medicine (National Academy of Sciences—NAS), Dietary Intake Reference Tables: Vitamins Table, http://www.iom.edu/Object.File/Master/7/296/0.pdf.

———, Dietary Intake Reference Tables: Elements Table, http://www .iom.edu/Object.File/Master/7/294/0.pdf

Gaby, Alan R., "Vitamin C and E Effective Against Endometriosis Pain," *Townsend Letter for Doctors and Patients*, August–September 2004.

Huggins, Charnicia E., "Calcium, Vitamin D May Help Prevent PMS," *Reuters Health*, http://www.nlm.nih.gov/medlineplus/news/fullstory _25180.html.

Johnson, Kate, "Improved Endometriosis Pain Tied to Vitamins: Small Study of Short-Term Use," *OB/GYN News*, December 15, 2003.

Krapp, Kristine, and Jacqueline L. Longe (eds.), *The Gale Encyclopedia of Alternative Medicine*, vols. 1–4, Detroit: Gale Group, 2001.

Lark, Susan M., "Supplements and Herbs for Endometriosis and Fibroids," http://dev1.drlark.com/nc/fe_supplements.asp.

Mayo Clinic Staff, "Herb and Drug Interactions: 'Natural' Products Not Always Safe," http://www.mayoclinic.com/invoke.cfm?id=SA00039.

———, "Herbal Supplements: What to Know Before You Buy," http://www.mayoclinic.com/invoke.cfm?id=SA00044.

———, "Vitamin and Mineral Supplements: Use with Care," http://www.mayoclinic.com/invoke.cfm?id=NU00198.

National Center for Complementary and Alternative Medicine (NCCAM), "Backgrounder—Biologically Based Practices: An Overview," http://nccam.nih.gov/health/backgrounds/biobasedprac.pdf.

———, "Get the Facts—Are You Considering Complementary and Alternative Medicine?" http://nccam.nih.gov/health/decisions/considering.pdf.

———, "Get the Facts—What Is Complementary and Alternative Medicine," http://nccam.nih.gov/health/whatiscam/pdf/whatiscam.pdf.

Office of Dietary Supplements (ODS), "Dietary Supplement Fact Sheet: Calcium," http://ods.od.nih.gov/factsheets/calcium.asp.

———, "Dietary Supplement Fact Sheet: Magnesium," http://ods.od.nih.gov/factsheets/magnesium.asp.

———, "Dietary Supplement Fact Sheet: Selenium," http://ods.od.nih.gov/factsheets/selenium.asp.

———, "Facts About Dietary Supplements: Zinc," http://ods.od.nih.gov/factsheets/cc/zinc.html.

———, "Questions and Answers About Black Cohosh and the Symptoms of Menopause," http://ods.od.nih.gov/factsheets/BlackCohosh.asp.

"Vitamin E May Relieve Menstrual Pain," http://www.endometriosis.org/vitaminE.html.

WholeHealthMD.com, "Calcium/Magnesium," http://www.wholehealthmd.com/refshelf/substances_view/1,1525,937,00.html.

———, "Chasteberry," http://www.wholehealthmd.com/refshelf/substances_view/1,1525,767,00.html.

———, "Dandelion," http://www.wholehealthmd.com/refshelf/substances_view/1,1525,10021,00.html.

————, "Dong Quai," http://www.wholehealthmd.com/refshelf/substances_view/1,1525,774,00.html.

————, "Evening Primrose Oil," http://www.wholehealthmd.com/refshelf/substances_view/1,1525,779,00.html.

————, "Flaxseed Oil," http://www.wholehealthmd.com/print/view/1,1560,SU_783,00.html

————, "Lipotropic Combination," http://www.wholehealthmd.com/refshelf/substances_view/1,1525,861,00.html.

————, "Natural Progesterone Cream," http://www.wholehealthmd.com/refshelf/substances_view/1,1525,10099,00.html.

————, "Turmeric," http://www.wholehealthmd.com/refshelf/substances_view/1,1525,10062,00.html.

————, "Wild Yam," http://www.wholehealthmd.com/refshelf/substances_view/1,1525,10070,00.html.

Chapter 10

Anandarjah, Gowri, and Ellen Hight, "Spirituality and Medical Practice: Using the HOPE Questions as a Practical Tool for Spiritual Assessment," *American Family Physician*, January 1, 2001, http://www.aafp.org/afp/20010101/81.html.

"Dietary Modification to Alleviate Endometriosis Symptoms," http://www.endozone.org/display.asp?page=congress_ASRM2002-Mills02.

"Exercise Lowers Endometriosis Risk—Live Healthy," *Shape Magazine*, January 2004.

"Fish Oils," http://www.herbs2000.com/miss/fish_oils.htm.

"Italian Research Links Diet with Endometriosis Risk," http://www.eurekalert.org/pub_releases/2004-07/esfh-ir/071204.php.

Lark, Susan M., "Diet for Endometriosis and Fibroids," http://dev1.drlark.com/nc/fe_diet.asp.

Lee, John, *What Your Doctor May Not Tell You About Menopause*, New York: Warner Books, 2005.

Mayo Clinic Staff, "Acupuncture: Sharp Answers to Pointed Questions," http://www.mayoclinic.com/invoke.cfm?id=SA00086.

————, "Biofeedback: Using the Power of Your Mind to Improve Your Health," http://www.mayoclinic.com/invoke.cfm?id=SA00083.

———, "Chronic Pain: Exercise Can Bring Relief," http://www.mayo clinic.com/invoke.cfm?id=AR00017.

———, "Massage: A Relaxing Way to Relieve Muscle Tension," http://www.mayoclinic.com/invoke.cfm?id=SA00082.

———, "Meditation: Focusing Your Mind to Achieve Relaxation," http://www.mayoclinic.com/invoke.cfm?id=HQ01070.

———, "Relax: Techniques to Help You Achieve Tranquility," http://www.mayoclinic.com/invoke.cfm?id=SR00007.

———, "Tai Chi," http://www.mayoclinic.com/invoke.cfm?id=SA00087.

———, "Yoga: Moving and Breathing Your Way to Relaxation," http://www.mayoclinic.com/invoke.cfm?id=CM00004.

Morin, Richard, "Calling Dr. God," July 8, 2001, http://www.washington post.com/ac2/wp-dyn?pagename=article&contentId=A30449-2001Jul7&notFound=true.

National Center for Complementary and Alternative Medicine (NCCAM), "Backgrounder—Energy Medicine: An Overview," http://nccam.nih.gov/health/backgrounds/energymed.pdf.

———, "Backgrounder—Manipulative and Body-Based Practices: An Overview," http://nccam.nih.gov/health/backgrounds/manipulative.pdf.

———, "Backgrounder—Mind-Body Medicine: An Overview," http://nccam.nih.gov/health/backgrounds/mindbody.pdf.

———, "Get the Facts: Acupuncture," http://nccam.nih.gov/health/acupuncture/acupuncture.pdf.

National Women's Health Information Center (NWHIC), "Stress and Your Health," http://www.4woman.gov/faq/stress.htm.

"Nutrients and Endometriosis," OBGYN.net Conference Coverage from Endometriosis 2000—7th Biennial World Congress, London, May 2000, http://www.obgyn.net/infertility/infertility.asp?page=/avtranscripts/wce2klondon_mills.

"Prayer and Spirituality in Health: Ancient Practices, Modern Science," CAM at the NIH: Focus on Complementary and Alternative Medicine, vol. XII, no. 1, Winter 2005, http://nccam.nih.gov/news/newsletter/2005_winter/prayer.htm.

Shepperson Mills, Dian, "Nutritional Support for Endometriosis and Fertility," http://www.obgyn.net/endo/articles/nutrient.htm.

Smyth, Joshua M., et al., "Effects of Writing About Stressful Experiences on Symptom Reduction in Patients with Asthma or Rheumatoid Arthritis," *Journal of the American Medical Association*, vol. 281, no. 14, April 14, 1999.

"Spirituality and Health," *American Family Physician*, January 1, 2001, http://www.aafp.org/afp/20010101/89ph.html.

University of Iowa Health Science Relations and Donald Black, "Laughter: It Does More Than Improve Your Mood," *Health Prose: A One-Minute Update for Your Health*, December 2004, http://www.vh.org/adult/patient/psychiatry/prose/laughter.html.

WholeHealthMD.com, "Acupuncture," http://www.wholehealthmd.com/refshelf/substances_view/1,1525,663,00.html.

———, "Biofeedback," http://www.wholehealthmd.com/refshelf/substances_view/1,1525,675,00.html.

———, "Guided Imagery," http://www.wholehealthmd.com/refshelf/substances_view/1,1525,699,00.html.

———, "Fish Oils," http://www.wholehealthmd.com/refshelf/substances_view/1,1525,781,00.html.

———, "Massage," http://www.wholehealthmd.com/refshelf/substances_view/1,1525,716,00.html.

———, "Meditation," http://www.wholehealthmd.com/refshelf/substances_view/1,1525,717,00.html.

———, "Writing Therapy," http://www.wholehealthmd.com/refshelf/substances_view/1,1525,745,00.html.

Woolston, Chris, "Writing for Therapy Helps Erase Effects of Trauma," http://archives.cnn.com/2000/HEALTH/03/16/health.writing.wmd.

Chapter 12

Abrao, Mauricio Simoes, et al., "Microlaparoscopy for an Intact Ectopic Pregnancy and Endometriosis with the Use of a Diode Laser: Case Report," *Journal of Human Reproduction*, vol. 15, no. 6, June 2000.

Bedaiwy, Mohamed A., and Tommaso Falcone, "Laboratory Testing for Endometriosis," *Clinica Chimica Acta*, February 2004.

Blumenthal, Rosalyn D., et al., "Unique Molecular Markers in Human Endometriosis: Implications for Diagnosis and Therapy," *Expert Reviews in Molecular Medicine*, http://www-ermm.cbcu.cam.ac.uk/01003763h.htm.

Brosens, Ivo, et al., "Transvaginal Laparoscopy," *Clinical Obstetrics and Gynecology*, vol. 46, no.1, March 2003.

Bulletini, Carlo, et al., "Endometriosis: Absence of Recurrence in Patients After Endometrial Ablation," *Journal of Human Reproduction*, vol. 16, no. 12, December 2001.

Cook, Andrew, "Ask Dr. Cook—Conscious Pain Mapping," http://www.drcook.com/adca23.html.

———, "Ask Dr Cook—Surgical Techniques in the Treatment of Endometriosis—To Excise or Not to Excise," http://www.drcook.com/adca3.html.

Demco, Larry, "Patient Information—Pain Mapping," http://www.obgyn.net.

"Endometrial Ablation," http://www.ivf.com/eablate.html.

Endometriosis Research Center (ERC), "The Laparoscopy," http://www.endocenter.org/.

Falcone, Tommaso, and Edward Mascha, "The Elusive Diagnostic Test for Endometriosis," *Fertility and Sterility*, vol. 80, no. 4, October 2003.

Gagne, Daniele, et al., "Development of a Non-Surgical Diagnostic Tool for Endometriosis Based on the Detection of Endometrial Leukocyte Subsets and Serum CA-125 Levels," *Fertility and Sterility*, vol. 80, no. 4, October 2003.

Gruppo Italiano per lo Studio dell'Endometriosi, "Ablation of Lesions or No Treatment in Minimal–Mild Endometriosis in Infertile Women: A Randomized Trial," *Journal of Human Reproduction*, vol. 14, no. 5, May 1999.

Harada, Tatsuya, et al., "Usefulness of CA-19-9 versus CA-125 for the Diagnosis of Endometriosis," *Fertility and Sterility*, vol. 78, no.4, October 2002.

Hill, D. Ashley, "Issues and Procedures in Women's Health—Laparoscopy," http://www.obgyn.net/women/women.asp?page=/women/articles/lap_dah.

Medina, Marelyn, "Laparoscopic Surgery," http://www.laparoscopy.org/i4a/pages/index.cfm?pageid=3294.

"Microlaparoscopy," http://www.obgyn.net/displaytranscript.asp?page=/avtranscripts/sls2000_almeida.

"Microlaparoscopy for Women with Chronic Pelvic Pain and Pain Mapping," http://www.obgyn.net/displaytranscript.asp?page=/avtranscripts/aagl98-demco.

Redwine, David, "Should Laser Vaporization and Electrocoagulation of Endometriosis Be Banned?," *St. Charles Medical Center Endometriosis*

Newsletter, Spring/Summer 2004, http://www.endometriosistreatment
.org/html/laser_vaporization.html.

"Safety in Laparoscopy," http://www.obgyn.net/displaytranscript.asp?page=/
avtranscripts/israel2k_turner.

Spaczynski, Robert Z., and Antoni J. Duleba, "Diagnosis of Endometriosis," *Seminars in Reproductive Medicine*, vol. 21, no. 2, February 2003.

"Transvaginal Laparoscopy in the Diagnosis and Treatment of Endometriosis," http://www.endometriosiszone.org/display.asp?page=/congress_ISGE
2003-Gordts.htm.

"What Is Microlaparoscopy?" http://www.ivf.com/microlap.html.

Winkel, Craig A., "Evaluation and Management of Women with Endometriosis," *Obstetrics and Gynecology*, vol. 102, no.2, August 2003.

Chapters 13 and 14

"ACOG's Physician Directory," http://acog.org/member-lookup/disclaimer
.cfm.

Akerkar, S. M., and L. S. Bichile, "Doctor-Patient Relationship: Changing
Dynamics in the Information Age," *Journal of Postgraduate Medicine*,
vol. 50, issue 2, June 2004.

———, "Health Information on the Internet: Patient Empowerment or Patient Deceit?" *Indian Journal of Medical Sciences*, vol. 58, no. 8, August
2004.

American Board of Medical Specialists (ABMS), "Which Medical Specialists for You?" http://www.abms.org/which.asp.

Bertakis, Klea D., Peter Franks, and Rahman Azari, "Effects of Physician
Gender on Patient Satisfaction," *Journal of the American Medical
Women's Association*, vol. 58, no. 2, 2003.

Emanuel, Ezekiel J., and Linda L. Emanuel, "Fair Models of the Physician-
Patient Relationship," *Journal of the American Medical Association*, vol.
267, no. 16, April 1992.

Endometriosis Association (EA), http://www.killercramps.org/press3.html.

Erickson, Dave, "New Study: Patient Empowerment Is Real, Are Your Physicians Ready for It?" http://mm.meetingsnet.com/ar/meetings_new_study
_patient/.

Fox, Susannah, and Lee Rainie, "Pew Internet and American Life Project:
The Online Health Care Revolution—How the Web Helps Americans

Take Better Care of Themselves," Washington, D.C., 2000, http://www.pewinternet.org/pdfs/PIP_Health_Report.pdf.

———, "Pew Internet and American Life Project: Vital Decisions—How Internet Users Decide What Information to Trust When They or Their Loved Ones Are Sick," Washington D.C., 2002, http://www.pewinternet.org/pdfs/PIP_vital_Decisions_May2002.pdf.

Fox, Susannah, and Deborah Fallows, "Pew Internet and American Life Project: Internet Health Resources," Washington D.C., 2003, http://www.pewinternet.org/pdfs/PIP_health_report_july_2003.pdf.

Guidone, Heather, "The Encounter or How to Get Your Doctor to Listen," http://www.hcgresources.com/talkdoctor.html.

———, "How the Internet Is Improving the Doctor-Patient Relationship, Part 1: The Internet Patient," http://www.obgyn.net/women/women.asp?page=/women/articles/inet_pat.

Harvard Medical School, "Specialists," *The Harvard Medical School Family Health Guide*, http://www.health.harvard.edu/fhg/specialists.shtml.

Hummelshøj, Lone, "Meeting Expectations in the Chronically Ill Patient by Extending the Therapeutic Network." Paper presented at the 5th World Congress on Controversies in Obstetrics, Gynecology and Infertility, Las Vegas, USA, June 3–6, 2004, http://www.endometriosiszone.com/content/PDF/cogi2004-61-Hummelshoj.pdf.

Johns Hopkins University and American Healthways, *Defining the Patient-Physician Relationship for the 21st Century: 3rd Annual Disease Management Outcomes Summit, October 30–November 2, 2003, Phoenix, Arizona*, http://www.patient-physician.com/.

Johnson, Ellen T., "Finding an Endometriosis Specialist," http://www.endometriosis.org/finding-a-specialist.html.

———, "When Others Don't Understand," http://www.endometriosis.org/understand.html.

Medical Library Association (MLA), "A User's Guide to Finding and Evaluating Health Information on the Web," http://www.mlanet.org/resources/userguide.html.

Roter, Debra S., "How Physician Gender Shapes the Communication and Evaluation of Medical Care," *Mayo Clinic Proceedings*, vol. 76, July 2001.

Shanahan, Kelly, "How the Internet Is Improving the Doctor-Patient Relationship, Part 2: The Internet Doctor," http://www.obgyn.net/displayarticle.asp?page=/english/pubs/roberta/rr_03-04-98.

Smeal College of Business, Penn State University, "Bedside Manner Makes a Difference in Patient Relationship with Physician," Press Release, Penn State University Smeal College of Business, February 22, 2001.

Speyer, Roberta, "The Changing Face of Patient-Doctor Interaction Online," http://www.obgyn.net/avtranscripts/med%20forum_speyer.htm.

"Talking with Your Doctor: Selecting a Physician to Care for You," http://www.endometriosistreatment.org/html/talking.html.

Taylor, Humphrey, "The Harris Poll #19, April 18, 2001," http://www.harrisinteractive.com.harris_poll/index.as?PID=229.

———, "The Harris Poll #21, May 1, 2002," http://www.harrisinteractive.com/harris_poll/index.asp?PID=299.

"WebMD Health Guide: Medical Specialists," http://my.webmd.com/hw/health_guide_atoz/ps2269.asp.

WholeHealthMD.com, "Chinese Herbal Medicine," http://www.wholehealthmd.com/refshelf/substances_view/1,1525,10147,00.html.

———, "Nutritionist," http://www.wholehealthmd.com/refshelf/substances_view/1,1525,10130,00.html.

INDEX

Page numbers in *italics* refer to charts, illustrations, and tables.

WANT TO LIVE WELL?

LIVING WELL WITH MIGRAINE DISEASE AND HEADACHES
What Your Doctor Doesn't Tell You . . . That You Need to Know
by Teri Robert, Ph.D.
0-06-076685-9 (trade paperback)
A holistic, patient-centered guide to the diagnosis, side effects and treatments for headaches and Migraine disease.

LIVING WELL WITH MENOPAUSE
What Your Doctor Doesn't Tell You . . . That You Need To Know
by Carolyn Chambers Clark, ARNP, Ed.D.
0-06-075812-0 (trade paperback)
A complete holistic guide and self-care manual to menopause.

LIVING WELL WITH HYPOTHYROIDISM
What Your Doctor Doesn't Tell You . . . That You Need to Know
by Mary J. Shomon
0-06-074095-7 (trade paperback)
An expanded and updated edition of the hugely successful *Living Well with Hypothyroidism*.

LIVING WELL WITH GRAVES' DISEASE AND HYPERTHYROIDISM
What Your Doctor Doesn't Tell You . . . That You Need to Know
by Mary J. Shomon
0-06-073019-6 (trade paperback)
Here is a holistic road map for diagnosis, treatment, and recovery from Graves' disease and hyperthyroidism.

LIVING WELL WITH EPILEPSY AND OTHER SEIZURE DISORDERS
An Expert Explains What You Really Need to Know
by Carl W. Bazil. M.D., Ph.D
0-06-053848-1 (trade paperback)
A much-needed book of information, support, and lifestyle strategies for this surprisingly common problem.

LIVING WELL WITH ENDOMETRIOSIS
What Your Doctor Doesn't Tell You . . . That You Need to Know
by Kerry-Ann Morris
0-06-084426-4 (trade paperback)
A complete guide to the side effects and treatments—both conventional and alternative—for endometriosis.

LIVING WELL WITH CHRONIC FATIGUE SYNDROME AND FIBROMYALGIA
What Your Doctor Doesn't Tell You . . . That You Need to Know
by Mary J. Shomon
0-06-052125-2 (trade paperback)
A comprehensive guide to the diagnosis and treatment of chronic fatigue syndrome and fibromyalgia.

LIVING WELL WITH AUTOIMMUNE DISEASE
What Your Doctor Doesn't Tell You . . . That You Need to Know
by Mary J. Shomon
0-06-093819-6 (trade paperback)
A complete guide to understanding the mysterious disorders of the immune system.

LIVING WELL WITH ANXIETY
What Your Doctor Doesn't Tell You . . . That You Need to Know
by Carolyn Chambers Clark, ARNP, Ed.D.
0-06-082377-1 (trade paperback)
A complete guide to the side effects and treatments for anxiety disorders.